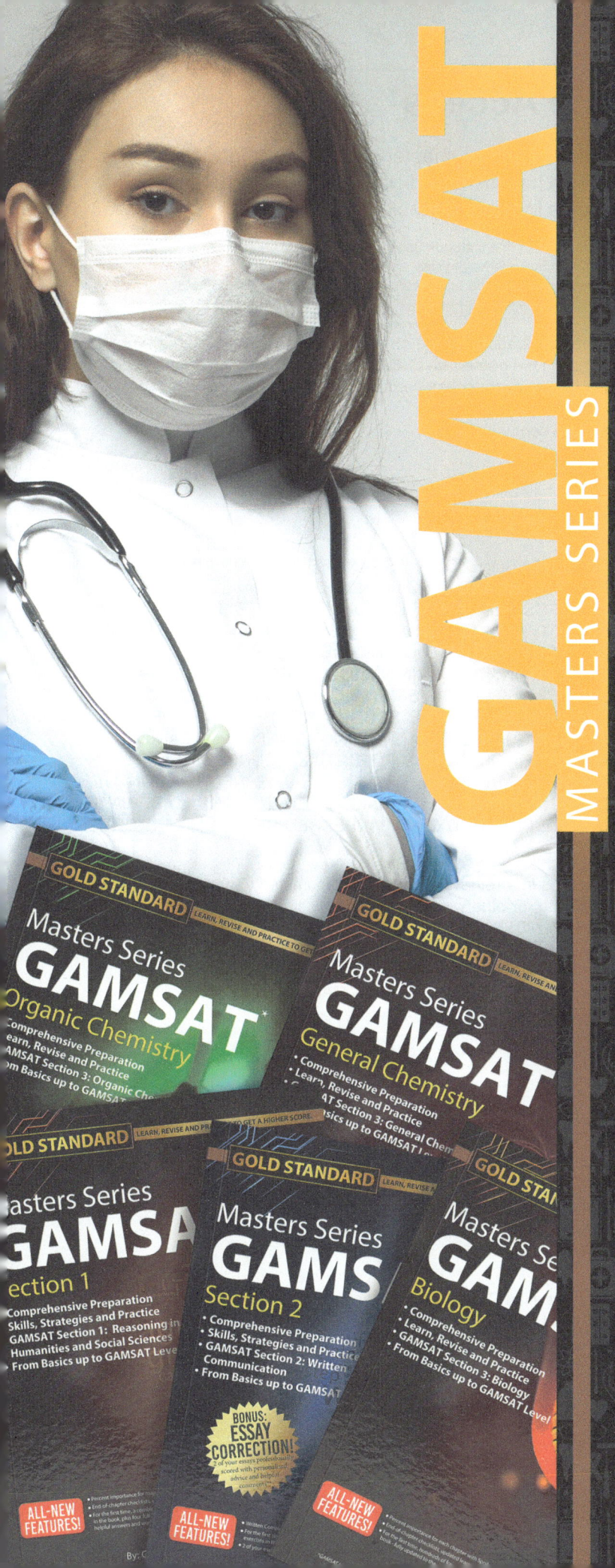

GAMSAT
MASTERS SERIES

GOLD S

01 Editor and Author
Brett Ferdinand BSc MD-CM

02 Contributors
Lisa Ferdinand BA MA
Sean Pierre BSc MD
Kristin Finkenzeller BSc MD
Ibrahima Diouf BSc MSc PhD
Charles Haccoun BSc MD-CM
Timothy Ruger BA MA
Jeanne Tan Te

03 Illustrators
Harvie W. Gallatiera BS CompE
Gilbert Rafanan BSc

GOLD STANDARD — LEARN, REVISE AND PRACTICE TO GET A HIGHER SCORE.

Masters Series
GAMSAT*
Maths and Physics

- Comprehensive Preparation
- Learn, Revise and Practice
- GAMSAT Section 3: Maths and Physics
- From Basics up to GAMSAT Level

ALL-NEW FEATURES!
- Percent importance for each chapter with Spoiler Alerts listing official sources
- End-of-chapter checklists, updated learning objectives, and extensive cross-referencing
- For the first time, hundreds of foundational and GAMSAT-level practice questions in the book - fully updated to the current standard - with helpful answers and worked solutions online**

By: Gold Standard GAMSAT

*GAMSAT is administered by the Australian Council for Education Research (ACER) which is not associated with this product.
**One year of continuous online access for the original owner consistent with our Terms of Use; not transferable.

Free Online Access*

Answers and detailed worked solutions for hundreds of end-of-chapter practice questions, as well as the full-length practice test GS-Free which has the new digital GAMSAT format and cross-references to this Masters Series book.

*One year of continuous access for the original owner of this textbook upon online registration at www.gamsat-prep.com/gamsat-maths-physics
If you purchased this textbook or the eBook directly from www.gamsat-prep.com, then your online access is automated.

Please note: Benefits last for one year from the date of online registration, for the original book owner only, and are not transferable; unauthorized access and use outside the Terms of Use posted on GAMSAT-prep.com may result in account deletion; if you are not the original owner, you can purchase your virtual access card separately at GAMSAT-prep.com.

Visit The Gold Standard's Education Center at www.gold-standard.com.

Copyright (c) 2021 RuveneCo (Worldwide), 1st Edition

ISBN 978-1-927338-55-1

THE PUBLISHER AND THE AUTHORS MAKE NO REPRESENTATIONS OR WARRANTIES WITH RESPECT TO THE ACCURACY OR COMPLETENESS OF THE CONTENTS OF THIS WORK AND SPECIFICALLY DISCLAIM ALL WARRANTIES, INCLUDING WITHOUT LIMITATION WARRANTIES OF FITNESS FOR A PARTICULAR PURPOSE. NO WARRANTY MAY BE CREATED OR EXTENDED BY SALES OR PROMOTIONAL MATERIALS. THE ADVICE AND STRATEGIES CONTAINED HEREIN MAY NOT BE SUITABLE FOR EVERY SITUATION. THIS WORK IS SOLD WITH THE UNDERSTANDING THAT THE PUBLISHER IS NOT ENGAGED IN RENDERING LEGAL, ACCOUNTING, MEDICAL, DENTAL, CONSULTING, OR OTHER PROFESSIONAL SERVICES. IF PROFESSIONAL ASSISTANCE IS REQUIRED, THE SERVICES OF A COMPETENT PROFESSIONAL PERSON SHOULD BE SOUGHT. NEITHER THE PUBLISHER NOR THE AUTHORS SHALL BE LIABLE FOR DAMAGES ARISING HEREFROM. THE FACT THAT AN ORGANIZATION OR WEBSITE IS REFERRED TO IN THIS WORK AS A CITATION AND/OR A POTENTIAL SOURCE OF FURTHER INFORMATION DOES NOT MEAN THAT THE AUTHORS OR THE PUBLISHER ENDORSES THE INFORMATION THE ORGANIZATION OR WEBSITE MAY PROVIDE OR RECOMMENDATIONS IT MAY MAKE. READERS SHOULD BEWARE THAT INTERNET WEBSITES LISTED IN THIS WORK MAY HAVE CHANGED OR DISAPPEARED BETWEEN WHEN THIS WORK WAS WRITTEN AND WHEN IT IS READ.

All rights reserved. No part of this book may be reproduced, stored in a retrieval system, or transmitted in any form or by any means, electronic or mechanical, including photocopying, recording, or otherwise, without permission in writing from the publisher. Images in the public domain: Brandner, D. and Withers, G. (2013). The Cell: An Image Library, www.cellimagelibrary.org, CIL numbers 197, 214, 240, 9685, 21966, ASCB.

Address all inquiries, comments, or suggestions to the publisher. For Terms of Use go to: www.GAMSAT-prep.com

Gold Standard GAMSAT Product Contact Information

Distribution in Australia, NZ, Asia	**Distribution in Europe**	**Distribution in North America**
Woodslane Pty Ltd 10 Apollo Street Warriewood NSW 2102 Australia ABN: 76 003 677 549 learn@gamsat-prep.com	Central Books 99 Wallis Road LONDON, E9 5LN, United Kingdom orders@centralbooks.com	RuveneCo Publishing 334 Cornelia Street # 559 Plattsburgh, New York 12901, USA buy@gamsatbooks.com

RuveneCo Inc. is neither associated nor affiliated with the Australian Council for Educational Research (ACER) who has developed and administers the Graduate Medical School Admissions Test (GAMSAT). Printed in Australia.

GAMSAT-Prep.com

GAMSAT (Graduate Medical School Admissions Test)
Computer-based exam held at test centres internationally for graduate-entry medicine

Section I
Reasoning in Humanities and Social Sciences

multiple-choice section with stimulus materials requiring comprehension and analysis of non-science content

poetry • proverbs cartoons • novels or play excerpts • travel and/or medical journal entries • social science graphs

Section II
Written Communication (Writing Tasks A & B)

2 essays responding to 2 different themes using sound reasoning and competent English-writing skills (essays must be typed)

Writing Task A: sociocultural theme (e.g., free speech, justice, social media)
Writing Task B: personal-social themes (e.g., humour, love, happiness)

Section III
Reasoning in Biological and Physical Sciences

multiple-choice section with questions mostly based on science passages that require problem-solving and graph analysis

first-year undergraduate level Biology (40%), General Chemistry (20%) & Organic Chemistry (20%) • A-level/Leaving Certificate/- Year 12 level Physics (20%)

Top GAMSAT Score: 100
Average GAMSAT Score: 57

Summary of the new Digital-format GAMSAT Exam Day

	KEY POINTS	EVENT	DURATION
Arrival and Sitting of Exam	Bring only the acceptable ID documents and permitted items to the test centre as specified in ACER's GAMSAT Information Booklet	Security, identification, health protocols	45-60 minutes
Section 1: Reasoning in Humanities and Social Sciences	Key skills are reading speed and comprehension of information within socio-cultural contexts	47 MCQs* (the test centre will provide you with 2 sheets of A4 scratch paper to be used for both Section 1 and 2)	70 minutes
Section 2: Written Communication	Produce ideas in writing with clarity and soundness; essays are typed with no copy/paste function	2 essays typed on a computer (for all sections including the essays: no longer is there a formal, dedicated reading time)	65 minutes
Lunch	Consider packing your own lunch to avoid queues with nervous chatter	–	30 minutes
Section 3: Reasoning in Biological and Physical Sciences	Analyse and solve problems: 40% Biology, 40% Chemistry (equally split between General and Organic); 20% Physics	75 MCQs* (the test centre will provide you with 2 new sheets of A4 scratch paper to be used only for Section 3)	150 minutes
Total Test Time	–	–	4 hours, 45 minutes
Total Appointment Time	Success requires stamina; stamina improves with practice.	–	Approximately 6 hours**

*MCQs: multiple-choice questions, 4 options per question with only 1 best answer. Note that the 'old' GAMSAT had a dedicated 'reading time' of 10 minutes for each of Section 1 and 3, and 5 minutes for Section 2. During that reading time, students were not permitted to write or mark their exam paper in any way. The new digital GAMSAT has added time for each of the 3 exam sections as a legacy to 'reading time'; however, in practice, you can use your exam time in any way that you see fit.

**It might be a good idea to allocate a whole day to sit the GAMSAT test to allow for any contingencies and/or technical issues that you might encounter. Before the 2020 sittings, the exam-day experience lasted more than 7 hours excluding added traffic and queues at the larger testing centres (i.e. Sydney, Melbourne, Brisbane, Perth, London, Dublin). Safety measures and health protocols should be carefully anticipated when making travel arrangements and accommodations to and from the testing centre.

<u>Common formula for acceptance</u>:

GPA + GAMSAT score + Interview = Medical School Admissions

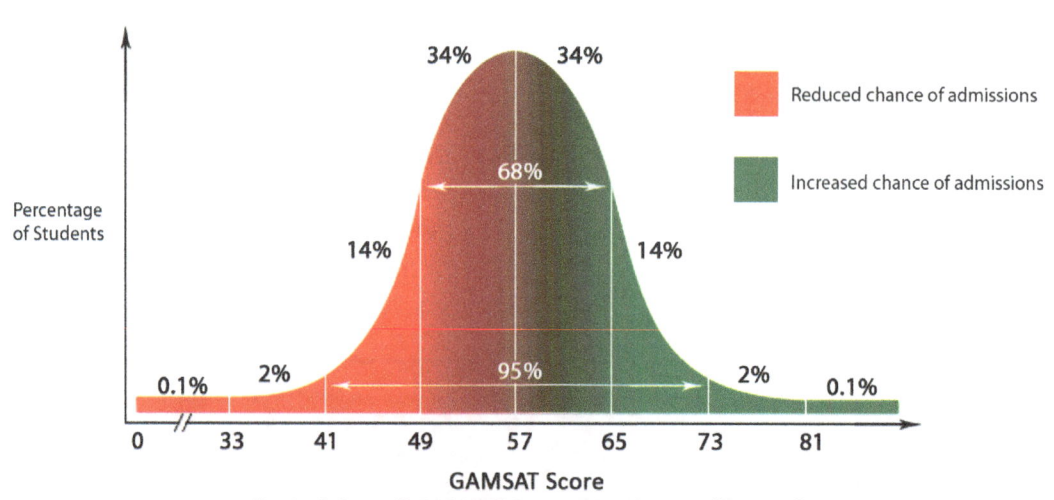

Typical Overall GAMSAT Score Distribution (Approx)

GAMSAT-Prep.com

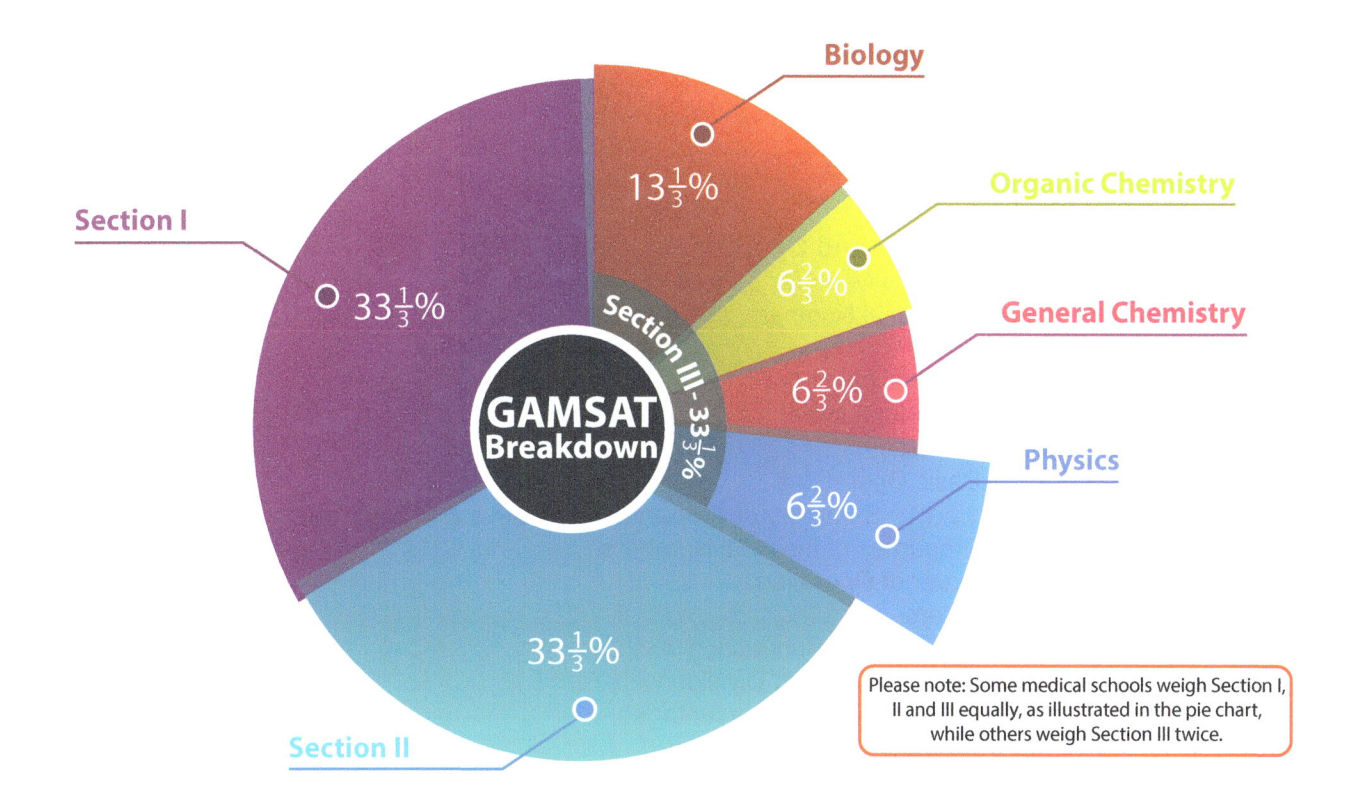

GAMSAT Breakdown

- **Biology**: $13\frac{1}{3}\%$
- **Organic Chemistry**: $6\frac{2}{3}\%$
- **General Chemistry**: $6\frac{2}{3}\%$
- **Physics**: $6\frac{2}{3}\%$
- **Section III**: $33\frac{1}{3}\%$
- **Section I**: $33\frac{1}{3}\%$
- **Section II**: $33\frac{1}{3}\%$

Please note: Some medical schools weigh Section I, II and III equally, as illustrated in the pie chart, while others weigh Section III twice.

GAMSAT is challenging, get organised.
gamsat-prep.com/free-GAMSAT-study-schedule

1. How to study
- Learn, revise and practice using the GAMSAT Masters Series book(s) and/or videos.
- Complete all exercises and multiple-choice practice questions in this book.
- Consolidate: create and study from your personal summaries (= Gold Notes) daily.

2. Once you have completed your studies
- Sit a full-length GAMSAT practice test.
- Analyse mistakes and all worked solutions.
- Consolidate: Revise all your Gold Notes and create more.

3. Sit multiple mock exams
- ACER GAMSAT practice exams with free Gold Standard worked solutions on YouTube
- Free full-length Gold Standard (GS) mock exam GS-Free with helpful, detailed worked solutions
- HEAPS: 10 full-length exams, 5 in the book and 5 online with the new, digital GAMSAT format

4. How much time do you need to study?
- On average, 3-6 hours per day for 3-6 months; depending on life experiences, 2 weeks may be enough and 8 months could be insufficient.
- Try to study full on for 1-2 weeks and then adjust your expectations for the required time.

5. Recommended GAMSAT Communities
- All countries (mainly Australia): pagingdr.net, reddit.com/r/GAMSAT/
- Mainly the UK: thestudentroom.co.uk (Medicine Community Discussion)
- Mainly Ireland: boards.ie (GAMSAT and GEM forum)

Is there something in the Masters Series that you did not understand? Don't get frustrated, get online:
gamsat-prep.com/forum

Introduction GM-06

GAMSAT MATHS AND PHYSICS

GAMSAT MATHS

Chapter 1. Numbers and Operations **GM-17**
1.0   GAMSAT Has a *Need for Speed*! GM-18
1.1   Integers, Rational Numbers, and the Number Line GM-20
    1.1.1   Integers GM-20
    1.1.2   Rational Numbers GM-20
    1.1.3   Real Numbers and the Number Line GM-21
1.2   Basic Arithmetic GM-21
    1.2.1   Basic Operations GM-21
        1.2.1.1   Summary of Properties of Positive and Negative Integers . . . GM-23
    1.2.2   Properties of the Real Numbers GM-24
    1.2.3   Order of Operations GM-24
1.3   Rules on Zero GM-26
    1.3.1   Addition and Subtraction with Zero GM-26
    1.3.2   Multiplication and Division with Zero GM-26
1.4   Fractions, Decimals, and Percentages GM-27
    1.4.1   Fractions GM-27
    1.4.2   Manipulating Fractions GM-28
    1.4.3   Decimals and Percentages GM-33
1.5   Roots and Exponents GM-37
    1.5.1   Properties of Exponents GM-37
    1.5.2   Scientific Notation GM-38
    1.5.3   Types of Exponents GM-39
    1.5.4   Zero and Exponents GM-40
    1.5.5   Summary of the Rules for Exponents GM-41
    1.5.6   Recognising Number Patterns GM-41
1.6   Ratio and Proportion GM-42
    1.6.1   What is a Ratio? GM-42
    1.6.2   Solving Proportions GM-42
Chapter 1: Gold Standard Warm-Up Exercises GM-43
Chapter 1: Worked Solutions GM-45

Chapter 2. Scientific Measurement and Dimensional Analysis **GM-51**
2.0   GAMSAT Has a *Need for Speed*! GM-52
2.1   Systems of Measurement GM-53
    2.1.1   British Units (Imperial System of Measurement) GM-53
    2.1.2   Metric Units GM-54
    2.1.3   SI Units GM-56
2.2   Mathematics of Conversions (Dimensional Analysis) GM-60
    2.2.1   Dimensional Analysis with Numeric Calculations GM-60
    2.2.2   Dimensional Analysis with Variables GM-66
Chapter 2: Gold Standard Warm-Up Exercises GM-67
Chapter 2: Worked Solutions GM-69

Note that: H = High-level Importance; M = Medium-level Importance; L = Low-level Importance.

Chapter 3. Algebra and Graph Analysis **GM-73**
3.0   GAMSAT Has a *Need for Speed*! GM-74
3.1   Equation Solving and Functions GM-76
    3.1.1   Algebraic Equations GM-76
    3.1.2   Addition and Subtraction of Polynomials GM-78
    3.1.3   Simplifying Algebraic Expressions GM-78
3.2   Simplifying Equations GM-78
    3.2.1   Combining Terms GM-79
    3.2.2   Variables in Denominators GM-79
    3.2.3   Factoring GM-80
3.3   Linear Equations GM-80
    3.3.1   Linearity GM-80
    3.3.2   Solving Linear Equations with Multiple Variables GM-81
3.4   Graphing Linear Functions GM-84
    3.4.1   Linear Equations and Functions GM-84
    3.4.2   Cartesian Coordinates in 2D GM-84
    3.4.3   Graphing Linear Equations GM-85
    3.4.4   Slope-Intercept Form GM-85
3.5   Basic Graphs GM-86
    3.5.1   The Graph of a Linear Equation GM-86
    3.5.2   Illustrations of Common Graphs GM-87
    3.5.3   Common Graphs Found in Other Sections or Chapters GM-88
    3.5.4   Tangential Slope and Area under a Curve GM-89
    3.5.5   Breaking Axes and Error Bars GM-92
3.6   Cartesian Coordinates in 3D GM-94
3.7   Logarithms GM-99
    3.7.1   Log Rules and Logarithmic Scales GM-99
3.8   Exponential and Logarithmic Curves GM-101
3.9   Nomograms: The Art of Unusual Graphs GM-107
Chapter 3: Gold Standard Warm-Up Exercises GM-118
Chapter 3: Worked Solutions GM-123

Chapter 4. Geometry **GM-131**
4.1   Points, Lines and Angles GM-132
    4.1.1   Points and Distance GM-132
    4.1.2   Line Segments GM-133
    4.1.3   Angles GM-134
4.2   2D Figures GM-138
    4.2.1   Rectangles and Squares GM-138
    4.2.2   Types of Triangles GM-138
    4.2.3   Circles GM-142
    4.2.4   Trapezoids and Parallelograms GM-142
4.3   3D Solids GM-144
    4.3.1   Boxes GM-144
    4.3.2   Spheres GM-145
    4.3.3   Cylinders GM-145
Chapter 4: Gold Standard Warm-Up Exercises GM-146
Chapter 4: Worked Solutions GM-148

Note that: H = High-level Importance; M = Medium-level Importance; L = Low-level Importance.

GAMSAT MATHS (cont'd)

Chapter 5. Trigonometry **GM-153**
- 5.1 Basic Trigonometric Functions GM-154
  - 5.1.1 Sine GM-154
  - 5.1.2 Cosine GM-155
  - 5.1.3 Tangent GM-155
  - 5.1.4 Secant, Cosecant, and Cotangent GM-156
- 5.2 The Unit Circle GM-156
  - 5.2.1 Trig Functions on a Circle GM-156
  - 5.2.2 Degrees and Radians GM-157
  - 5.2.3 Graphing Trig Functions GM-159
- 5.3 Trigonometric Problems GM-160
  - 5.3.1 Inverse Trig Functions GM-160
- Chapter 5: Gold Standard Warm-Up Exercises GM-161
- Chapter 5: Worked Solutions GM-162

Chapter 6. Probability and Statistics **GM-165**
- 6.1 Probability GM-166
  - 6.1.1 What is Probability? GM-166
  - 6.1.2 Combining Probabilities GM-167
- 6.2 Statistics GM-169
  - 6.2.1 Averages GM-169
  - 6.2.2 Mode, Median, Mean GM-169
- 6.3 More Tools for Probability and Statistics GM-170
  - 6.3.1 The Correlation Coefficient GM-170
  - 6.3.2 The Standard Deviation GM-172
  - 6.3.3 Variance GM-173
  - 6.3.4 Simple Probability Revisited GM-174
- Chapter 6: Gold Standard Warm-Up Exercises GM-175
- Chapter 6: Worked Solutions GM-176

GAMSAT PHYSICS

Chapter 1. Translational Motion **PHY-03**
- 1.0 GAMSAT has a *Need for Speed*! PHY-04
- 1.1 Scalars and Vectors PHY-06
  - 1.1.1 Trigonometric Functions: A Quick Reminder PHY-08
  - 1.1.2 Common Values of Trigonometric Functions PHY-09
- 1.2 Distance and Displacement PHY-10
- 1.3 Speed and Velocity PHY-10
  - 1.3.1 Displacement, Time and Velocity PHY-11
- 1.4 Acceleration, Deceleration: Speeding Up, Slowing Down PHY-12
  - 1.4.1 Average and Instantaneous Acceleration PHY-12
- 1.5 Uniformly Accelerated Motion PHY-14
- 1.6 Equations of Kinematics PHY-14
- Chapter 1: Gold Standard Foundational GAMSAT Practice Questions PHY-15
- Chapter 1: Gold Standard GAMSAT-Level Practice Questions PHY-17

Note that: H = High-level Importance; M = Medium-level Importance; L = Low-level Importance.

Chapter 2. Force, Motion, and Gravitation **PHY-21**
- 2.0 GAMSAT has a *Need for Speed*! PHY-22
- 2.1 Mass, Centre of Mass, Weight PHY-23
- 2.2 Newton's Second Law PHY-23
- 2.3 Newton's Third Law PHY-24
- 2.4 The Law of Gravitation PHY-24
- 2.5 Free-fall Motion PHY-25
- 2.6 Projectile Motion PHY-26
    - 2.6.1 Projectile Motion Problem (Imperial units) PHY-27
- Chapter 2: Gold Standard Foundational GAMSAT Practice Questions PHY-29
- Chapter 2: Gold Standard GAMSAT-Level Practice Questions PHY-31

Chapter 3. Particle Dynamics **PHY-35**
- 3.1 GAMSAT has a *Need for Speed*! PHY-36
- 3.2 Frictional Forces PHY-36
    - 3.2.1 Incline Plane Problem with Friction (SI units) PHY-37
- 3.3 Uniform Circular Motion PHY-38
- 3.4 Pulley Systems PHY-39
- Chapter 3: Gold Standard Foundational GAMSAT Practice Questions PHY-40
- Chapter 3: Gold Standard GAMSAT-Level Practice Questions PHY-42

Chapter 4. Equilibrium **PHY-47**
- 4.0 GAMSAT has a *Need for Speed*! PHY-48
- 4.1 Translational, Rotational and Complex Motion PHY-48
    - 4.1.1 Torque Problem (SI units) PHY-50
- 4.2 Newton's First Law PHY-51
- 4.3 Momentum PHY-51
    - 4.3.1 Understanding Conservation PHY-51
- 4.4 Collisions PHY-52
    - 4.4.1 Collision Problem (CGS units) PHY-53
- Chapter 4: Gold Standard Foundational GAMSAT Practice Questions PHY-54
- Chapter 4: Gold Standard GAMSAT-Level Practice Questions PHY-56

Chapter 5. Work and Energy **PHY-61**
- 5.0 GAMSAT has a *Need for Speed*! PHY-62
- 5.1 Work PHY-62
- 5.2 Energy PHY-63
- 5.3 Kinetic Energy PHY-63
- 5.4 Potential Energy PHY-63
- 5.5 Conservation of Energy PHY-64
    - 5.5.1 Conservation of Energy Problem (SI units) PHY-64
- 5.6 Conservative Forces PHY-65
- 5.7 Power PHY-65
- Chapter 5: Gold Standard Foundational GAMSAT Practice Questions PHY-66
- Chapter 5: Gold Standard GAMSAT-Level Practice Questions PHY-68

Chapter 6. Fluids and Solids **PHY-73**
- 6.0 GAMSAT has a *Need for Speed*! PHY-74
- 6.1 Fluids PHY-74
    - 6.1.1 Density, Specific Gravity PHY-74

Note that: H = High-level Importance; M = Medium-level Importance; L = Low-level Importance.

GAMSAT PHYSICS (cont'd)

- 6.1.2 Hydrostatic Pressure, Buoyancy, Archimedes' Principle ... PHY-75
  - 6.1.2.1 Atmospheric Pressure ... PHY-77
  - 6.1.2.2 Gauge Pressure ... PHY-78
- 6.1.3 Fluids in Motion, Continuity Equation, Bernoulli's Equation ... PHY-79
- 6.1.4 Fluid Viscosity and Determining Turbulence ... PHY-80
- 6.1.5 Surface Tension ... PHY-81
- 6.2 Solids ... PHY-82
  - 6.2.1 Elastic Properties of Solids ... PHY-82
- 6.3 The Effect of Temperature on Solids and Liquids ... PHY-83
- Chapter 6: Gold Standard Foundational GAMSAT Practice Questions ... PHY-84
- Chapter 6: Gold Standard GAMSAT-Level Practice Questions ... PHY-84

Chapter 7. Wave Characteristics and Periodic Motion ... PHY-89
- 7.1 Wave Characteristics ... PHY-90
  - 7.1.1 Transverse and Longitudinal Motion ... PHY-90
  - 7.1.2 Wavelength, Frequency, Velocity, Amplitude, Intensity ... PHY-90
  - 7.1.3 Superposition of Waves, Phase, Interference, Addition ... PHY-91
  - 7.1.4 Resonance ... PHY-94
  - 7.1.5 Standing Waves, Pipes and Strings ... PHY-94
- 7.2 Periodic Motion ... PHY-95
  - 7.2.1 Hooke's Law ... PHY-95
  - 7.2.2 Features of SHM and Hooke's Law ... PHY-96
  - 7.2.3 SHM Problem: The Simple Pendulum ... PHY-96
- Chapter 7: Gold Standard Foundational GAMSAT Practice Questions ... PHY-99
- Chapter 7: Gold Standard GAMSAT-Level Practice Questions ... PHY-100

Chapter 8. Sound ... PHY-107
- 8.1 Production of Sound ... PHY-108
- 8.2 Relative Velocity of Sound in Solids, Liquids, and Gases ... PHY-108
- 8.3 Intensity, Pitch ... PHY-108
  - 8.3.1 Calculation of the Intensity Level ... PHY-109
- 8.4 Beats ... PHY-109
- 8.5 Doppler Effect ... PHY-110
  - 8.5.1 Doppler Effect Problem (SI units) ... PHY-111
- Chapter 8: Gold Standard Foundational GAMSAT Practice Questions ... PHY-112
- Chapter 8: Gold Standard GAMSAT-Level Practice Questions ... PHY-113

Chapter 9. Electrostatics and Electromagnetism ... PHY-117
- 9.0 GAMSAT has a *Need for Speed*! ... PHY-118
- 9.1 Electrostatics ... PHY-118
  - 9.1.1 Charge, Conductors, Insulators ... PHY-118
  - 9.1.2 Coulomb's Law, Electric Force ... PHY-119
  - 9.1.3 Electric Field, Electric Field Lines ... PHY-120
  - 9.1.4 Potential Energy, Absolute Potential ... PHY-122
  - 9.1.5 Equipotential Lines, Potential Difference, Electric Dipoles ... PHY-122

9.2 Electromagnetism PHY-124
    9.2.1 Notion of Electromagnetic Induction PHY-124
    9.2.2 Magnetic Field Vector PHY-124
    9.2.3 The Lorentz Force PHY-125
    9.2.4 Electromagnetic Spectrum, Radio, Infrared, X-rays PHY-126
Chapter 9: Gold Standard Foundational GAMSAT Practice Questions PHY-127
Chapter 9: Gold Standard GAMSAT-Level Practice Questions PHY-128

Chapter 10. Electric Circuits PHY-135
10.0 GAMSAT has a *Need for Speed*! PHY-136
10.1 Current PHY-137
10.2 Resistance, Resistivity, Series and Parallel Circuits PHY-138
    10.2.1 Resistance Problem in Series and Parallel PHY-139
10.3 Batteries, Electromotive Force, Voltage, Internal Resistance PHY-140
    10.3.1 Kirchoff's Laws and a Multiloop Circuit Problem PHY-141
10.4 Capacitors and Dielectrics PHY-143
10.5 Root-Mean-Square Current and Voltage PHY-145
Chapter 10: Gold Standard Foundational GAMSAT Practice Questions PHY-146
Chapter 10: Gold Standard GAMSAT-Level Practice Questions PHY-147

Chapter 11. Light and Geometrical Optics PHY-151
11.0 GAMSAT has a *Need for Speed*! PHY-152
11.1 Generalities PHY-154
11.2 Polarisation PHY-154
11.3 Reflection, Mirrors PHY-155
11.4 Refraction, Dispersion, Refractive Index, Snell's Law PHY-158
11.5 Thin Lens, Diopters PHY-160
    11.5.1 Lens Aberrations PHY-162
11.6 Light vs. Sound PHY-162
Chapter 11: Gold Standard Foundational GAMSAT Practice Questions PHY-163
Chapter 11: Gold Standard GAMSAT-Level Practice Questions PHY-165

Chapter 12. Atomic and Nuclear Structure PHY-171
12.0 GAMSAT has a *Need for Speed*! PHY-172
12.1 Protons, Neutrons, Electrons PHY-172
12.2 Isotopes, Atomic Number, Atomic Weight PHY-173
12.3 Nuclear Forces, Nuclear Binding Energy, Stability, Radioactivity PHY-175
12.4 Nuclear Reaction, Radioactive Decay, Half-Life PHY-176
12.5 Quantised Energy Levels For Electrons, Emission Spectrum PHY-179
12.6 Fluorescence PHY-181
Chapter 12: Gold Standard Foundational GAMSAT Practice Questions PHY-182
Chapter 12: Gold Standard GAMSAT-Level Practice Questions PHY-184

Note that: H = High-level Importance; M = Medium-level Importance; L = Low-level Importance.

INTRODUCTION

GAMSAT Section 3, Reasoning in Biological and Physical Sciences, is the longest of the 3 subtests on exam day. 'Biological Sciences' refers to Organic Chemistry and Biology. 'Physical Sciences' refers to Physics and General (Inorganic, not Organic) Chemistry. In our experience, most students with a non-science background (NSB) can successfully learn the assumed knowledge for GAMSAT independently, while a smaller number may need to enrol in a short tertiary-level science course, or use a video series to supplement their learning.

Essentially, 20% of Section 3 is Physics. The level of assumed knowledge is A-Level/Leaving Certificate/Year 12 Physics.

For a typical secondary or tertiary-level exam, you could read all the chapters in the relevant book, commit as much to memory as possible, walk into the exam room, match the questions with your knowledge, and reply. Your training: study anytime, even the night before the exam since you might encounter something that is word-for-word on exam day, replicate what you read, and you can ace the exam, in fact, you are brilliant!

The GAMSAT: study all you want even the night before, extremely unlikely to be able to identify something word-for-word on exam day, no feeling of being brilliant (this is true even for many students who actually 'ace' the exam). The actual exam includes 2 atypical sensations: **1)** you must learn a lot of new information *during* the exam; **2)** the topics and questions almost seem random. In some ways, these atypical sensations emulate life as a doctor!

In summary, you have been trained to focus on 'knowledge' as a priority to succeed in university studies. Frankly, for some exams, 'understanding' is secondary. If you had both knowledge and understanding, you would likely ace any exam – except GAMSAT. We will continually try to adjust the way you study while you read chapters herein.

Why is there so much GAMSAT Maths content in this textbook?

GAMSAT is designed and administered by ACER. Here is ACER's quote about the structure and content of the exam:

"The purpose of GAMSAT is to assess the ability to understand and analyse material, to think critically about issues ... to read and think about a passage of writing, to interpret graphical displays of information, to use mathematical relationships and to apply reasoning skills to tables of data."

https://gamsat.acer.org/about-gamsat/structure-and-content (2021)

In their very first paragraph regarding the exam's structure and content, ACER embedded at least 3 phrases that link directly to GAMSAT Maths: 'analyse', 'interpret graphical displays', and 'use mathematical relationships'. Maths is not even a formal GAMSAT subject, shocking!

GAMSAT Maths is the foundation for all GAMSAT Section 3, except perhaps GAMSAT Organic Chemistry. The other 3 sciences follow ACER's quote very closely. In GAMSAT Masters Series Organic Chemistry, you will discover ACER's emphasis on geometric (spatial) reasoning and pattern recognition which are, essentially, unique to GAMSAT Organic Chemistry. The other 3 sciences have a laser-like focus on equation manipulation – with or without exponential or logarithmic relationships – and the interpretation and analysis of diagrams, graphs, tables and flow charts.

Note that not every student has the same exam experience - even if they sit the GAMSAT on the same day. After all, experience is subjective in addition to the fact that not all students sitting the exam will have identical questions. ACER makes such modifications across GAMSAT sittings for exam security, statistical aims, and to try 'test questions' for research purposes. Nonetheless, Gold Standard GAMSAT has completed an extensive analysis of ACER's official GAMSAT practice materials. We can lay the data in your lap to hopefully guide you towards more efficient studies.

We placed the step-by-step worked solutions to all of the over 400 multiple-choice Section 3 official ACER GAMSAT practice questions on YouTube for free access in the Gold Standard GAMSAT Channel. Then we re-examined all of ACER's practice materials multiple times and compared the data generated with students' experiences as publicly reported in online forums. If we have erred, it is on the side of conservative estimates.

We can confirm that most students will experience more than 50% of GAMSAT Section 3 questions as intimately related to Maths: in other words, either based on

"MATHS!!! You do not need to know advanced maths or anything, but you need to be very confident and quick in your maths calculations as many, perhaps most, questions involved it in some form or other"
"Lots of equation manipulation; lots of maths"
"i think if you are good at recognising mathematical and logical relationships quickly you'd do well… stuff like ratios and exponents"
"… some really crazy and confusing graphs"
"50% of the test was graphs"
"So. Many. Graphs. I pretty much felt like the exam was graphs/diagrams, maths (disguised as physics) …"
"Lots of random passages/tables/graphs that required little science background"

Student "Debriefs": Comments from recent GAMSAT sittings left in online forums about GAMSAT Section 3 shortly after the real exam.

graphs, calculations, equation manipulation with little or no background, etc. As a consequence, GAMSAT Maths is a more important component to GAMSAT Section 3 success than any other standard science subject.

Despite being a digital exam, GAMSAT will have many numerical calculations and equation manipulations requiring the use of scratch paper which will be provided to you by an attendant at your exam centre (two A4 sheets for the entirety of Section 3). No calculator is permitted, just old-fashioned longhand calculations. Keeping your scratch paper organised using lines separating the work from different questions, and neat so that all work remains crystal clear to you, is paramount. Feel free to use A4 scratch paper for the multiple-choice questions at the end of chapters in this book to become accustomed to the experience.

What is Physics?

Physics is largely concerned with the nature and properties of matter (= *physic*al substances) and energy. This includes mechanics (= movement and forces), heat, light and other radiation, sound, electricity, magnetism, and the structure of atoms.

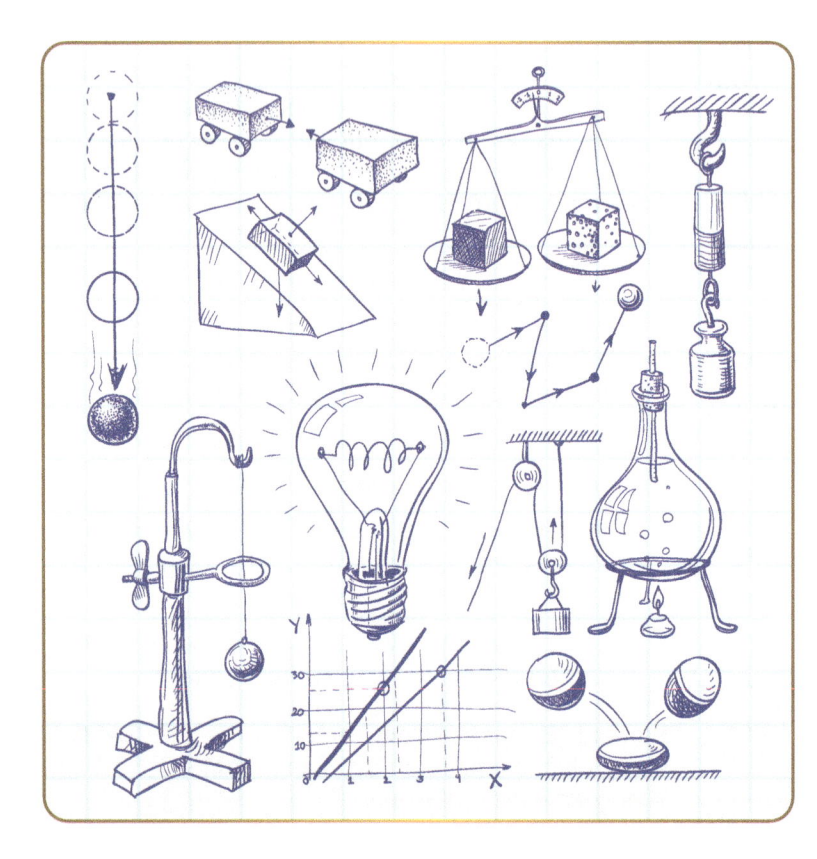

Elements of Classical and GAMSAT Physics. Along the top row: A ball dropping (*free-fall motion*) with a downward arrow (*vector*) which could represent the acceleration due to gravity; a collision between vehicles (*momentum, impulse*); a block sliding down a sloping ramp (*inclined plane*); a balance and a stretching spring hung from the ceiling (*weight = force*); an atom of gas in random collisions (*momentum, vectors*). Along the bottom row starting on the left: A string with a weight swinging back and forth (*the simple pendulum*), where the time period T = 1/(frequency); a globe or lightbulb (*electricity, Ohm's Law*); two graphs with different, positive slopes; a pulley system (*vectors showing the direction of the tension in the cord or string*); fire boiling a liquid creating a gas under pressure (*fluids; pressure = force/area*); a rubber ball strikes the ground with temporary deformation and change in direction but no change in the energy of movement (*kinetic energy; elastic collision*).

Physics is not just about sending rocket ships to the moon. Physics includes walking (gait), running, surfing, throwing, blood circulation, heart defibrillation, bungee jumping, vision, etc. In fact, all of the preceding have been publicly reported as past GAMSAT Physics topics on the real exam. From common every day events to the strange behaviour of tiny things (subatomic particles, PHY Chapter 12), all can be described by graphs and/or equations.

As Latin was the language of ancient Romans, Maths is the language of Physics. In fact, there have been branches of Maths that have been 'invented' simply to describe occurrences in the physical world.

How do I study GAMSAT Maths and Physics?

We do not believe that it would be an efficient use of your time to plan to read all chapters in this textbook multiple times, nor to attempt to read straight through from the beginning to the end in one go. Ideally, you would plan to read each chapter once while taking very brief notes (less than 1 page per chapter). Either before or after reading a chapter – where applicable – you may choose to watch some online videos relevant to that chapter while also taking very brief notes. Revise your notes often according to your GAMSAT study schedule which you can modify from the one we created (gamsat-prep.com/free-GAMSAT-study-schedule).

What is so *new* about the new GAMSAT Masters Series?

The trifecta: We have introduced 3 new tools to increase your study efficiency comprising of Percent Importance, Spoiler Alerts and Chapter Checklists.

Percent importance

'Importance' deals with the classic-student conundrum: How much effort should I invest in studying this or that chapter? How relevant is it to the GAMSAT?

After an exhaustive analysis of ACER's materials, we converted our previous Importance boxes to reveal percentages so students are better informed as to what they should emphasise when studying.

Again, we went back and assessed all Maths-related questions in all of the released official GAMSAT practice materials from ACER and then cross-referenced that information to content that would have been specifically helpful to solve those particular questions. Here are the results for the 6 GAMSAT Maths chapters in this book:

Chapter	1	2	3	4	5	6
Percent Importance	13%	11%	65%	7%	2.5%	1%
Relative Importance	HIGH	HIGH	HIGH	MEDIUM	LOW	LOW

The data is clear. The labels representing 'relative importance' is, of course, subjective. We will always remind you of the percentages on the first page of each chapter so that you do not have to accept our judgement as to the level of importance, you can decide for yourself. Note that approximately 90% of GAMSAT Maths is covered in the first 3 chapters. We regard 10% or more as 'High-level Importance' although, clearly, Chapter 3 is stratospheric in importance.

Here is the summary of Importance for the 12 GAMSAT Physics chapters in this book:

Chapter	1	2	3	4	5	6	7	8	9	10	11	12
Percent Importance	10%	6%	2%	12%	5%	12%	6%	1%	10%	7%	14%	15%
Relative Importance	H	M	L	H	M	H	M	L	H	M	H	H

The data is real, but again, the labels representing 'relative importance' are subjective. Note that 80% of GAMSAT Physics lies within 7 of the 12 chapters: 1, 4, 6, 9, 10, 11 and 12.

Spoiler Alert!

And for those who only believe if they can see for themselves: Spoiler Alert! This feature is at the end of each chapter and provides specific cross-references to ACER official practice materials. This way, you may choose to either check our work through specific examples from official content, or continue your studies for that particular chapter. Please note: 1-2% of official ACER practice questions either change or are moved every year.

Chapter Checklists

Part 3 of the trifecta to improve study efficiency: At the end of each chapter, we encourage you to participate in a reassessment of your understanding based on the learning objectives for that chapter, to take appropriate notes, to engage in multimedia learning, and more.

More changes?

In addition to the trifecta, for the first time, this book contains many other features with the sole aim of increasing your study efficiency and understanding: *Need for Speed* exercises at the beginning of most chapters, improved quality and quantity of practice questions, detailed worked solutions, re-editing of each and every page, and more online discussion boards to ensure that you have access to resolve any question you may have regarding the content in this book.

Practice questions

We have 3 levels of multiple-choice practice questions, the first two are at the back of each chapter:

1) Foundational practice questions: Basic, understanding questions to ensure that you have read the chapter; if you have a NSB, if you do not know the answer, it would be better to treat these questions as 'open-book' questions rather than just looking at the worked solutions in your online account;

2) GAMSAT-level practice questions: Reasoning, application questions with the normal GAMSAT dosage of graphs, tables, diagrams and algebraic manipulations;

3) Full-length practice tests which span the depth and breadth of a simulation of the real exam. Be warned: We do not replicate real-exam questions, we replicate real-exam reasoning. You can start with GS-Free which is a full-length Gold Standard (GS) GAMSAT mock exam with the new digital format, with free answers and worked solutions at gamsat-prep.com. GS-Free is one of 15 GS/HEAPS full-length mock exams.

For GAMSAT Sciences, "Study, practice, then full-length testing" should be your mantra for success!

Note for NSB students: If you read poems for months, you will increase your comfort reading poems. Reading science chapters is quite similar. It will feel bewildering at times, but less so as you progress. The real GAMSAT will have some articles that even the best science students do not fully grasp during the exam. However, they can still manage to obtain top GAMSAT scores by focusing on the minimum required in order to answer the questions correctly. This is a skill you can develop but it will not always feel comfortable.

A word about your online access . . .

The GS Online Access has saved thousands of trees and have reduced the cost of this book to you. It is not just the hundreds of online answers and worked solutions that you get access to with your gamsat-prep.com account, it is the fact that we do not have to limit the length of our worked solutions because of printing cost restrictions. It permits this textbook to sell for less than most with the same production value, while at the same time, providing you with more detailed worked solutions than any other GAMSAT publication, ever. You will also find that many of the solutions include videos.

Cross-references!

Wherever possible, we will identify another chapter, section or subsection of the book where you can find more information regarding a particular topic. For the most part, each book is self-contained but there are some exceptional cases where we cross-reference between different Masters Series books. The following table contains a summary of the abbreviations used throughout the Masters Series.

Cross-references to the Masters Series books, videos, apps, etc.

Abbreviation	Subject	Theme, Book
RHSS	Reasoning in Humanities & Social Sciences	Section 1, Book 1
WC	Written Communication	Section 2, Book 2
GM	GAMSAT Maths	Physical Sciences, Book 3
PHY	Physics	Physical Sciences, Book 3
CHM	General Chemistry	Physical Sciences, Book 4
ORG	Organic Chemistry	Biological Sciences, Book 5
BIO	Biology	Biological Sciences, Book 6

For example, CHM 2.4 means that you will find more information by looking at the Masters Series textbook, Chapter 2 General Chemistry, in the section 2.4. After a few chapters, you will find the system to be quite straightforward and, often, helpful.

GAMSAT-Prep.com

Note: Despite the many new additions throughout this textbook, including over 100 pages of brand-new content, it remains 99% error-free. Should you have any doubts, join us at gamsat-prep.com/forum.

Good luck!

- BF, MD

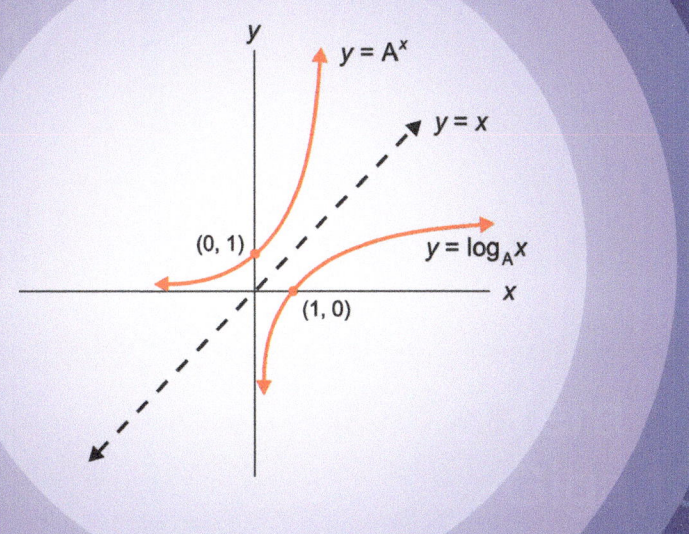

GAMSAT-Prep.com

GAMSAT MATHS

NUMBERS AND OPERATIONS
Chapter 1

Memorise
* Properties of Real Numbers
* Order of Operations
* Rules on Zero
* Important Fraction-Decimal Conversions
* Properties of Exponents
* Common squares and cubes of integers

Understand
* Integer, Rational, and Real Numbers
* Absolute Value
* Basic Operations and Definitions
* Fractions, Mixed Numbers, Decimals and Percentages; Scientific Notation
* Root and Exponent Manipulations
* Ratios and Proportions

Importance
High level: 13% of GAMSAT Section 3 maths-based questions released by ACER are related to content in this chapter (in our estimation).
* Note that approximately 90% of such questions are related to just 3 chapters: 1, 2, and 3.

GAMSAT-Prep.com

Introduction

Maths is not specifically a section of the GAMSAT but basic, secondary-school maths is necessary for most GAMSAT Physical Sciences (i.e. Physics and General Chemistry), and a surprising amount of GAMSAT Biological Sciences (particularly logs and graph analysis in Biology). Thus GAMSAT Section 3 preparation must begin with maths.

There will never be a GAMSAT question where you would need to know mathematical terms in order to get the right answer (i.e. terms such as 'rational numbers' or 'integers' or 'associative laws', etc.). However, if we are to have an understanding of 'GAMSAT Maths' then, for some students, we will need to start with the basics. If the maths is too basic for you, either skim through until it gets to your level, or at least complete the *Need for Speed* exercises at the beginning of chapters and the multiple-choice questions at the end of chapters. As for your entire Section 3 studies, please take very brief notes ('Gold Notes') and study from them frequently according to your GAMSAT study schedule.

Additional Resources

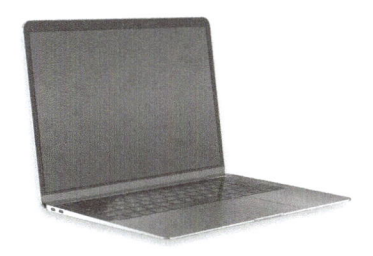

Open Discussion Boards

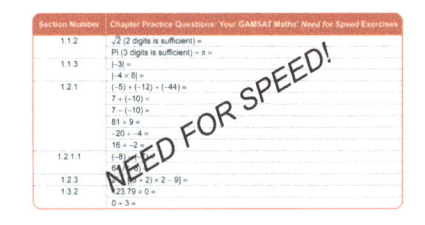

Special Guest

GAMSAT-Prep.com
GOLD STANDARD MATHS

1.0 GAMSAT Has a *Need for Speed*!

High-level Importance

Yes, this is the cart before the horse! This new section is intended to help you quickly assess your level of GAMSAT Maths. Answer any or all of the questions. If it has been a really long time since you have completed longhand calculations, do what you can and then begin studying Chapter 1 sequentially. After completing this chapter, return to the table below to ensure that you can complete all entries. Then you can proceed to answer the additional multiple-choice questions at the end of this chapter.

For those of you who are able to answer quickly but get stuck at some point, take note of the section number associated with the problem, and then you can skip forward to that particular section. We used a pink highlighter throughout the chapter so that you can quickly identify the practice questions from the table in order to check your answers and to find the worked solutions. We are not teaching you maths. We are teaching GAMSAT Maths: Skills specifically required to answer GAMSAT questions.

Section Number	Chapter Practice Questions: Your GAMSAT Maths' *Need for Speed* Exercises
1.1.2	$\sqrt{2}$ (2 digits is sufficient) =
	Pi (3 digits is sufficient) = π =
1.1.3	$\lvert -3 \rvert$ =
	$\lvert -4 \times 8 \rvert$ =
1.2.1	$(-5) + (-12) + (-44)$ =
	$7 + (-10)$ =
	$7 - (-10)$ =
	$81 \div 9$ =
	$-20 \div -4$ =
	$16 \div -2$ =
1.2.1.1	$(-8) - (-7)$ =
	$64 / (-8)$ =
1.2.3	$2^2 + [(3 + 2) \times 2 - 9]$ =
1.3.2	123.79×0 =
	$0 \div 3$ =
1.4.2A	$\dfrac{2}{3} \times \dfrac{4}{5}$ =
1.4.2B	$3 / (4 / 3)$ =
	$(3 / 4) / 3$ =
1.4.2C	$\dfrac{3}{5} - \dfrac{1}{5}$ =
	$\dfrac{2}{3} + \dfrac{2}{7}$ =
1.4.2D	Circle the higher fraction: $\dfrac{4}{5}$ or $\dfrac{3}{7}$
	Circle the lowest fraction: $\dfrac{4}{5}$ or $\dfrac{3}{7}$ or $\dfrac{9}{13}$

GAMSAT MASTERS SERIES

1.4.2E (reduce each expression)	$\dfrac{20}{28} =$
	$\dfrac{5}{9} \times \dfrac{6}{25} =$
1.4.2F (convert to a fraction)	$6\dfrac{2}{5} =$
1.4.3B	$3.33 + 23.6 =$
	$3.03 \times 1.2 =$
	$\dfrac{4.4}{1.6} =$
	Consider the number 5.3618: Round to the nearest tenth = Round to the nearest hundredth = Fraction Decimal Fraction Decimal 1/2 1/6 1/3 1/8 1/4 1/10 1/5
1.4.3C	What is 25% of 40?
	What percentage of 50 is 23?
1.5.1 (simplify)	$4^3 =$ $\qquad$ $2^x \times 3^x =$
	$a^2 \times a^3 =$ $\qquad$ $\dfrac{6^x}{2^x} =$
	$\dfrac{x^5}{x^3} =$ $\qquad$ $(x^3)^4 =$
1.5.2 (simplify)	$2.0 \times 10^4 \times 10 \times 10^2 =$
	$34.5 \times 10^{-5} + 6.7 \times 10^{-4} =$
1.5.3 (simplify)	$2^4 =$
	$8^{\frac{2}{3}} =$
1.5.4 (simplify)	$3^{-2} =$
	$\left[1.2 + \left(37 - \sqrt{5}\right) \times 2.331\right]^0 =$
1.5.6 (squares and cubes of common numbers; fill in the 22 empty cells)	(table with x = 1,2,3,4,5,6,7,8,9,10,11,12,13,14,15,20; rows for x^2 and x^3)
1.6.2	Solve for x: $\dfrac{2}{3} = \dfrac{5}{x}$
2.2.1, EXAMPLE 3	Calculate the number of seconds in a day.

High-level Importance

GAMSAT-Prep.com
GOLD STANDARD MATHS

1.1 Integers, Rational Numbers, and the Number Line

1.1.1 Integers

Integers are whole numbers without any decimal or fractional portions. They can be any number from negative to positive infinity including zero.

EXAMPLES   −2, −1, 0, 1, 2, 3 etc.

1.1.2 Rational Numbers

Rational numbers are numbers that can be written as fractions of integers. "Rational" even contains the word "ratio" in it, so if you like, you can simply remember that these are ratio numbers.

EXAMPLES

$$\frac{1}{2}$$

$$-5 \left(-5 = \frac{-5}{1} \right)$$

$$1.875 \left(1.875 = \frac{15}{8} \right)$$

NOTE

Every integer is also a rational number, but not every rational number is an integer. You can write them as fractions simply by dividing by 1.

Make sure you are extra careful when ratios and fractions are involved because they are notorious for causing mistakes.

Irrational numbers are numbers that cannot be written as fractions of integers. Irrational numbers are normally numbers that have a decimal number that goes on forever with no repeating digits.

EXAMPLES

$\sqrt{2} = 1.4142135623730950...$

$Pi = \pi = 3.14159265358979...$

$e = 2.718281828459045...$

For GAMSAT Maths, it is expected that you have memorised pi to 3.14 and you will work faster during the exam if you recognise root 2 as 1.4 and root 3 as 1.7.

We will discuss the number e in context (natural logs) in Chapter 3.

1.1.3 Real Numbers and the Number Line

Real numbers are all numbers that can be represented on the number line. These include both rational and irrational numbers.

EXAMPLES

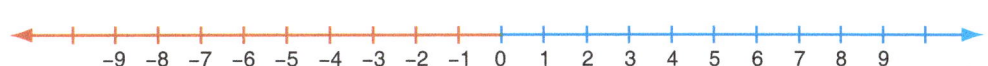

$0, -\dfrac{1}{3}, \sqrt{2}$, etc.

The **number line** is an infinite straight line on which every point corresponds to a real number. As you move up the line to the right, the numbers get larger, and down the line to the left, the numbers get smaller.

$$-9\ -8\ -7\ -6\ -5\ -4\ -3\ -2\ -1\ 0\ 1\ 2\ 3\ 4\ 5\ 6\ 7\ 8\ 9$$

Absolute value refers to how far a real number is from zero on the number line and it is indicated by a bar "|" placed on either side of a number or expression. For GAMSAT purposes, "absolute value" means to remove any negative sign in front of a number, thus the number must be positive (or zero). Thus |−3| = 3, and |8| = 8, and |−4×8| = 32. {This simple concept is needed for: ACER's current *GAMSAT Practice Questions* "Red" booklet, Section 3, Unit 12, Question 33.}

1.2 Basic Arithmetic

1.2.1 Basic Operations

An **operation** is a procedure that is applied to numbers. The fundamental operations of arithmetic are addition, subtraction, multiplication, and division.

A **sum** is the number obtained by adding numbers.

EXAMPLE

The sum of 7 and 2 is 9 since 2 + 7 = 9.

A **difference** is the number obtained by subtracting numbers.

EXAMPLE

In the equation 7 − 2 = 5, 5 is the difference of 7 and 2.

A **product** is the number obtained by multiplying numbers.

GAMSAT-Prep.com
GOLD STANDARD MATHS

High-level Importance

EXAMPLE

The product of 7 and 2 is 14 since 7 × 2 = 14.

A **quotient** is the number obtained by dividing numbers.

EXAMPLE

In the equation 8 ÷ 2 = 4, 4 is the quotient of 8 and 2.

> Unlike a sum or a product, difference and quotient can result in different numbers depending on the order of the numbers in the expression:
>
> 10 − 2 = 8 while 2 − 10 = −8
> 20 ÷ 5 = 4 while 5 ÷ 20 = 0.25

The sum and difference of positive numbers are obtained by simple addition and subtraction, respectively. The same is true when adding negative numbers, except that the sum takes on the negative sign.

EXAMPLES

(-3) + (-9) = -12

(-5) + (-12) + (-44) = -61

On the other hand, when adding two integers with unlike signs, you need to ignore the signs first, and then subtract the smaller number from the larger number. Then follow the sign of the larger number in the result.

EXAMPLES

(-6) + 5 ⇒ 6 − 5 = 1 ⇒ -1

7 + (-10) ⇒ 10 − 7 = 3 ⇒ -3

When subtracting two numbers of unlike signs, start by changing the minus sign into its reciprocal, which is the plus sign. Next reverse the sign of the second number. This will make the signs of the two integers the same. Now follow the rules for adding integers with like signs.

EXAMPLES

(-6) − 5 = (-6) + (-5) = -11

7 − (-10) = 7 + 10 = 17

Multiplication and division of integers are governed by the same rules: If the numbers have like signs, the product or quotient is positive. If the numbers have unlike signs, the answer is negative.

EXAMPLES

5 × 6 = 30
−5 × −3 = 15
81 ÷ 9 = 9
−20 ÷ −4 = 5
7 × −4 = −28
−9 × 6 = −54
−15 ÷ 3 = −5
16 ÷ −2 = −8

GM-22   CHAPTER 1: NUMBERS AND OPERATIONS

An **expression** is a grouping of numbers and mathematical operations.

EXAMPLE

2 + (3 × 4) × 5 is a mathematical expression.

An **equation** is a mathematical sentence consisting of two expressions joined by an equals sign. When evaluated properly, the two expressions must be equivalent.

EXAMPLE

$2 \times (1+3) = \frac{16}{2}$ is an equation since the expressions on both sides of the equals sign are equivalent to 8.

> **NOTE**
>
> Whenever you see simple calculations in these chapters, take the time to make sure that you are able to make the presented calculations quickly and efficiently. We know that you have learnt all of these skills before, we just want to firmly rebuild your foundation for more complex, speed-driven, GAMSAT-level maths.

1.2.1.1 Summary of Properties of Positive and Negative Integers

Positive + Positive = Positive
$$5 + 4 = 9$$

Negative + Negative = Negative
$$(-6) + (-2) = -8$$

Positive + Negative = Sign of the highest number and then subtract
$$(-5) + 4 = -1$$
$$(-8) + 10 = 2$$

Negative − Positive = Negative
$$(-7) - 10 = -17$$

Positive − Negative = Positive + Positive = Positive
$$6 - (-4) = 6 + 4 = 10$$

Negative − Negative = Negative + Positive = Sign of the highest number and then subtract
$$(-8) - (-7) = (-8) + 7 = -1$$

Negative × Negative = Positive
$$(-2) \times (-5) = 10$$

Positive/Positive = Positive
$$8/2 = 4$$

Negative × Positive = Negative
$$(-9) \times 3 = -27$$

Positive/Negative = Negative
$$64/(-8) = -8$$

GAMSAT-Prep.com
GOLD STANDARD MATHS

1.2.2 Properties of the Real Numbers

High-level Importance

Whenever you are working within the real numbers, these properties hold true. It isn't necessary to memorise the name of each property, but you must be able to apply them all.

Symmetric Property of Equality: The right and left hand sides of an equation are interchangeable, so if $a = b$, then $b = a$.

Transitive Property of Equality: If $a = b$ and $b = c$, then $a = c$. This means that if you have two numbers both equal to one other number, those two numbers are also equal.

Commutative Property of Addition: When adding numbers, switching the position of the numbers will not change the outcome, so $a + b = b + a$.

Associative Property of Addition: When adding more than two numbers, it doesn't matter what order you do the addition in, so $(a + b) + c = a + (b + c)$.

Commutative Property of Multiplication: When multiplying numbers, switching the position of the numbers will not change the outcome, so $a \times b = b \times a$.

Associative Property of Multiplication: When multiplying more than two numbers, it doesn't matter what order you do the multiplication in, so $(a \times b) \times c = a \times (b \times c)$.

Identity Property of Addition: When zero is added or subtracted to any number, the answer is the number itself, so $10b - 0 = 10b$.

Identity Property of Multiplication: When a number is multiplied or divided by 1, the answer is the number itself, so $6a \times 1 = 6a$.

Distributive Property of Multiplication: When multiplying a factor on a group of numbers that are being added or subtracted, the factor may be distributed by multiplying it by each number in the group, so $a(b - c) = ab - ac$.

> Subtraction and division do not follow associative laws.

1.2.3 Order of Operations

Knowing the order of operations is fundamental to evaluating numerical expressions. If you follow it properly, you will always come up with the correct answer! Here it is in list form, to be followed from the top down:

Parentheses
Exponents (including square roots)
Multiplication
Division
Addition
Subtraction

GAMSAT MASTERS SERIES

This forms the simple acronym **PEMDAS**, which is a great way to keep the operations straight. Alternatively, some people find it easier to remember the phrase "**P**lease **E**xcuse **M**y **D**ear **A**unt **S**ally."

If you don't like either of these techniques, feel free to come up with your own, or use BODMAS which is described in the NOTE below. It's important to have this clear because, as simple as it may seem, being able to carry out the order of operations quickly is crucial.

Using PEMDAS, let's evaluate this expression composed only of integers.

$$2^2 + [(3 + 2) \times 2 - 9]$$

First, evaluate the expression contained in the inner set of parentheses.

$$= 2^2 + [(5) \times 2 - 9]$$

You can then choose to strictly follow the PEMDAS order by evaluating the exponent next. Alternatively, you can perform the operations within the square brackets, working your way outward, for a more organised procedure as follows:

> **NOTE**
> Don't like PEMDAS? BODMAS is equally helpful! BODMAS stands for "B"rackets, "O"f or "O"rder, "D"ivision, "M"ultiplication, "A"ddition and "S"ubtraction. As long as you have the order correct, the means to help you remember can be whatever is easiest for you.

First, perform the multiplication.

$$= 2^2 + (10 - 9)$$

Then, perform the subtraction.

$$= 2^2 + 1$$

Now evaluate the exponent.

$$= 4 + 1$$

Finally, evaluate the remaining expression.

$$= 5$$

> **NOTE**
> - Multiplication and division have the same rank. It is generally recommended to do them in order from left to right as they appear in the expression, but you can also do them in whatever order that makes most sense to you.
> - The same goes for addition and subtraction. Execute them from left to right, or in the order that feels most comfortable.
> - When you encounter nested parentheses, evaluate the innermost ones first then work your way outward.

High-level Importance

GAMSAT-Prep.com
GOLD STANDARD MATHS

1.3 Rules on Zero

1.3.1 Addition and Subtraction with Zero

Zero is a unique number, and it has special properties when it comes to operations.

Zero is known as the **additive identity** of the real numbers since whenever it is added to (or subtracted from) a number, that number does not change.

Let's examine a simple expression.

$$(3 + 2) - 4$$

We can add or subtract zero anywhere within the expression and the value will not change:

$$(3 - 0 + 2) - 4 + 0$$
$$= (3 + 2) - 4$$

The addition or subtraction of the two zeros has no effect whatsoever on the outcome.

1.3.2 Multiplication and Division with Zero

When adding zero in an expression, it is easy to come up with a practical picture of what the operation represents; you begin with a collection of things and add zero more things to them. When multiplying and dividing with zero, however, such a conceptualisation is more difficult. The idea of using zero in this manner is far more abstract.

Fortunately, you don't need to wrestle with trying to picture what multiplication or division with zero looks like. You can simply remember these easy rules:

Multiplying by Zero: The result of multiplying any quantity by zero is *always* equal to zero.

Remember that by the commutative property of multiplication, $a \times b = b \times a$, so if we let $b = 0$, then we have $a \times 0 = 0 \times a$. This means that instead of trying to imagine multiplying a number by zero, you can reverse the thought and consider multiplying zero by a number instead. This second statement is more natural to visualise. You start with nothing, and then no matter how many times you duplicate that nothing, you still end up with nothing.

EXAMPLE

$3 \times 0 = 0$
$123.79 \times 0 = 0$
$\left[1.2 + \left(37 - \sqrt{5}\right) \times 2.331\right] \times 0 = 0$

In the last example, there is no need to go through the order of operations and evaluate the expression inside the parentheses. Because you can see immediately that the entire parenthetical expression is being multiplied by zero, you know that the end result will be zero.

Zero Divided by a Number: The result of dividing zero by any quantity is *always* equal to zero. As with multiplication by zero, if you start with nothing and then take a portion of that nothing, you still end up with nothing.

EXAMPLE

$0 \div 3 = 0$

$0 \div 123.79 = 0$

$0 \div \left[1.2 + \left(37 - \sqrt{5} \right) \times 2.331 \right] = 0$

Just like with the multiplication by zero example, you do not need to evaluate the parenthetical expression in order to know that the solution is zero.

Dividing by Zero: Dividing any nonzero quantity by zero results in a solution that is not defined and is therefore undefined.

You should never have to deal with this case on the GAMSAT. If you end up with division by zero in a calculation, you have probably made a mistake. Similarly, you should never end up with zero divided by zero (an undefined quantity). If you do, you should go back and check your work.

1.4 Fractions, Decimals, and Percentages

1.4.1 Fractions

A **fraction** is the quotient of two numbers. It represents parts of a whole and may be seen as a proportion. The number on top is the *numerator*, and the one on the bottom is the *denominator*. Another way of understanding fractions is to consider one as the number of parts present (*numerator*) and the amount of parts it takes to make up a whole (*denominator*). These values can be divided by each other, and this fraction is the quotient.

EXAMPLE

$$\frac{2}{7}$$

In this fraction, 2 is the numerator and 7, the denominator.

Remember, all rational numbers (including integers) can be written as fractions.

GAMSAT-Prep.com
GOLD STANDARD MATHS

1.4.2 Manipulating Fractions

A. Fraction Multiplication

To multiply fractions, simply multiply the numerators together (this will be the new numerator) and then multiply the denominators together (this will be the new denominator).

EXAMPLE

$$\frac{2}{3} \times \frac{4}{5}$$

Multiply the numerators and denominators separately.

$$= \frac{(2 \times 4)}{(3 \times 5)}$$

$$= \frac{8}{15}$$

B. Fraction Division

A **reciprocal** is the number obtained by switching the numerator with the denominator of a fraction. For example, the reciprocal of $\frac{2}{3}$ is $\frac{3}{2}$.

To divide a number by a fraction, multiply that number by the reciprocal of the fraction. {"*Dividing fractions is easy as pie, flip the second fraction then multiply.*"}

EXAMPLE

$$3/(4/3) = 3 \div \frac{4}{3}$$

Switch the numerator and the denominator in the fraction and multiply. Remember that 3 is really 3 ÷ 1 so the new denominator would be the product of 1 × 4.

$$= \frac{3}{1} \times \frac{3}{4}$$

$$= \frac{9}{4}$$

Note: 3/(4/3) is not the same as (3/4)/3. Using the rule for fraction division, (3/4)/3 = 3/4 × 1/3 = 3/12 = 1/4.

C. Fraction Addition and Subtraction

With fractions, addition and subtraction are not so easy. You can only add or subtract fractions from each other if they have the same denominator. If they satisfy this condition, then to add or subtract, you do so with the numerators only and leave the denominator unchanged.

EXAMPLE

$$\frac{1}{5} + \frac{3}{5}$$

Both fractions have the same denominator, so add the numerators.

$$= \frac{1 + 3}{5}$$

$$= \frac{4}{5}$$

EXAMPLE

$$\frac{3}{5} - \frac{1}{5}$$

High-level Importance

GM-28   CHAPTER 1: NUMBERS AND OPERATIONS

Both fractions have the same denominator, so subtract the numerators.

$$= \frac{3-1}{5}$$

$$= \frac{2}{5}$$

What if the denominators of two fractions you are adding or subtracting are not the same? In this case, you must find the Lowest Common Denominator (LCD), the smallest number that is divisible by both of the original denominators.

Ideally, you would like to find the smallest common denominator because smaller numbers in fractions are always easier to work with. But this is not always easy to do, and usually it isn't worth the extra time it will take to do the necessary calculation. The simplest way to find a common denominator is to multiply each fraction by a new fraction in which the numerator and denominator are both the same as the denominator of the other fraction.

EXAMPLE

$$\frac{2}{3} + \frac{2}{7}$$

Don't be confused by the fact that the numerators are the same. We still need to find a common denominator because the denominators are different.

$$= \left(\frac{2}{3} \times \frac{7}{7}\right) + \left(\frac{2}{7} \times \frac{3}{3}\right)$$

$$= \frac{14}{21} + \frac{6}{21}$$

Now that we have the same denominator, we can add the numerators.

$$= \frac{20}{21}$$

This method of finding common denominators utilises the fact that any number multiplied by 1 is still the same number. The new fractions we introduce are always made of equivalent numerators and denominators, which make the fraction equal to 1, so the values of the original fractions do not change.

D. Comparing Fractions

Another method with which you should be familiar when manipulating fractions is comparing their values (i.e., which of the given fractions is greater than or lesser than the other) when they have different denominators. We will show you three ways to do this.

When you are confronted with only two fractions, finding their common denominator makes the task of evaluating the values easier.

1. Similar to the preceding discussion on adding or subtracting fractions that have different denominators, the fastest way to come up with a common denominator is to multiply both the numerator and denominator of each fraction by the other's denominator.

Let's say you are given the two fractions:

$$\frac{4}{5} \text{ and } \frac{3}{7}$$

GAMSAT-Prep.com
GOLD STANDARD MATHS

High-level Importance

Multiply the first fraction by 7 over 7 and the second fraction by 5 over 5. (The 7 comes from the fraction $\frac{3}{7}$ while 5 from $\frac{4}{5}$.)

$$\frac{4}{5} \times \frac{7}{7} = \frac{28}{35}$$

$$\frac{3}{7} \times \frac{5}{5} = \frac{15}{35}$$

With both fractions having 35 as the common denominator, you can now clearly see that 28 must be greater than 15. Therefore, $\frac{4}{5}$ is greater than $\frac{3}{7}$.

2. Another way to go about this is through cross-multiplication. Using the same fractions as examples, you first multiply the numerator of the first fraction by the denominator of the second fraction. The product will then serve as the new numerator of the first fraction.

$$\frac{4}{5} \searrow \frac{3}{7} \Rightarrow 4 \times 7 = 28$$

Next, multiply the denominators of the two fractions. The product will now serve as the new denominator of the first fraction.

$$\frac{4}{5} \rightarrow \frac{3}{7} \Rightarrow 5 \times 7 = 35$$

The resulting new fraction would be $\frac{28}{35}$.

Now, let's work on the second fraction. To get its new numerator, this time, multiply the numerator of the second fraction by the denominator of the first fraction. Then multiply the denominators of both fractions.

$$\frac{4}{5} \swarrow \frac{3}{7} \Rightarrow 3 \times 5 = 15$$

$$\frac{4}{5} \leftarrow \frac{3}{7} \Rightarrow 7 \times 5 = 35$$

The second fraction will now become $\frac{15}{35}$. Thus comparing the first and second fractions, we get the same result as we had in the first method.

Because $\frac{28}{35}$ is greater than $\frac{15}{35}$, therefore $\frac{4}{5}$ is greater than $\frac{3}{7}$.

Both procedures follow the same basic principles and prove to be efficient when dealing with two given fractions. But what if you were given three or four fractions (since the GAMSAT is multiple choice, this will happen from time to time)?

3. A much simpler way is to convert each fraction to decimals, and then compare the decimals. All you have to do is divide the numerator of the fraction by its own denominator. With a little practice, you can actually train your brain to work fast with arithmetic.

Now let's say a third fraction is introduced to our previous examples: $\frac{4}{5}, \frac{3}{7}, \frac{9}{13}$. Working on the first fraction, simply divide 4 by 5; on the second fraction, 3 by 7; and on

GM-30   CHAPTER 1: NUMBERS AND OPERATIONS

the last, 9 by 13 (you should try this yourself to ensure that you can perform these basic calculations quickly and correctly).

$$\frac{4}{5} = 4 \div 5 = 0.8$$

$$\frac{3}{7} = 3 \div 7 = 0.43$$

$$\frac{9}{13} = 9 \div 13 = 0.69$$

Comparing the three fractions in their decimal forms, 0.43 ($\frac{3}{7}$) is the smallest, 0.69 ($\frac{9}{13}$) is the next, and the largest is 0.8 ($\frac{4}{5}$). Comparing multiple fractions is a skill required for several questions from official ACER GAMSAT practice materials (examples in the Spoiler Alert section at the end of this chapter).

> **NOTE**
> For the GAMSAT, decimals should be the recourse of last resort. When needed, try to complete calculations using fractions which will improve your speed.

E. Reduction and Cancelling

To make calculations easier, you should always avoid working with unnecessarily large numbers. To reduce fractions, you can cancel out any common factors in the numerator and denominator.

EXAMPLE

$$\frac{20}{28}$$

First, factor both the numerator and denominator.

$$= \frac{(4 \times 5)}{(4 \times 7)}$$

Since both have a factor of four, we can cancel.

$$= \frac{5}{7}$$

When multiplying fractions, it is possible to cross-cancel like factors before performing the operation. If there are any common factors between the numerator of the first fraction and the denominator of the second fraction, you can cancel them. Likewise, if there are common factors between the numerator of the second and the denominator of the first, cancel them as well.

EXAMPLE

$$\frac{5}{9} \times \frac{6}{25}$$

First, factor the numerators and denominators.

$$= \frac{5}{(3 \times 3)} \times \frac{(2 \times 3)}{(5 \times 5)}$$

GAMSAT-Prep.com
GOLD STANDARD MATHS

Now, we see that we can cross-cancel 5's and 3's.

$$= \frac{1}{3} \times \frac{2}{5}$$

$$= \frac{2}{15}$$

F. Mixed Numbers

You may encounter numbers on the GAMSAT that have both an integer part and a fraction part. These are called mixed numbers.

EXAMPLE

$$3\frac{1}{2}$$

Mixed numbers should be thought of as addition between the integer and the fraction.

EXAMPLE

$$3\frac{1}{2} = 3 + \frac{1}{2}$$

Now in order to convert a mixed number back to a fraction, all you have to do is consider the integer to be the fraction of itself over 1 and perform fraction addition.

EXAMPLE

$$3\frac{1}{2}$$

$$= \frac{3}{1} + \frac{1}{2}$$

Obtain a common denominator.

$$= \left(\frac{3}{1}\right)\left(\frac{2}{2}\right) + \frac{1}{2}$$

$$= \frac{6}{2} + \frac{1}{2}$$

$$= \frac{7}{2}$$

To add or subtract mixed numbers, you can deal with the integer and fraction portions separately. {Notice above that parentheses (brackets) side by side is shorthand for multiplication.}

EXAMPLE

$$3\frac{1}{2} - 2\frac{1}{2}$$

$$= (3-2) + \left(\frac{1}{2} - \frac{1}{2}\right)$$

$$= 1$$

> **NOTE**
>
> To convert a mixed number to a fraction, keep the denominator of the fraction while multiplying the integer part of the mixed number by the denominator. Then add to the numerator of the mixed number.
>
> #### EXAMPLE
>
> $$6\frac{2}{5} = (6 \times 5) + \frac{2}{5} = 30 + \frac{2}{5} = \frac{32}{5}$$

G. Fractions: Summary

Multiplying $\quad \left(\dfrac{a}{b}\right)\left(\dfrac{c}{d}\right) = \dfrac{ac}{bd}$ $\qquad$ Addition $\quad \dfrac{a}{b} + \dfrac{c}{d} = \dfrac{ad + bc}{bd}$

Dividing $\quad \dfrac{\left(a/b\right)}{\left(c/d\right)} = \dfrac{ad}{bc}$ $\qquad$ Subtraction $\quad \dfrac{a}{b} - \dfrac{c}{d} = \dfrac{ad - bc}{bd}$

High-level Importance

1.4.3 Decimals and Percentages

There are two other ways to represent non-integer numbers that you will encounter on the GAMSAT: As decimals and as percentages.

A. Decimals

Decimal numbers can be recognised by the decimal point (a period) that they contain. Whatever digits are to the left of the decimal point represent a whole number, the integer portion of the number. The digits to the right of the decimal point are the decimal portion.

EXAMPLE

12.34

The integer portion of the number is 12, and .34 is the fractional portion.

The value of the decimal portion of a number operates on a place-value system just like the integer portion. The first digit to the right of the decimal point is the number of tenths (1/10 is one tenth), two digits over is the number of hundredths (1/100 is one hundredth), three digits over is the number of thousandths, then ten-thousandths, etc.

For example, in the decimal 0.56789:
- the 5 is in the tenths position;
- the 6 is in the hundredths position;
- the 7 is in the thousandths position;
- the 8 is in the ten thousandths position;
- the 9 is in the one hundred thousandths position.

Thus, to convert a decimal into a fraction, just drop the decimal point and divide by the power of ten of the last decimal digit. To convert a fraction to a decimal, simply perform the long division of the numerator divided by the denominator.

EXAMPLE

$$0.34 = \dfrac{34}{100}$$

GAMSAT MATHS $\qquad$ GM-33

B. Operations with Decimals

Addition and Subtraction: Adding and subtracting decimals is the same as with integers. The only difference is that you need to take care to line up the decimal point properly. Just like with integers, you should only add or subtract digits in the same place with each other.

EXAMPLE

Add 3.33 to 23.6.

$$\begin{array}{r} 23.60 \\ + \ 03.33 \end{array}$$

Notice how we have carried the decimal point down in the same place. Also, to illustrate the addition more clearly, we have added zeros to hold the empty places. Now perform the addition as if there were no decimal points.

$$\begin{array}{r} 23.60 \\ + \ 03.33 \\ \hline 26.93 \end{array}$$

Multiplication: You can multiply numbers with decimals just as you would with integers, but placing the decimal point in the solution is a little tricky. To decide where the decimal point goes, first count the number of significant digits after the decimal points in each of the numbers being multiplied. Add these numbers together to obtain the total number of decimal digits. Now, count that number of digits in from the right of the solution and place the decimal point in front of the number at which you end.

EXAMPLE

Multiply 3.03 by 1.2.

$$\begin{array}{r} 3.03 \\ \times \ 1.20 \end{array}$$

We have written in a zero as a placeholder at the end of the second number, but be careful not to include it in your decimal count. Only count up to the final nonzero digit in each number (the 0 in the first number counts because it comes before the 3). Thus our decimal digit count is 2 + 1 = 3, and we will place our decimal point in the solution 3 digits in from the right; but first, perform the multiplication while ignoring the decimal.

$$\begin{array}{r} 3.03 \\ \times \ 1.20 \\ \hline 606 \\ + \ 3030 \\ \hline 3636 \end{array}$$

Now, insert the decimal point to obtain the final solution.

$$= 3.636$$

When counting significant digits, remember to consider the following:

1. all zeros between nonzero digits

EXAMPLE

0.45078 → 5 significant figures

2. all zeros in front of a nonzero number

EXAMPLE

0.0056 → 4 significant figures

3. ignore all zeros after a nonzero digit

EXAMPLE

0.2500 → 2 significant figures

> **NOTE**
>
> Unfortunately, this last maths rule is not so simple because in science labs, significant figures (= significant digits = sig figs) represent the accuracy of measurement. The good news is that if there were ever a question on the GAMSAT involving significant figures, they would clarify which rule to apply before asking questions.

Division: We can use our knowledge of the equivalence of fractions to change a decimal division problem into a more familiar integer division problem. Simply multiply each number by the power of ten corresponding to the smallest significant digit out of the two decimal numbers being divided, and then, perform the division with the integers obtained.

This operation is acceptable because it amounts to multiplying a fraction by 1.

EXAMPLE

Divide 4.4 by 1.6

$$\frac{4.4}{1.6}$$

Since the smallest decimal digit in either number is in the tenth place, we multiply the top and bottom by 10.

$$= \frac{4.4}{1.6} \times \frac{10}{10}$$

$$= \frac{44}{16}$$

$$= \frac{11}{4}$$

If you like, you can convert this back to a decimal.

$$= 2.75$$

Rounding Decimals: Rounding decimals to the nearest place value is just like rounding an integer. Look at the digit one place further to the right of the place to which you are rounding. If that digit is 5 or greater, add 1 to the previous digit and drop all the subsequent digits. If it is 4 or less, leave the previous digit alone and simply drop the subsequent digits.

Consider the number 5.3618:

(a) Round to the nearest tenth.

$$= 5.4$$

Since the digit after the tenth place is a 6, we add 1 tenth and drop every digit after the tenth place.

(b) Round to the nearest hundredth.

$$= 5.36$$

GAMSAT-Prep.com
GOLD STANDARD MATHS

Since the digit after the hundredth place is a 1, we do not change any digits. Just drop every digit after the hundredth place.

Fraction-Decimal Conversions to Know: Having these common conversions between fractions and decimals memorised will help you save valuable time on the test.

Fraction	Decimal
1/2	.5
1/3	~ .33
1/4	.25
1/5	.2
1/6	~.167
1/8	.125
1/10	.1

C. Percentages

Percentages are used to describe fractions of other numbers. One percent (written 1%) simply means 1 hundredth. This is easy to remember since "percent" can literally be broken down into "per" and "cent", and we all know that one cent is a hundredth of both a dollar and a euro.

We can use this conversion to hundredths when evaluating expressions containing percents of numbers, but a percentage has no real meaning until it is used to modify another value. For example, if you see 67% in a problem you should always ask "67% of what?"

EXAMPLE

What is 25% of 40?

$$= .25 \times 40$$
$$= 10$$

To find what percentage a certain part of a value is of the whole value, you can use what is known as the **percentage formula**:

$$\text{Percent} = (\text{Part/Whole}) \times 100$$

EXAMPLE

What percentage of 50 is 23?

$$\text{Percentage} = (23/50) \times 100$$
$$= (46/100) \times 100$$
$$= 46\%$$

Combining percentages requires some nuance (i.e. 'it depends on the question' thus there are several possibilities). Although GAMSAT scores are not percentages, since they are scaled scores out of 100, they can be used as an analogy.

To calculate your *average* (GM 6.2.1) GAMSAT score, you would add the scaled score for each of the 3 sections and divide by 3, thus (S1 + S2 + S3)/3. To get a weighted score, since most medical programmes weight Section 3 twice: (S1 + S2 + 2 x S3)/4. However, no programme weights each question equally: (total correct)/(total number of questions). We will calculate average percentages when we look at ternary nomograms (GM 3.9).

1.5 Roots and Exponents

1.5.1 Properties of Exponents

An exponent is simply shorthand for multiplying that number of identical factors. So 4^3 is the same as $(4)(4)(4) = 64$, three identical factors of 4. Thus x^2 (i.e. 'x squared') is two factors of x, $(x)(x)$, while x^3 (i.e. 'x cubed') is three factors of x, $(x)(x)(x)$.

To multiply exponential values with the same base, keep the base the same and add the exponents.

EXAMPLE

$$a^2 \times a^3 = a^{2+3} = a^5$$

To divide exponential values with the same base, keep the base the same and subtract the exponent of the denominator from the exponent of the numerator.

EXAMPLE

$$\frac{x^5}{x^3} = x^{5-3} = x^2$$

To multiply exponential values with different bases but the same exponent, keep the exponent the same and multiply the bases.

EXAMPLE

$$2^x \times 3^x = (2 \times 3)^x = 6^x$$

To divide exponential values with different bases but the same exponent, keep the exponent the same and divide the bases.

EXAMPLE

$$\frac{6^x}{2^x} = \left(\frac{6}{2}\right)^x = 3^x$$

To raise an exponential value to another power, keep the base the same and multiply the exponents.

EXAMPLE

$$(x^3)^4 = x^{(3 \times 4)} = x^{12}$$

Even though all of the preceding examples use only positive integer exponents, these properties hold true for all three of the types described in section 1.5.3.

1.5.2 Scientific Notation

Scientific notation, also called exponential notation, is a convenient method of writing very large (or very small) numbers. Instead of writing too many zeroes on either side of a decimal, you can express a number as a product of a power of ten and a number between 1 and 10. For example, the number 8,765,000,000 can be expressed as 8.765×10^9.

The first number 8.765 is called the coefficient. The second number should always have a base of ten with an exponent equal to the number of zeroes in the original numbers. Moving the decimal point to the left makes a positive exponent while moving to the right makes a negative exponent.

In multiplying numbers in scientific notation, the general rule is as follows:

$$(a \times 10^x)(b \times 10^y) = ab \times 10^{x+y}$$

EXAMPLE

To multiply 2.0×10^4 and 10×10^2

{Whenever possible, when you see a practice question like the one above, consider using a sheet of paper or Post-It note to cover the worked solution while you try to answer the question yourself.}

(i) Find the product of the coefficients first.

$2.0 \times 10 = 20$

(ii) Add the exponents.

$4 + 2 = 6$

(iii) Construct the result.

20×10^6

(iv) Make sure that the coefficient has only one digit to the left of the decimal point. This will also adjust the number of the exponent depending on the number of places moved.

2.0×10^7

Dividing numbers in scientific notation follows this general rule:

$$\frac{(a \times 10^x)}{(b \times 10^y)} = \frac{a}{b} \times 10^{x-y}$$

Going back to our preceding example, let's divide 2.0×10^4 and 10×10^2 this time:

(i) Divide the coefficients.

$2.0 \div 10 = 0.2$

(ii) Subtract the exponents.

$4 - 2 = 2$

(iii) Construct the result and adjust the values to their simplest forms.

$0.2 \times 10^2 = 2 \times 10 = 20$

In adding and subtracting numbers written in scientific notation, you need to ensure that all exponents are identical. You would need to adjust the decimal place of one of the numbers so that its exponent becomes equivalent to the other number.

EXAMPLE

Add 34.5×10^{-5} and 6.7×10^{-4}

(i) Choose the number that you want to adjust so that its exponent is equivalent to the other number. Let's pick 34.5 and change it into a number with 10^{-4} as its base-exponent term.

$3.45 \times 10^{-4} + 6.7 \times 10^{-4}$

(ii) Add the coefficients together:

$3.45 + 6.7 = 10.15$

(iii) The exponents are now the same, in this case 10^{-4}, so all you have to do is plug it in:

10.15×10^{-4}

(iv) Adjust the end result so that the coefficient is a number between 1 and 10:

1.015×10^{-3}

The same procedure basically applies to subtraction.

> **NOTE**
>
> Notice in the examples in this section, when you lower the power from the coefficient (i.e. by moving the decimal to the left), you must add to the exponent, and vice-versa.

1.5.3 Types of Exponents

Positive Integer Exponents: This is the type of exponent you will encounter most often. Raising a base number *b* to a positive integer exponent *x* is equivalent to making *x* copies of *b* and multiplying them together.

EXAMPLE

$2^4 = 2 \times 2 \times 2 \times 2 = 16$

Fractional Exponents: Fractional exponents are also known as roots. Let *x* be the fraction. To raise a base number *b* to the *x* power we make use of the fifth property of exponents in section 1.5.1.

We can write $b^{\frac{n}{d}}$ as $\left(b^{\frac{1}{d}}\right)^n$. The value $b^{\frac{1}{d}}$ is known as the *d*-th root of *b*. So the base *b* raised to the *x* power is the same as the *d*-th root of *b* raised to the *n* power.

GAMSAT-Prep.com
GOLD STANDARD MATHS

High-level Importance

EXAMPLE

$$8^{\frac{2}{3}}$$

$$= \left(8^{\frac{1}{3}}\right)^2$$

The expression inside the parentheses is the cube root of 8. Since 2 × 2 × 2 = 8, the cube root of 8 is 2.

$$= 2^2$$
$$= 4$$

Consider the following: What is the cube root of 125, and separately, what is the cube root of -125? The number 5 multiplied by itself 3 times equals 125. Similarly, the number -5 multiplied by itself 3 times equals -125. Thus the answers are 5 and -5, respectively.

Negative Exponents: The value of a base raised to a negative power is equal to the reciprocal of the base, raised to a positive exponent of the same value. For any exponential value b^{-x}, b^{-x} is equivalent to $\frac{1}{(b^x)}$.

EXAMPLE

$$3^{-2}$$

Take the reciprocal and invert the sign of the exponent.

$$= \frac{1}{(3^2)}$$
$$= \frac{1}{(3 \times 3)}$$
$$= \frac{1}{9}$$

1.5.4 Zero and Exponents

Raising a Number to the Zero: Any number raised to the zero power is equal to 1.

We can see that this follows the rules of exponents (*see* section 1.5), because $a^0 = a^1 \times a^{-1} = a/a = 1$.

> **NOTE**
>
> The quantity 0^0 (read as zero to the zero power) is 1.

EXAMPLES

$$3^0 = 1$$
$$123.79^0 = 1$$
$$\left[1.2 + \left(37 - \sqrt{5}\right) \times 2.331\right]^0 = 1$$

As with multiplication and division, you should not waste time evaluating the parenthetical expression.

GM-40 CHAPTER 1: NUMBERS AND OPERATIONS

1.5.5 Summary of the Rules for Exponents

$$a^0 = 1 \qquad\qquad a^1 = a$$

$$a^n a^m = a^{n+m} \qquad\qquad a^n/a^m = a^{n-m}$$

$$(a^n)^m = a^{nm} \qquad\qquad a^{\frac{1}{n}} = \sqrt[n]{a} \quad \{\text{note that } a^{\frac{1}{2}} \text{ is simply } \sqrt{a}\}$$

1.5.6 Recognising Number Patterns

It is possible to save a lot of time during the real GAMSAT by avoiding unnecessary calculations by the recognition of certain patterns. One helpful way to achieve this is by knowing at least the following relationships that are typically memorised in primary school maths class (*see* table below).

Test makers choose their numbers carefully. The moment you see 1.44 on the GAMSAT, there would be a high likelihood that taking the square root, which gives 1.2, would be required (because, of course, the square root of 144 is 12, the square root of 1.44 must be 1.2). Likewise, the square root of 1.7, being an approximation of 1.69, must be 1.3 (the square root of 169 being 13).

x	1	2	3	4	5	6	7	8	9	10	11	12	13	14	15	20
x^2	1	4	9	16	25	36	49	64	81	100	121	144	169	196	225	400
x^3	1	8	27	64	125	-	-	-	-	1000	-	-	-	-	-	-

Table 1: Common squares and cubes that are helpful to know. Applying the rules of exponents (GM 1.5.3, 1.5.5), $5^2 = 25$, $5^3 = 125$; square root of $121 = (121)^{1/2} = \sqrt[2]{121} = \sqrt{121} = 11$; cube (= 3rd) root of $64 = (64)^{1/3} = \sqrt[3]{64} = 4$. These basic manipulations are commonly required for the real exam.

> **NOTE**
>
> Try to complete all the chapter review warm-up exercises as quickly as possible and, of course, without the use of a calculator.

GAMSAT-Prep.com
GOLD STANDARD MATHS

1.6 Ratio and Proportion

1.6.1 What is a Ratio?

A **ratio** is the relation between two numbers. There are multiple ways they can be written, but ratios can always be denoted as fractions.

These are all ways to represent the same ratio:

$$3 \text{ to } 4 = 3:4 = \frac{3}{4} = 3/4$$

If a ratio is written out in words, the first quantity stated should generally be placed in the numerator of the equivalent fraction and the second quantity in the denominator. Just make sure you keep track of which value corresponds to which category.

1.6.2 Solving Proportions

A **proportion** is a statement of equality between two or more ratios.

Solving for an unknown variable is the most common type of proportion problem. If you have just a ratio on either side of an equation, you can rewrite the equation as the numerator of the first times the denominator of the second equal to the denominator of the first times the numerator of the second. This allows you to find the missing information more easily.

EXAMPLE

Solve for x in the following equation.

$$\frac{2}{3} = \frac{5}{x}$$

Cross multiply to eliminate fractions.

$$2 \times x = 3 \times 5$$
$$2x = 15$$
$$x = \frac{15}{2} = 7\frac{1}{2}$$

This means that the ratio 2 to 3 is equivalent to the ratio 5 to $7\frac{1}{2}$.

Unless it is stated, a proportion does not describe a specific number of things. It can only give you information about quantities in terms of other quantities. But if it is explicitly stated what one of the two quantities is, the other quantity can be determined using the proportion.

GOLD STANDARD WARM-UP EXERCISES

CHAPTER 1: Numbers and Operations (answers and worked solutions are at the end of this chapter)

High-level Importance

1. What is the approximate value of
   $$0.125 + \sqrt{\frac{1}{9}}?$$

   A. 0.40
   B. 0.46
   C. 0.50
   D. 0.45

2. 0.8 is to 0.9 as 80 is to:

   A. 9
   B. 100
   C. 8
   D. 90

3. If you invest in Bank A, you will receive 19% interest on the amount you invest. If you invest in Bank B, you will receive 21% interest. The maximum amount you can invest in Bank A is $6,430, and the maximum amount you can invest in Bank B is $5,897. How much more interest will you earn if you invest the maximum amount in Bank B than if you invest the maximum amount in Bank A?

   A. $16.67
   B. $16.30
   C. $101.27
   D. $111.93

4. Board C is 3/4 as long as Board B. Board B is 4/5 as long as Board A. What is the sum of the lengths of all three Boards if Board A is 100 m long?

   A. 255 m
   B. 225 m
   C. 240 m
   D. 235 m

5. The proportion of the yellow marbles in a jar of yellow and green jars is 7 out of 9. If there are 999 marbles in the jar, how many of these are yellow?

   A. 111
   B. 777
   C. 2
   D. 222

6. If 0.25 months is equal to one week, what fraction of a month is equal to one day?

   A. 1/7
   B. 4/7
   C. 1/30
   D. 1/28

7. Which of the following is 6.4% of 1,000?

   A. $64^{\frac{3}{4}}$
   B. $256^{\frac{3}{4}}$
   C. $\left(\frac{64}{100}\right)^2$
   D. 6.4 / 100

8. $2 + \left[71 - 8\left(\frac{6}{2}\right)^2\right]$ is what percent of $\sqrt{2500}$?

   A. 50%
   B. 1%
   C. 44%
   D. 2%

9. Which is the largest?

   A. 0.636
   B. 0.136
   C. 0.46
   D. 0.163

10. Determine the sum of 9, -5, and 6.

    A. 20
    B. -20
    C. -10
    D. 10

GAMSAT-Prep.com
GOLD STANDARD MATHS

High-level Importance

11. Determine the value of 1.5×10^7 divided by 3.0×10^4.
    A. 5.0×10^3
    B. 5.0×10^2
    C. 5.0×10^{-2}
    D. 0.5×10^{-3}

12. Determine the value of 1.5×10^7 subtracted by 3.0×10^4.
    A. 1.497×10^7
    B. -1.5×10^3
    C. 1.2×10^3
    D. 1.47×10^7

13. Determine the value of $|(-3)(6)|$.
    A. 3
    C. 18
    B. -3
    D. -18

14. Determine the value of $-|2-5|$.
    A. 3
    C. 7
    B. -3
    D. -10

15. Try to complete the following calculation in under 30 seconds: Determine the value of $.333 \times .125$. {Reminder: all calculations in this book should be performed without the use of a calculator.}
    A. 0.02
    C. 0.04
    B. 0.03
    D. 0.05

16. Which of the following is the greatest number?
    A. $\frac{31}{50}$
    C. $\frac{3}{5}$
    B. $\frac{31}{51}$
    D. $\frac{16}{25}$

17. Which of the following is the greatest number?
    A. $\frac{96}{5}$
    C. $\frac{230}{15}$
    B. $\frac{53}{3}$
    D. $\frac{147}{9}$

18. Simplify the expression: $(x^2)(y^2)(x^3)(y)(x^0)$.
    A. 0
    C. x^5y^3
    B. x^6y^3
    D. x^5y^2

19. Simplify the expression: $(x^{2a+b})(x^{a-2b})/(x^{2a-b})$.
    A. x^a
    B. x^{ab}
    C. x^{5a-2b}
    D. x^{5a+2b}

20. Let $x = 4$ and $y = 8$. Evaluate the expression: $((y^{-2/3})^{1/2})/(x^{-1/2})$.
    A. 8
    C. 2
    B. 1
    D. 1/2

> **NOTE**
>
> No matter what your previous experience has been, please keep in mind: ==Maths skills improve with practice.== Each GAMSAT Maths chapter has practice questions. You will be exposed repeatedly to all of the common maths manipulations required for the real exam. Persistent effort will eventually meet reward.

Chapter 1 Worked Solutions

Question 1   B

See: GM 1.2.3, 1.4.3

According to the rules of order of operations, we work with the square root first: $0.125 + \sqrt{\frac{1}{9}} = 0.125 + \frac{1}{3}$.

Since the answers are in decimal form, this problem is easiest to solve if all values are in decimal form. From the list of fraction-to-decimal conversions, $\frac{1}{3} \approx 0.33$, and so, $0.125 + \frac{1}{3} \approx 0.125 + 0.33 = 0.455$. All of the answers have only two decimal places, so we must round this answer off to the hundredths decimal place. The digit in the thousandths decimal place is a 5, and so the digit in the hundredths decimal place increases by 1 to become 6. 0.455 therefore rounds off to 0.46.

Quick Solution:

$$0.125 + \sqrt{\frac{1}{9}} = 0.125 + \frac{1}{3} \approx 0.125 + 0.333$$

$$= 0.458 \approx 0.46.$$

Question 2   D

See: GM 1.6.2

This is a proportion problem, so there will be two equivalent ratios. We construct the first ratio as $\frac{0.8}{0.9}$ and the second as $\frac{80}{x}$. If we set them equal, we get $\frac{0.8}{0.9} = \frac{80}{x}$, and cross-multiplication gives us $0.8x = (0.9)(80)$, or $0.8x = 72$. Therefore, $x = \frac{72}{0.8} = 90$.

> **Quick Solution:** 80 differs from 0.8 by a factor of 100. This means that the answer must be related to 0.9 by the same factor: $x = 100(0.9) = 90$

Question 3   A

See: GM 1.4.3

The interest earned by investing $5,897 in Bank B is 21% of $5,897, or $(0.21)(\$5,897) = \$1238.37$. The interest earned by investing $6,430 in Bank A is 19% of $6,430, or $(0.19)(\$6,430) = \$1221.70$. Subtracting the smaller from the larger, we get $\$1238.37 - \$1221.70 = \$16.67$.

Though you won't be asked about interest for GAMSAT Section 3 (though it is possible for Section 1), the words will be different but the maths will be the same. Also, you must be quick and precise with your calculations.

Question 4   C

See: GM 1.4.2

We must work backwards to find the lengths of boards B and C. Board B is 4/5 as long as Board A, which is $\frac{4}{5}(100m) = 80m$. Board C is 3/4 as long as this, which is $\frac{3}{4}(80m) = 60m$. To find the sum of these lengths, we add the three values: $100m + 80m + 60m = 240m$.

Question 5   B

See: GM 1.6.2

This is a proportion problem in which the following are given: The proportion of the yellow marbles in the jar of yellow and green marbles is 7 out of 9. This makes the ratio of the number of yellow marbles to green marbles 7:2. The total number of marbles is 999. Therefore, the number of yellow marbles = $(7/9) \times 999 = 777$ marbles.

Question 6   D

See: GM 1.6.1

This is a ratio problem involving different units. The given ratio is 0.25 months per week. We need to re-write this as a fraction: 0.25 months per week = $\frac{25}{100}$ months/week = $\frac{1}{4}$ months/week. This ratio tells us that there are four weeks in

GAMSAT-Prep.com
GOLD STANDARD MATHS

one month. We can express the number of months corresponding to one day using an intermediate relationship. There are 7 days in one week, which we can express with the ratio $\frac{1}{7}$ weeks/day. To express the number of months per day, we must multiply the first ratio by the second: ($\frac{1}{4}$ months/week) ($\frac{1}{7}$ weeks/day) = $\frac{1}{28}$ months/day. Notice that the weeks units cancel so that the only units left are months and days. If we had used a ratio expressing the number of days per week (the reciprocal of weeks per day), $\frac{7}{1}$ days/week, this cancellation would not occur and the final answer would not have the correct units of months per day.

> **Quick Solution:** To convert a ratio that expresses a relationship between months and weeks to one that expresses a relationship between months and days, multiply it by a ratio that expresses a relationship between weeks and days:
>
> ($\frac{1}{4}$ months/week) ($\frac{1}{7}$ weeks/day) = $\frac{1}{28}$ months/day.

We will link the process to solve the problem above to 'dimensional analysis' in Chapter 2 (GM 2.2).

Question 7   B
See: GM 1.2.3, 1.4.3, 1.5.2
The first step in this problem is to find the value of 6.4% of 1,000. We convert the percentage to a decimal (0.064) and multiply by one thousand: 0.064(1,000) = 64. Next, we find which of the answer choices is equal to this value. Choice A is obviously incorrect because 64 taken to any power besides 1 does not equal 64. The order of operations tells us that we must perform the calculation inside the parentheses first in choice C, which is a decimal (0.64). Squaring this value does not give us 64. Choice D begins with a small number (6.4) and divides it by a much larger number, so we know that the answer will be even smaller, and therefore not equal to 64. The correct choice is B. To check this, note that $256^{3/4} = (256^{1/4})^3 = (4)^3$ (because 4 × 4 × 4 × 4 = 256) and $(4)^3 = 64$.

Question 8   D
See: GM 1.2.3, 1.4.3
First, simplify the expressions according to the rules of the order of operations:

$$2 + \left[71 - 8\left(\frac{6}{2}\right)^2\right] = 2 + (71 - 8(3)^2)$$
$$= 2 + (71 - 8(9))$$
$$= 2 + (71 - 72)$$
$$= 2 + (-1) = 1$$

and $\sqrt{2500} = 50$. So, we need to find the percentage of 50 that is constituted by 1. Using the formula

Percent = Part/Whole × 100

$$\frac{1}{50} \times 100 = 0.02 \times 100 = 2,$$

we see that the answer is 2%.

Question 9   A
See: GM 1.4.3
The tenths decimal place is the largest occupied in each number. Comparing the digits in this decimal place, it is clear that the .6 in .636 is the largest.

Question 10   D
See: GM 1.2.1
Following the rule of adding like and unlike signs:

= 9 + −5 + 6
= 4 + 6
= 10

Question 11   B
See: GM 1.5.2
Dividing the coefficients 1.5 and 3.0 gives an answer of 0.5. Then the correct exponent value is determined by subtracting the exponents involved, which are 7 and 4. The final answer in scientific notation is $0.5 \times 10^3 = 5.0 \times 10^2$.

High-level Importance

Question 12   A
See: GM 1.5.1, 1.5.2
Convert so that both numbers have the same power of 10, then and only then can subtraction (or addition) be accomplished.

$$1.5 \times 10^7 = 1500 \times 10^4$$
$$1500 \times 10^4 - 3.0 \times 10^4 =$$
$$1497 \times 10^4 = 1.497 \times 10^7$$

Question 13   C
See: GM 1.2.1.1, 1.1.3
Vertical bars mean 'absolute value'. First we calculate what is within the vertical bars, then to take the absolute value, we convert to a positive number.

$$|(-3)(6)| = |-18| = 18$$

Question 14   B
See: GM 1.2.1.1, 1.1.3
Vertical bars mean 'absolute value'. First we calculate what is within the vertical bars, then to take the absolute value, we convert to a positive number. Note that there is a negative symbol *outside* the vertical lines which will ensure that the answer becomes negative.

$$-|2-5| = -|-3| = -|3| = -3$$

{Recall: $2-5 = -3$, $|-3| = 3$, and then the first minus gets you -3}

Question 15   C
See: GM 1.4.3
It is usually easier to calculate using fractions than decimals. You should instantly recognise .333 as 1/3 and .125 as 1/8 (GM 1.4.3).

$1/3 \times 1/8 = 1/24$ which is approximately $1/25 = 4/100 = 0.04$.

You may be surprised at how often the test makers for the GAMSAT choose numbers to give you the option to work faster with fractions.

Question 16   D
See: GM 1.4.2D
When comparing answer choice A and B, you can immediately notice that answer choice B has the same numerator but a slightly larger denominator which means that 31/51 is a smaller number than 31/50. Answer choice C can be converted to a form that can easily be compared to the highest number so far (answer choice A): so 3/5 = 30/50 which has a smaller numerator but the same denominator as answer choice A, thus B is smaller. Now let's convert answer choice D so we can compare with A: 16/25 = 32/50 which is slightly higher than 31/50 and thus D is the winner.

Question 17   A
See: GM 1.4.2D
Choose the method that you are most comfortable with. As decimals: A is 19.2, B is 17.7, C is 15.3, D is 16.3. Thus the answer is A. If you did not complete the decimal calculations, see if you can do them now with speed. If you did not try reducing (as below), also see if you can do that now with speed.

You could choose to reduce: A = 96/5 = 19 1/5 (notice that 96 is close to 100 and 100/5 is clearly 20; so you could try 19 x 5 to get to 95 with 1 remainder); B = 53/3 (again, 60/3 is easily 20 but we are a few 3's below 60: try 17 x 3 = 51 with 2 remainder thus 17 2/3; C = 230/15 = 15 5/15 = 15 1/3 (recall that 15 x 15 is on your list for rote learning, GM 1.5.6, and is 225); D = 147/9 = 16 1/3. And so answer choice A has the greatest number.

Please note: there are dozens of other ways to solve these questions (including estimating to achieve rounder numbers). Choose your technique.

Question 18   C
See: GM 1.5
First rearrange the expression and group like terms:

$$(x^2)(y^2)(x^3)(y)(x^0) = (x^2 \, x^3 \, x^0)(y^2 y)$$

When multiplying powers with the same base, you can combine them by adding the exponents. For example:

$$y^2 y = (y)(y)(y) = y^{2+1} = y^3$$

So the expression becomes:

$(x^2 \, x^3 \, x^0)(y^2 y)$

$= x^{2+3+0} y^{2+1}$

$= x^5 y^3$

Question 19   A
See: GM 1.5
First simplify the numerator:

$(x^{2a+b})(x^{a-2b}) / (x^{2a-b})$

$= (x^{2a+b+a-2b}) / (x^{2a-b})$

$= (x^{3a-b}) / (x^{2a-b})$

Then combine the numerator and denominator using the properties of exponent division.

$= (x^{3a-b-2a+b})$

$= x^a$

Question 20   B
See: GM 1.5
First combine the exponents where possible, and rearrange so they are all positive:

$((y^{-2/3})^{1/2}) / (x^{-1/2})$

$= (y^{-1/3}) / (x^{-1/2})$

$= (x^{1/2}) / (y^{1/3})$

Now plug in $x = 4$ and $y = 8$. Notice that $4 = 2^2$ and $8 = 2^3$.

$= (4^{1/2}) / (8^{1/3})$

$= (2^{(2)1/2}) / (2^{(3)1/3})$

$= 2^1 / 2^1$

$= 1$.

GAMSAT MASTERS SERIES

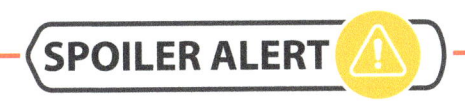

> **SPOILER ALERT** ⚠
>
> Gold Standard has cross-referenced the content in this chapter to examples from ACER's official GAMSAT practice materials (note that only ACER sells their eBooks brand new). It is for you to decide when you want to explore these questions since you may want to preserve some of ACER's materials for timed mock-exam practice.
>
> | Number | 1 | 2 | 3 | 4 | 5 |
> |---|---|---|---|---|---|
> | Title | GAMSAT Practice Questions | GAMSAT Sample Questions | GAMSAT Practice Test | GAMSAT Practice Test 2 | GAMSAT Practice Test 3 |
> | Colour | Orange/Red | Blue | Green | Purple | Pink |
>
> **Examples** – Absolute value: Q33 of 1; proportions/fractions: Q13, Q34 of 1; fractions with assumed knowledge (voltage = current x resistance, V = IR; Ohm's Law, PHY 10.1): Q21 of 5; fractions (add/subtract/multiply): Q37-39 of 5; proportions: Q53 of 5. Determining the highest fraction, examples: Q50 of 1, Q16 of 2, Q61 of 5. Calculations involving scientific notation, examples: Q49 of 1, Q68 of 3, Q32 and Q46 of 4, Q87 of 5. Note that "Q" is followed by the question number, and, for example, "of 1" refers to booklet number 1 in the table above. Also note that your gamsat-prep.com Masters Series online account has direct links to the step-by-step worked solutions for all of ACER's Section 3 practice questions (the solutions can also be found in the Gold Standard GAMSAT YouTube Channel). The 10 full-length HEAPS GAMSAT practice tests (by Gold Standard and MediRed), exams 1 through 10, contain specific cross-references to this chapter within the worked solutions. Note that the HEAPS exams and the GAMSAT-level practice questions in Physics (at the end of chapters after GAMSAT Maths in this book) and Chemistry will continually have you exposed to the content in Chapter 1 at the rate that you can expect on the real exam.

High-level Importance

Chapter Checklist

- ☐ Reassess your 'learning objectives' for this chapter: Go back to the first page of this chapter and re-evaluate the top 3 boxes and the Introduction.
  - ☐ Please be sure that you have completed the *Need for Speed* exercises at the beginning of this chapter.
- ☐ Complete a maximum of 1 page of notes using symbols/abbreviations to represent the entire chapter based on your learning objectives. These are your Gold Notes.
- ☐ Consider your multimedia options based on your optimal way of learning:
  - ☐ Download the free Gold Standard GAMSAT app for your Android device or iPhone.
  - ☐ Create your own, tangible study cards or try the free app: Anki.
  - ☐ Record your voice reading your Gold Notes onto your smartphone (MP3s) and listen during exercise, transportation, etc.
  - ☐ Try out the Gold Standard GAMSAT Physics online videos at gamsat-prep.com which have heaps of calculations, or you can try other maths options on YouTube like Khan Academy or Leah4sciMCAT playlist for Maths Without a Calculator (the latter was produced for MCAT preparation but it remains helpful for GAMSAT).
- ☐ Schedule your full-length GAMSAT practice tests: ACER and/or HEAPS exams. Schedule one full day to complete a practice test and 1-2 days for a thorough assessment of worked solutions while adding to your abbreviated Gold Notes.
- ☐ Schedule and/or evaluate stress reduction techniques such as regular exercise (sports), yoga, meditation and/or mindfulness exercises (*see* YouTube for suggestions).

High-level Importance

GOLD NOTES

SCIENTIFIC MEASUREMENT AND DIMENSIONAL ANALYSIS
Chapter 2

Memorise	Understand	Importance
* SI units and prefixes	* Dimensional analysis	**High level: 11%** of GAMSAT Section 3 maths-based questions released by ACER are related to content in this chapter (in our estimation). * Note that approximately **90%** of such questions are related to just 3 chapters: 1, 2, and 3.

GAMSAT-Prep.com

Introduction

It is extremely important to know the SI system of measurement for the GAMSAT. The metric system is very much related to the SI system. The British system, though familiar, does not need to be memorised for the GAMSAT (related questions would only be asked if relevant conversion factors were provided). **'Dimensional analysis'** is a technique whereby **simply paying attention to units and applying the basic algebra** we covered in GM Chapter 1, you will be able to solve several real exam questions in GAMSAT Physics, Chemistry and Biology – even without previous knowledge in those subjects.

Additional Resources

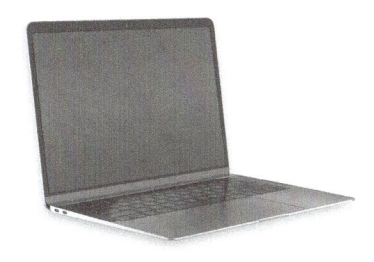

Open Discussion Boards

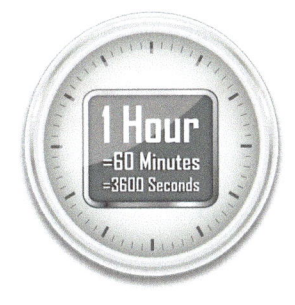

Special Guest

GAMSAT MATHS GM-51

GAMSAT-Prep.com
GOLD STANDARD MATHS

2.0 GAMSAT Has a *Need for Speed*!

High-level Importance

A 'unit' is any standard used for making comparisons in measurements. Units form an important part of the foundation of science and GAMSAT Section 3.

For non-science students, this is a new language to learn but the vocabulary is incredibly small. The units below can all be found in this chapter, and throughout GAMSAT Physics and Chemistry. Your familiarity with these units will make your study of Physics easier. It is normal if you cannot fill out the tables now, but please return to this page after you have studied this chapter so you can complete all entries below.

Science students? Do your best, be quick, note that some entries that appear simple may surprise you! ACER has exam questions directly dependent on your understanding of SI units and prefixes, so let's get started…

Section	Units		
2.1.3 Table 1: SI Base Units	length:		electric current:
	mass:		thermodynamic temperature:
	time:		amount of substance:

Section	Units	
2.1.3 Table 2: Examples of SI Derived Units	area:	speed, velocity:
	volume:	acceleration:

Section	Units	
2.1.3 Table 3: SI Derived Units with Special Names and Symbols	frequency:	power:
	force:	electric charge, quantity of electricity:
	pressure, stress:	electric potential difference, electromotive force:
	energy, work, quantity of heat:	

Section	Base 10	
2.1.3 Table 4: Important SI prefixes for GAMSAT, A closer look	tera:	deci:
	giga:	centi:
	mega:	milli:
	kilo:	micro:
	hecto:	nano:
	deca:	pico:

CHAPTER 2: SCIENTIFIC MEASUREMENT AND DIMENSIONAL ANALYSIS

2.1 Systems of Measurement

2.1.1 British Units (Imperial System of Measurement)

You are probably already familiar with several of these units of measurement, but we recommend reviewing them at least once.

A. Length: These units are used to describe things like the length of physical objects, the displacement of a physical object, the distance something has traveled or will travel, etc. Area and volume are also measured as the square and cube (respectively) of these units.

Inches	The *inch* is the smallest measurement of length in the British System.
Feet	There are 12 inches in every foot. 1 ft. = 12 in.
Yards	There are 3 feet in every yard. 1 yd. = 3 ft.
Miles	The *mile* is the largest unit of length in the British System. There are 5,280 feet in every mile. 1 mi. = 5,280 ft.

B. Time: These units describe the passage of time.

Seconds	The *second* is the smallest unit of time in the British System.
Minutes	There are 60 seconds in every minute. 1 min. = 60 s.
Hours	There are 60 minutes in every hour. 1 h. = 60 min.
Days	There are 24 hours in every day. 1 day = 24 h.
Years	The *year* is the largest unit of time in the British System. There are 365 days in every year. 1 yr. = 365 days

C. Mass/Weight: These terms are not technically the same and we will discuss the differences in Physics. The following units describe the amount of matter in an object.

Ounces	The *ounce* is the smallest unit of mass in the British System.
Pounds	There are 16 ounces (oz.) in every pound (lb.). 1 lb. = 16 oz.
Tons	The *ton* is the largest unit of mass in the British System. There are 2,000 lbs. in an American ton, and 2,240 lbs. in a British tonne. Neither should be committed to memory.

GAMSAT-Prep.com
GOLD STANDARD MATHS

2.1.2 Metric Units

Measuring with Powers of 10: Unlike the British System, the Metric System has only one unit for each category of measurement. In order to describe quantities that are much larger or much smaller than one of the base units, a prefix is chosen from a variety of options and added to the front of the unit. This changes the value of the unit by some power of 10, which is determined by what the prefix is. The following are the most common of these prefixes (with the representative symbols in brackets):

Milli (m) One thousandth (10^{-3}) of the base unit

Centi (c) One hundredth (10^{-2}) of the base unit

Deci (d) One tenth (10^{-1}) of the base unit

Deca (da) Ten (10^{1}) times the base unit

Kilo (k) One thousand (10^{3}) times the base unit

There is a mnemonic that may be used to identify these prefixes:

King	Kilometre	Kilo
Henry	Hectometre	Hecto (h)
Died	Decametre	Deca
Unexpectedly	Unit Base	Unit
Drinking	Decimetre	Deci
Chocolate	Centimetre	Centi
Milk	Milimetre	Milli

As you go down, you divide by 10 and as you go up, you multiply by 10 in order to convert between the units.

EXAMPLE

How many metres is 1 kilometre?

$$1 \text{ km} = 1000 \text{ m}$$

From general knowledge, we know that kilo means one thousand. This means there are 1000 metres in a kilometre. But just in case you get confused, you can also use the clue from the mnemonic. Now we know that Kilo is three slots upward from the Unit base. Hence we multiply 3 times by 10: $10 \times 10 \times 10 = 1000$.

An even less confusing way to figure out how to do the metric conversions quickly and accurately, is to use a metric conversion line. This is quite handy with any of the common units such as the *metre*, *litre*, and *grams*.

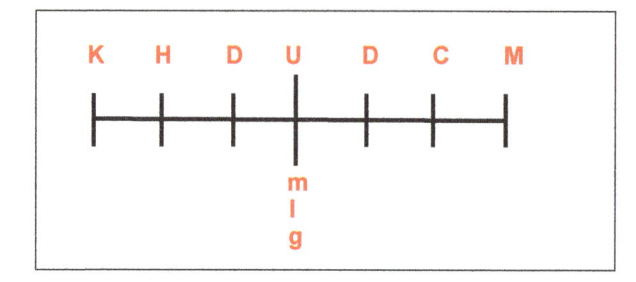

Figure GM 2.1: The Metric Conversion Line. The letters on top of the metric line stands for the "King Henry" mnemonic. On the other hand, the letters below the metric line - **m**, **l**, **g** – stand for the unit bases, **m**etre, **l**itre, or **g**ram, respectively.

GM-54   CHAPTER 2: SCIENTIFIC MEASUREMENT AND DIMENSIONAL ANALYSIS

To use this device, draw out the metric line as shown in Fig GM 2.1. From the centremost point **U**, the prefixes going to the left represent those that are larger than the base unit (kilo, hecto). These also correspond to the decimal places that you will be moving from the numerical value of the unit to be converted. Those going to the right are for the ones smaller than the unit (deci, centi, milli).

EXAMPLE

How much is 36 litres in millilitres?
Step 1: Place your pen on the given unit, in this case L (litre). Then count the number of places it takes you to reach the unit being asked in the problem (millilitre).

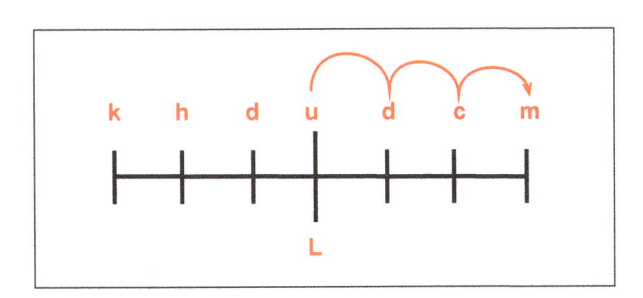

```
k   h   d   u   d   c   m
                    L
```

Fig GM 2.2: Converting litre to millilitre using the metric conversion line.

Step 2: Because it took you three places going to the right to move from the litre to the millilitre units, you also need to add three places from the decimal point of the number 36.0.

36 L = 36,000 ml

Now, let's try converting centimetre to kilometre: What is 6.3 cm in km?

1. Place your pen on the **c** (centi) point in the metric line.

2. Moving from **c** to **k** (kilo) takes five places going to the left. This also means moving five places from the decimal point of the number 6.3.
6.3 cm = .000063 km

Using this method definitely makes doing the metric conversions so much faster than the fraction method!

There are other prefixes that are often used scientifically:

Tera (T) 10^{12} times the base unit
Giga (G) 10^{9} times the base unit
Mega (M) 10^{6} times the base unit
Micro (μ) 10^{-6} of the base unit
Nano (n) 10^{-9} of the base unit
Pico (p) 10^{-12} of the base unit

A. Length: As with British length units, these are used to measure anything that has to do with length, displacement, distance, etc. Area and volume are also measured as the square and cube (respectively) of these units.

Metres	The *metre* is the basic unit of length in the Metric System.
Other Common Forms	millimetre, centimetre, kilometre

B. Time: These are units that quantify the passage of time.

Seconds	Just as in the British System, the *second* is the basic unit of time in the Metric System. Minutes, hours, and the other British units are not technically part of the Metric System, but they are often used anyway in problems involving metric units.
Other Common Forms	millisecond

C. Mass: These are units that describe the amount of matter in an object.

Grams	The *gram* is the basic metric unit of mass.
Other Common Forms	milligram, kilogram

High-level Importance

2.1.3 SI Units

SI units is the **International System of Units** (abbreviated **SI** from the French *Le Système International d'Unités*) and is a modern form of the metric system. SI units are used to standardise all the scientific calculations that are done anywhere in the world. Throughout this book, and during the real exam, you will see the application of base SI units and the units derived from the base SI units.

> **NOTE**
>
> Typically, because of Chemistry, students think that the litre (L) is an SI unit. It is not. The cubic metre is the SI unit for volume. It is important that you know that 1 L = 1000 cubic centimetres (= cc or mL) = 1 cubic decimetre.

Table 1: SI Base Units

Base quantity	Name	Symbol
	\multicolumn{2}{c}{SI base unit}	
length	metre	m
mass	kilogram	kg
time	second	s
electric current	ampere	A
thermodynamic temperature	kelvin	K
amount of substance	mole	mol

Table 2: Examples of SI Derived Units

	SI derived unit	
area	square metre	m^2
volume	cubic metre	m^3
speed, velocity	metre per second	m/s
acceleration	metre per second squared	m/s^2

Table 3: SI Derived Units with Special Names and Symbols

			SI base unit	
frequency	hertz	Hz	-	s^{-1}
force	newton	N	-	$m \cdot kg \cdot s^{-2}$
pressure, stress	pascal	Pa	N/m^2	$m^{-1} \cdot kg \cdot s^{-2}$
energy, work, quantity of heat	joule	J	$N \cdot m$	$m^2 \cdot kg \cdot s^{-2}$
power	watt	W	J/s	$m^2 \cdot kg \cdot s^{-3}$
electric charge, quantity of electricity	coulomb	C	-	$s \cdot A$
electric potential difference, electromotive force	volt	V	W/A	$m^2 \cdot kg \cdot s^{-3} \cdot A^{-1}$

> **NOTE**
>
> We will see all the units from these 3 tables in the Physics and Chemistry chapters.
>
> Do not try to memorise the last 2 columns in Table 3. However, if this is your second time studying from this page, you should be able to derive all the units displayed in the last 2 columns of Table 3. In fact, the derivation of units through dimensional analysis is a regular type of GAMSAT question. You will be tested on this point with the GAMSAT-level practice questions in Physics and Chemistry.

GAMSAT-Prep.com
GOLD STANDARD MATHS

High-level Importance

Table 4: Important SI prefixes for GAMSAT, A closer look

Prefix Name	Symbol	Base 10	Decimal	English Word
tera	T	10^{12}	1000000000000	trillion
giga	G	10^{9}	1000000000	billion
mega	M	10^{6}	1000000	million
kilo	k	10^{3}	1000	thousand
hecto	h	10^{2}	100	hundred
deca	da	10^{1}	10	ten
BASE UNIT	-	10^{0}	1	one
deci	d	10^{-1}	0.1	tenth
centi	c	10^{-2}	0.01	hundredth
milli	m	10^{-3}	0.001	thousandth
micro	μ	10^{-6}	0.000001	millionth
nano	n	10^{-9}	0.000000001	billionth
pico	p	10^{-12}	0.000000000001	trillionth

There exists more SI prefixes than those presented in Table 4 but, if needed, additional prefixes will be defined during the exam. However, Table 4 is considered 'assumed knowledge' and therefore must be memorised.

As we have seen in GM 2.1.2, each prefix name has a symbol (Table 4) that is used in combination with the symbols for units of measure (Tables 1-3). For example, the symbol for *kilo-* is 'k', and is used to produce 'km', 'kg', and 'kW', which are the SI symbols for kilometre, kilogram, and kilowatt, respectively. Even if you do not have a science background, you have likely heard of many SI prefixes because of your use of computers (a *byte* is a unit of digital memory): very small files like the text of an email = kilobytes, larger files like a good quality digital image = megabytes, storage space on a smartphone = gigabytes, but storage space on a computer is increasingly measured in terabytes.

The following practice questions do not require previous knowledge in Physics. For 'beginners', please feel free to consult Tables 1-4 to assist in solving the questions.

> **NOTE**
>
> As mentioned in Chapter 1, whenever possible, consider using a sheet of paper or Post-It note to cover the worked solution while you try to answer the question yourself. You will benefit from doing so for most of the practice questions in this chapter and subsequent chapters.

GAMSAT MASTERS SERIES

EXAMPLE 1

The power (P) of an electrical appliance can be calculated from the current (I) that flows through it and the potential difference (V) across it, such that P = IV (PHY 10.2).

Determine the power if the potential difference is 5 mV and the current is 5 mA.

A. 25 µW
B. 25 MW
C. 2.5×10^{-3} W
D. 2.5×10^{-3} mW

P = IV = 5 mA × 5 mV
= 5×10^{-3} A × 5×10^{-3} V

P = 25×10^{-6} A•V = 25 µW

- the latter is equivalent to 25×10^{-6} W = 25×10^{-3} mW, NOT 2.5×10^{-3} mW.
- Ref. Tables 1-4; PHY 10.2. Answer: A.

Note that the preceding question and those to follow have no science assumed knowledge other than the understanding of SI units. Also note that if the base units have prefixes, all but one of the prefixes must be expanded to their numeric multiplier, except when combining values with identical units (i.e. 'you can add apples to apples but you can't add apples to oranges').

Consider the following (if you are stuck, please consult any of the preceding tables – 1 to 4 – to try to work out the answer before looking at the worked solution).

EXAMPLE 2

What is the sum of 5.00 mV and 10 µV?

A. 15 µV
B. 5.1 mV
C. 5.01 mV
D. 5.001 mV

The common base unit is the volt (V, see Table 3).

We must ensure that the prefixes are the same in order to perform the addition (or subtraction if that had been the case). Thus 5.00 mV + 10 µV = 5.00 mV + 0.01 mV = 5.01 mV. Answer C.

When units are presented as exponents, for example, in square and cubic forms, the multiplication prefix must be considered part of the unit, and thus included as part of the exponent.

Consider the following cases:

- 1 km² means one square kilometre, or the area of a square of 1000 m by 1000 m and not 1000 square metres.

- 2 Mm³ means two cubic megametres, or the volume of two cubes of 1 000 000 m by 1 000 000 m by 1 000 000 m or 2×10^{18} m³, and not 2 000 000 cubic metres (2×10^{6} m³).

High-level Importance

GAMSAT MATHS GM-59

GAMSAT-Prep.com
GOLD STANDARD MATHS

EXAMPLE 3

Which of the following is NOT equivalent?

A. 3 MW = 3 × 1 000 000 W
B. 9 km^2 = 9 × 10^6 m^2
C. 5 cm = 5 × 0.01 m
D. Each option above represents an equivalence.

- 3 MW = 3 × 10^6 W = 3 × 1 000 000 W = 3 000 000 W

- 9 km^2 = 9 × (10^3 m)^2 = 9 × (10^3)^2 × m^2 = 9 × 10^6 m^2 = 9 × 1 000 000 m^2 = 9 000 000 m^2

- 5 cm = 5 × 10^{-2} m = 5 × 0.01 m = 0.05 m

- Answer: D.

2.2 Mathematics of Conversions (Dimensional Analysis)

2.2.1 Dimensional Analysis with Numeric Calculations

You are about to learn, or revise, a topic of enormous importance for your exam. In fact, the trick or skill of dimensional analysis will help you solve problems during the real GAMSAT even when you might not understand the question! How is this possible? ACER will give you the units in the question and the units for the answer choices. Even if the question is contorted, maths speaks. There is a step-by-step, logical technique to take you from one set of units to another.

The irony is that you have been using this technique all of your life for simple problems without necessarily applying rigid maths. Let's say that you had been working for Q dollars/pounds/euros per hour. After 5 hours, you want to remind yourself of your progress so you do a quick calculation to assess the money that you have earned: 5 × Q. Easy, but in science, that is a dangerous calculation.

Every day, in major hospitals around the world, the health of patients is at risk due to medication errors. One major issue is dosage. Patients sometimes receive the wrong dose because of human error: someone did not pay careful attention to the units.

Basically, a **dimension** is a measurement of length in one direction. Examples include width, depth and height. A line has one dimension, a square has two dimensions (2D), and a cube has three dimensions (3D). In Physics, 'dimensions' can also refer to any physical measurement such as length, time, mass, etc.

Dimensional analysis (also called 'factor-label method' or the 'unit-factor method') permits the solving of problems across the sciences simply by carefully analysing and manipulating units. Unlike the 'normal' equations which you have seen in Chapter 1, equations developed during the process of dimensional analysis require you to focus on numbers and units. ==Dimensional analysis uses the fact that any number or expression can be multiplied by one without changing its value.==

The Process: In order to convert a quantity from one type of unit to another type of unit, all you have to do is set up and execute multiplication between ratios. Each conversion from the preceding subsections of Chapter 2 is actually a ratio.

Consider the following equation that you would naturally feel is reasonable:

$$60 \text{ minutes} = 1 \text{ hour}$$

Divide both sides by 1 hour and you get:

$$\frac{60 \text{ minutes}}{1 \text{ hour}} = 1$$

But if we had divided both sides of the first equation by 60 minutes, you get:

$$1 = \frac{1 \text{ hour}}{60 \text{ minutes}}$$

Since both expressions are equal to 1, then both expressions are equal to each other:

$$1 = \frac{1 \text{ hour}}{60 \text{ minutes}} = \frac{60 \text{ minutes}}{1 \text{ hour}}$$

And, even more powerful is the idea that you can multiply any expression by 60 minutes / 1 hour, or, 1 hour / 60 minutes because it is the same as multiplying that expression by the number 1. But which expression should you use? It depends on your assessment of the units you have and the units you wish to end up with (this is the 'analysis' in dimensional analysis).

When you are performing a conversion, you should treat the units like numbers. This means that when you have a fraction with a certain unit on top and the same unit on bottom, you can cancel out the units leaving just the numbers.

You can multiply a quantity by any of your memorised conversions, and its value will remain the same as long as all of the units, but one, cancel out.

EXAMPLE 1

Given that there are 2.54 cm in an inch, and 12 inches in 1 foot, how many inches are there in 3 feet?

First, determine which conversion will help. We have been provided a conversion directly between feet and inches, so that is

GAMSAT-Prep.com
GOLD STANDARD MATHS

High-level Importance

what we'll use and we'll ignore the distractor (cm). {Yes, the real GAMSAT will deliver some distractors.}

Next, determine which of the two possible conversion ratios we should use. The goal is to be able to cancel out the original units (in this case, feet), so we want to use whichever ratio has the original units in the denominator (in this case, inches/feet).

$$3 \text{ ft} = 3 \text{ ft} \times \frac{12 \text{ in}}{1 \text{ ft}}$$

Now perform the unit cancellation.

$$= 3 \times \frac{12 \text{ in}}{1}$$
$$= 36 \text{ in}$$

In many instances, you will not have a direct conversion. All you have to do in such a case is multiply by a string of ratios instead of just one (we will be using this important technique in EXAMPLE 3).

Warning for science students: We know that some of you may feel this is all trivial, and you may have had a successful academic career looking at problems and just saying "divide by 60" or some such thing. ACER has special traps for those who skip steps. Careful attention to units, irrespective of familiarity, will get you a higher GAMSAT score.

EXAMPLE 2

How many inches are there in 5.08 metres? {Try the conversion yourself before looking at the solution. Please go back to the previous Example - or section - to find an appropriate conversion factor.}

We cannot convert metres directly into inches, but we can convert metres to centimetres and then centimetres into inches. We can set up both these conversions at the same time and evaluate.

$$5.08 \text{ m} = 5.08 \text{ m} \times \frac{100 \text{ cm}}{1 \text{ m}} \times \frac{1 \text{ in}}{2.54 \text{ cm}}$$

Next, cancel the units.

$$= 5.08 \times \frac{100}{1} \times \frac{1 \text{ in}}{2.54}$$
$$= \frac{508 \text{ in}}{2.54}$$
$$= 200 \text{ in}$$

EXAMPLE 3

Calculate the number of seconds in a day.

1) Check the units of the answer: Convert the English "seconds in a day" to the maths, seconds/day or s/day.

2) Next, assess what you already know. You know that there are 60 seconds in one minute, 60 minutes in an hour, and 24 hours in one day. But to convert to

maths, should you use, for example, 60 seconds/minute, or, 1 minute/60 seconds? They are equivalent expressions so we can use either, but only one of the two will help solve this problem.

3) Choose the conversion that takes you towards your answer. In our first step, we determined that seconds was in the numerator, so we must choose a matching conversion, 60 seconds/minute has the correct unit in the numerator. Let's begin to set up the equation:

$$\frac{60 \text{ seconds}}{\text{minute}} \times A \times B = \frac{X \text{ seconds}}{\text{day}}$$

4) Now the new problem that we have is to get rid of "minute" in the denominator and replace it with "day". Should "A" be 60 minutes/hour, or, 1 hour/60 minutes. Only if we choose a conversion with minutes in the numerator could it cancel the "minute" in the denominator. We do the same analysis for 24 hours/day and we get:

$$\frac{60 \text{ seconds}}{\text{minute}} \times \frac{60 \text{ minutes}}{\text{hour}} \times \frac{24 \text{ hours}}{\text{day}} = \frac{X \text{ seconds}}{\text{day}}$$

Now we can cancel the units to confirm that our analysis was correct (i.e. that the units on the left of the equal sign are exactly equal to the units on the right):

$$\frac{60 \text{ seconds}}{\cancel{\text{minute}}} \times \frac{60 \cancel{\text{ minutes}}}{\cancel{\text{hour}}} \times \frac{24 \cancel{\text{ hours}}}{\text{day}} = \frac{X \text{ seconds}}{\text{day}}$$

Since all is equal, we are left with the following calculation:

$$60 \times 60 \times 24 = X$$

Try to quickly complete the calculation above.

If your method gets you the correct answer, well done! When you have completed hundreds of practice questions in GAMSAT sciences, you will begin to notice number patterns. In the preceding calculation, you can set the 2 zeros aside, and complete $6 \times 6 \times 24$. In the next step, rather than calculating 36×24, which is perfectly fine, you might notice that 6×24 is 144. You might find 6×144 faster than 36×24. $6 \times 144 = 864$, now return those 2 zeros, and we have 86 400 seconds/1 day (8.64×10^4 s/day).

On the real exam, you will rarely need to be so precise. You will first assess the units of the answer choices, then assess how close the numbers are, then you would have determined the degree of precision necessary for your calculation (how much can you safely estimate in order to increase speed?). We will examine these issues in the next example.

> **NOTE**
>
> Make sure you check and see that all of your units cancel properly! A lot of unnecessary errors can be avoided simply by paying attention to the units.

GAMSAT-Prep.com
GOLD STANDARD MATHS

High-level Importance

The following are 2 typical GAMSAT-level dimensional analysis practice questions.

EXAMPLE 4

Consider the following diagram.

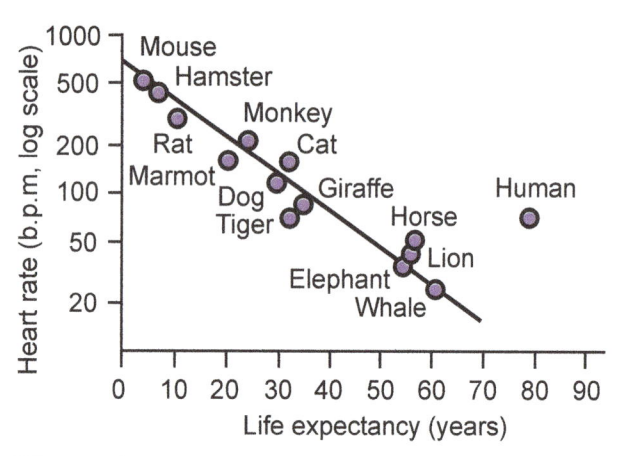

Figure 1: Heart rate in beats per minute (b.p.m.) on a log scale vs. life expectancy in years for various mammals.

Estimate the average number of heart beats over a lifetime for a person.

- A. 2.9×10^{11}
- B. 2.9×10^{9}
- C. 2.9×10^{7}
- D. 2.9×10^{5}

Please try the calculation before looking at the worked solution.

This question is asking for the number of heart beats per lifetime for a human being. If we can determine the rate of heart beats per minute from Figure 1, we could scale that quantity up to an hour, then a year, then a lifetime by estimating the average lifespan - also from Figure 1. You can easily estimate your heart rate by counting your pulse while watching a clock for a minute for comparison, but this question refers to Figure 1.

The heart rate for 'Human' on the graph is approximately 60-70 b.p.m. (= beats per minute as explained by the caption below the graph). Because the answers are far enough apart, which commonly occurs during the real exam, whether you estimate 60 or 70 (or even 80), you will approximate the same answer. We will examine the log scale in GM 3.8 at which point you will better understand why the heart rate is most likely less than 75 b.p.m. From Figure 1, we can estimate life expectancy of a person as 80 years/lifetime.

Putting all of the preceding together, we get:

$$\frac{70 \text{ beats}}{1 \text{ minute}} \cdot \frac{60 \text{ minutes}}{1 \text{ hour}} \cdot \frac{24 \text{ hours}}{1 \text{ day}} \cdot \frac{365 \text{ days}}{1 \text{ year}} \cdot \frac{80 \text{ years}}{1 \text{ lifetime}}$$

What happened to the units?

$$\frac{70 \text{ beats}}{1 \text{ ~~minute~~}} \cdot \frac{60 \text{ ~~minutes~~}}{1 \text{ ~~hour~~}} \cdot \frac{24 \text{ ~~hours~~}}{1 \text{ ~~day~~}} \cdot \frac{365 \text{ ~~days~~}}{1 \text{ ~~year~~}} \cdot \frac{80 \text{ ~~years~~}}{1 \text{ lifetime}}$$

As a result of the cancellations, the final units must be beats/lifetime, or in other words, heart beats over a lifetime.

We have completed the dimensional analysis, so what about the maths?

CHAPTER 2: SCIENTIFIC MEASUREMENT AND DIMENSIONAL ANALYSIS

Keeping in mind that the maths needs to be done quickly and efficiently by hand, we should seek ways to simplify the calculation. Fortunately, in terms of the order of operations (GM 1.2.3), we can perform the multiplications in any order that we want. In other words, we can choose to combine terms which create relatively simple answers.

For example: 70 × 60 is 4200 which is approximately 4000 (notice that we are rounding down to simplify the calculation, GM 1.4.3B; if we get an opportunity to round another calculation upward, it might restore a bit of balance). The 365 does not seem to be clearly simplified; however, 24 × 80 is approximately 25 × 80 which is 2000 (not only is it simpler than immediately using the 365, but it has the added advantage that we rounded upwards a small amount).

Thus, without performing any longhand calculations – only through observation – we have converted 4 factors to 4000 × 2000 = 8 000 000 = 8×10^6. Now we are left with $365 \times 8 \times 10^6$. If you have not already done it, you should complete 365 × 8 as a quick exercise.

Now we have $2920 \times 10^6 = 2.9 \times 10^9$, which is approximately 2.9 billion heart beats in a lifetime. If you did the calculation with a calculator (which is not permissible for the real exam), the result would still be approximately 2.9 billion heart beats per lifetime. Answer B.

With experience, you will not have to calculate 365 × 8 to get the correct answer.

Once you had determined $365 \times 8 \times 10^6$, without having done any longhand calculation, you could have observed that 365 is somewhere between 3×10^2 and 4×10^2. Thus $365 \times 8 \times 10^6$ = between 3 and $4 \times 10^2 \times 8 \times 10^6$ = between 24 and 32×10^8 = between 2.4 and 3.2×10^9. Answer B.

By observing how precise (or imprecise) the answer choices are, you will be able to gauge to what degree you can estimate in order to save time. Because suitable approximating is such a valuable skill for the time-pressured GAMSAT Section 3, we will be highlighting where it applies in the worked solutions for GAMSAT Maths and subsequent chapter-ending practice questions in GAMSAT Physics, Chemistry and Biology.

NOTE

On the real exam, sometimes there could be a question that is missing some data because ACER believes that you should be able to estimate the missing information within a reasonable error margin, as examples: the rate of growth of a part of your body, change in height or weight over time, your heart rate, etc. After all, if Example 3 did not have Figure 1, most people would guess that a resting heart rate is between 60 and 100 b.p.m. Even if a person chose a number between 30 and 200, it would not matter because the answer choices are 100 times apart, so they would still approximate the same answer. Expect that you could be asked the unexpected but that you are equipped with the tools to answer correctly.

2.2.2 Dimensional Analysis with Variables

There will be occasions on the real exam where you will need to apply dimensional analysis but there will not be any SI units, nor SI prefixes, nor numbers! This becomes a disciplined exercise to ensure that you understand how variables can be manipulated using basic maths.

EXAMPLE 5

Consider the Law of Gravitation where the force of gravity F is:

$$F = G(m_1 m_2 / r^2)$$

- F is the force between the masses;
- G is the gravitational constant;
- m_1 is the first mass;
- m_2 is the second mass;
- r is the distance between the centres of the masses.

{We will discuss the preceding Physics equation in PHY 2.4. If you have no background in Physics, please carefully consult Tables 1-3, GM 2.1.3, in order to remind yourself of the units for the various variables that are presented in this problem. Aside from a basic comfort with SI units, there is no assumed knowledge necessary to solve this question.}

The dimension of a physical quantity can be expressed as a product of the basic physical dimensions of mass (M), length (L) and time (T). For example, the dimension of the physical quantity speed or velocity (metres/second = m/s) is length/time (L/T).

Which of the following represents the gravitational constant G in the fundamental dimensions of mass (M), length (L) and time (T)?

A. $M^{-1}L^3T^{-2}$
B. $M^2L^3T^{-2}$
C. $M^{-1}L^{-3}T^{-2}$
D. $M^2L^3T^2$

This is a classic example of dimensional analysis. First, you should know that the unit of force is a newton which is also a kg•m/s² (see Tables 1-3, GM 2.1.3; in PHY 2.2, we will see the very important Newton's Law where F = ma so the units of F must be mass 'm' in kg multiplied by acceleration 'a' which is m/s²). Of course, according to the preamble for the question, the 2 m's in the Law of Gravitation represent masses (M) and the 'r' represents a distance or length (L). So we get:

$$F = G(m_1 m_2 / r^2)$$

Now transferring to the fundamental quantities except for G:

$$MLT^{-2} = GM^2 L^{-2}$$

In order to isolate G (our unknown), divide both sides by $M^2 L^{-2}$:

$$MLT^{-2} / M^2 L^{-2} = G$$

GAMSAT MASTERS SERIES

Remove the common M (GM 1.4.2):

$$LT^{-2} / ML^{-2} = G$$

Since the answer choices have no symbol for division, we can remove the denominator by following the rules for exponents (GM 1.5.1, 1.5.3, 1.5.5):

$$LT^{-2}M^{-1}L^{2} = G$$

Thus: $G = M^{-1}L^{3}T^{-2}$

Answer A. Note that in SI units, which is the other way you could be asked the same question on the exam, the preceding final answer is the same as $m^{3}kg^{-1}s^{-2}$ (Table 1, GM 2.1.3).

Of course, if it is your first time completing such a problem, it may seem quite challenging. Ideally, you will see this type of problem dozens of times before you sit the GAMSAT so that dimensional analysis, in its many forms, will become routine. Regarding the step where we isolated G: we will be doing many more practice questions isolating variables in the next chapter.

High-level Importance

GOLD STANDARD WARM-UP EXERCISES

CHAPTER 2: Scientific Measurement and Dimensional Analysis

1. How many millimetres are there in 75 metres?

   A. 750 mm
   B. 75 mm
   C. 7500 mm
   D. 75 000 mm

2. Which of the following is the shortest distance?

   A. 10 m
   B. 1000 mm
   C. 10 cm
   D. 0.1 km

3. A triathlon has three legs. The first leg is a 12 km run. The second leg is a 10 km swim. The third leg is a 15 km bike ride. How long is the total triathlon in metres?

   A. 37 000 m
   B. 3700 m
   C. 1000 m
   D. 37 m

4. If a paperclip has a mass of one gram and a staple has a mass of 0.05 g, how many staples have a mass equivalent to the mass of one paperclip?

   A. 10
   B. 100
   C. 20
   D. 25

5. Which of the following is the number of minutes equivalent to $17\frac{5}{6}$ hours?

   A. 1080
   B. 1056
   C. 1050
   D. 1070

GAMSAT-Prep.com
GOLD STANDARD MATHS

High-level Importance

6. The three children in a family weigh 67 lbs., 1 oz., 93 lbs., 2 oz., and 18 lbs., 5 oz. What is the total weight of all three children? {You may go back to section 2.1 to find an appropriate conversion factor.}

   A. 178.8 lbs.
   B. 178.5 lbs.
   C. 178.08 lbs.
   D. 179.8 lbs.

7. A lawyer charges clients $20.50 per hour to file paperwork, $55 per hour for time in court, and $30 per hour for consultations. How much will it cost for a 90-minute consultation, $\frac{8}{6}$ hours time filing paperwork, and 1 hour in court?

   A. $110.28
   B. $100.75
   C. $88.25
   D. $127.33

8. If a car moving at a constant speed travels 20 centimetres in 1 second, approximately how many feet will it travel in 25% of a minute? {You may go back to section 2.1 to find an appropriate conversion factor.}

   A. 10
   B. 15
   C. 12
   D. 9

9. The Dounreay Nuclear Power Station has been in operation for quite some time. Over the last six years, they have turned out a total of two megawatt-years of energy. Assuming that operations were continuous over a six year period at a constant rate, what was its power in watts (W)?

   A. 3.3×10^5 W
   B. 6.6×10^5 W
   C. 3.3×10^2 W
   D. 6.6×10^2 W

10. A novel medication is found to have a density of 7.8 µg/mL. What is the mass of 295 mL of the novel medication?

    A. 2.3 g
    B. 2.3 mg
    C. 2.3 µg
    D. 2.3 pg

11. What is the approximate number of minutes in 1 year?

    A. 5.3×10^3
    B. 5.3×10^5
    C. 5.3×10^7
    D. 5.3×10^9

12. The dimension of a physical quantity can be expressed as a product of the basic physical dimensions of mass (M), length (L) and time (T). For example, the dimension of the physical quantity speed or velocity (metres/second = m/s) is length/time (L/T).

    Given that $F = at^{-1} + bt^2$ where F is the force and t is the time, then the dimensions of a and b must be, respectively (note: this is a challenging question but it is at the level of the real GAMSAT. You can look at the table in section 2.1 to guide you to the dimensions that should apply to the force F but that would not be given to you on the real exam. Don't worry if you could not do this problem. We will revisit this question type throughout the GAMSAT Masters Series Physics practice problems at the end of chapters):

    A. LT^{-2}, T^{-2}
    B. T, T^{-2}
    C. LT^{-1}, T^{-2}
    D. MLT^{-1}, MLT^{-4}

CHAPTER 2: SCIENTIFIC MEASUREMENT AND DIMENSIONAL ANALYSIS

GAMSAT MASTERS SERIES

> **NOTE**
>
> If you have completed all of the practice questions with worked solutions in GAMSAT Maths Chapter 2, consider logging into your GAMSAT-prep.com account, clicking on Videos, Physics, and then the following virtual-classroom video: Dimensional Analysis, Reviewing and Manipulating Equations. If necessary, you can have Tables 1-3 in GM 2.1.3 open to consult during the video. Good luck!

Chapter 2 Worked Solutions

Question 1   D
See: GM 2.1, 2.2
Construct a ratio comparing millimetres to metres using the definition of the prefix "milli." Remember that we want to convert from metres to millimetres, so the denominator of the fraction we use for this ratio must contain the units of metres: $\frac{1000\,mm}{1\,m}$. Now multiply this ratio and the given value:

$$75\,m\left(\frac{1000\,mm}{1\,m}\right) = 75\,000\,mm.$$

Question 2   C
See: GM 2.1.2
Start with any of the choices and compare it to the rest:

$$0.1\,km = 100\,m > 10\,m$$
$$0.1\,km > 10\,m$$
$$10\,cm < 10\,m$$
$$1000\,mm = 1\,m > 10\,cm$$

Question 3   A
See: GM 2.2
The total length of the triathlon is 12 km + 10 km + 15 km = 37 km. Express the ratio of kilometres to metres as a fraction, with kilometres in the denominator to cancel the units of 37 km: $\frac{1000\,m}{1\,km}$. Now multiply:

$$37\,km\left(\frac{1000\,m}{1\,km}\right) = 37\,000\,m.$$

Question 4   C
See: GM 2.1
Construct an equation that expresses an unknown number of staples, times the weight of each, equals the weight of one paperclip:

$$0.05x = 1$$
$$x = \frac{1}{0.05} = 20$$

Question 5   D
See: GM 2.1, 2.2
Convert the mixed number to an improper fraction (which you should be able to 'do in your head' because 17 times 6 can be broken down to 10 times 6 = 60 PLUS 7 times 6 = 42 so SUBTOTAL = 102 PLUS 5 for a TOTAL = 107):

$$17\frac{5}{6} = \frac{107}{6}$$

Convert using the fact that 60 minutes equals 1 hour (notice that the number 6 cancels so the problem is reduced to 107 times 10 = 1070):

$$\left(\frac{107}{6}\,hours\right)\left(\frac{60\,minute}{1\,hour}\right) = 1070\,minutes$$

Question 6   B
See: GM 2.1, 2.2
Add like units:

$$67\,lbs. + 93\,lbs. + 18\,lbs. = 178\,lbs.$$
$$1\,oz. + 2\,oz. + 5\,oz. = 8\,oz.$$

Convert to pounds the part of the total weight that is in ounces and add to the rest of the weight:

$$(8 \text{ oz.}) \left(\frac{1 \text{ lbs.}}{16 \text{ oz.}} \right) = 0.5 \text{ lbs.}$$

178 lbs. + 0.5 lbs. = 178.5 lbs.

Question 7   D

See: GM 2.1.1, 2.2
Given that the charges are:

$20.50 per hour to file paper,
$55 per hour for time in court,
$30 per hour for consultations,

a 90-minute consultation = $30 + $15 = $45.
8/6 hours = 80 minutes time filing paper work = $20.50 + $6.83 = $27.33

Since 20 minutes = $6.83

1 hour in court = $55

Total charges = $45 + $27.33 + $55 = $127.33

Notice that the first and third charge add to $100 making the calculation trivial.

Question 8   A

See: GM 2.1, 2.2; dimensional analysis
Multiply by all ratios necessary to convert centimetres to feet (via inches) and seconds to minutes, and divide by 4 to calculate the speed for only 25% of a minute:

$$(20 \text{ cm/sec.}) \left(\frac{1}{2.54} \text{ in./cm} \right)$$

$$\left(\frac{1}{12} \text{ ft./in.} \right) (60 \text{ sec./min.}) \left(\frac{1}{4} \right) \approx 10 \text{ ft./min.}$$

Question 9   A

See: GM 2.1, 2.2; dimensional analysis
This problem is strictly a matter of dimensional analysis.
In the SI system, "mega" means 10^6
1 Megawatt = 10^3 kW = 10^6 W
Therefore, power in watts = (Total number of watt-years)/(Number of years)

Notice that the equation is constructed to allow "years" to cancel (i.e. it is in the numerator and in the denominator).
2×10^6 watt-years/6 years = 0.33×10^6 W = 3.3×10^5 W

Question 10   B

See: GM 2.1.3, 2.2
Even if you have never heard of 'density', even if you have never known that density is mass divided by volume (PHY 6.1.1), you can just examine the units provided and dimensional analysis (GM 2.2) will lead you to the correct answer. All of the answers are in a form of grams (GM 2.1.3), we are given µg/mL so in order to get g we need to multiply µg/mL by mL and then mL cancels and we will have µg. Then we can convert to mg by using our SI Unit Prefix knowledge. If you have not considered the preceding then try to answer the question before looking at the worked solution.

7.8 µg/mL × 295 mL = (7.8 × 295) µg = approx. (8 × 300) µg = 2400 µg = 2.4 mg

Notice that the answer choices are at least 1000 times apart and so small approximations can be done with confidence.

Question 11   B

See: GM 2.1, 2.2
X minutes/year = 60 minutes/hour × 24 hours/day × 365 days/year

Cancel units on the right side (hours, days) and we are left with:

X minutes/year = 60 × 24 × 365 minutes/year = approx. 60 × (25 × 400) m/y

X minutes/year = 60 × 10 000 = 600 000 m/y = 6×10^5 m/y which is a reasonable approximation of answer choice B, especially when all of the other choices are 100 times apart.

Question 12   D

See: GM 2.2; dimensional analysis
We will explore force in Physics. Force is in units called 'newtons' which is mass times acceleration, thus a newton is equivalent to a kg(m/s²) [*see* section 2.1] and since kg is M (mass), m is L (length) and s is T (time), we get that the force is dimensionally equivalent to ML/T². Now the terms

added on the right side of the equation must also be dimensionally equal to ML/T^2. Let's first solve for 'a' (note: most of the steps that we will show are really mental manipulations but we'll show the steps in case you are not used to it):

$$ML/T^2 = at^{-1} = aT^{-1} = a/T$$

To isolate 'a', multiply through by T:

$$(T)ML/T^2 = (T)a/T$$

Cancel T:

$$ML/T = a = MLT^{-1}$$

Now we solve for 'b':

$$ML/T^2 = bt^2 = bT^2$$

To isolate 'b', divide both sides by T^2:

$$ML/T^2/T^2 = ML/T^4 = b$$

SPOILER ALERT ⚠

Gold Standard has cross-referenced the content in this chapter to examples from ACER's official GAMSAT practice materials. It is for you to decide when you want to explore these questions since you may want to preserve some of ACER's materials for timed mock-exam practice.

Examples – Dimensional analysis: Q3, Q5, Q12 of 1; Q31 and 36 of 3; Q29 and Q87 of 5. Note that "Q" is followed by the question number, and, for example, "of 1" refers to booklet number 1 which is referenced in the Spoiler Alert table at the end of Chapter 1. The 10 full-length HEAPS GAMSAT practice tests (by Gold Standard and MediRed), exams 1 through 10, contain specific cross-references to this chapter within the worked solutions.

Chapter Checklist

- ☐ Reassess your 'learning objectives' for this chapter: Go back to the first page of this chapter and re-evaluate the top 3 boxes and the Introduction.
  - ☐ Please be sure that you have completed the *Need for Speed* exercises at the beginning of this chapter.
- ☐ Complete a maximum of 1 page of notes using symbols/abbreviations to represent the entire chapter based on your learning objectives. These are your Gold Notes.
- ☐ Consider your multimedia options based on your optimal way of learning:
  - ☐ Download the free Gold Standard GAMSAT app for your Android device or iPhone.
  - ☐ Create your own, tangible study cards or try the free app: Anki.
  - ☐ Record your voice reading your Gold Notes onto your smartphone (MP3s) and listen during exercise, transportation, etc.
  - ☐ Try out the Gold Standard GAMSAT Physics online videos at gamsat-prep.com which have heaps of calculations, or you can try other maths options on YouTube like Khan Academy or Leah4sciMCAT playlist for Maths Without a Calculator (the latter was produced for MCAT preparation but it remains helpful for GAMSAT).
- ☐ Reassess your schedule for your full-length GAMSAT practice tests: ACER and/or HEAPS exams. Ensure that you have scheduled one full day to complete a practice test and 1-2 days for a thorough assessment of worked solutions while adding to your abbreviated Gold Notes.
- ☐ Reassess your progress in scheduling and/or evaluating stress reduction techniques such as regular exercise (sports), yoga, meditation and/or mindfulness exercises (*see* YouTube for suggestions).

High-level Importance

GOLD NOTES

ALGEBRA AND GRAPH ANALYSIS
Chapter 3

Memorise
* The #1 Rule of Algebra
* Slope-Intercept Form for linear equations
* Rules of logarithms
* Gold Standard 5-step Graph Analysis Technique

Understand
* Basic equations and methods of problem-solving
* Simplifying equations
* Solving one or more linear equations
* Rules and graphs: logs and exponents
* Graph analysis, slopes, area under curves
* 2D (x, y) and 3D (x, y, z) graphs, nomograms

Importance
High level: 65% of GAMSAT Section 3 maths-based questions released by ACER are related to content in this chapter (in our estimation).
* Note that approximately 90% of such questions are related to just 3 chapters: 1, 2, and 3.

GAMSAT-Prep.com

Introduction

If Chapters 1 and 2 were High-level Importance then, truly, this chapter is Phenomenally High-level Importance! On ACER's webpage for the "Structure and Content" of the GAMSAT, apparently referring to both Section 1 and Section 3, they state: "GAMSAT questions ...typically require candidates to read and think about a passage of writing, to interpret graphical displays of information, to use mathematical relationships and to apply reasoning skills to tables of data." The core of that statement describes the title and essence of this chapter. Nowhere on ACER's webpage is there any inference for the need for rote learning of science facts. ==This one chapter is thus more important than any other single science chapter in the 4 standard sciences covered for this exam.== Of course, the concepts obtained herein will be tested and re-tested in the GAMSAT-level practice questions at the end of the great majority of science chapters in the GAMSAT Masters Series.

Additional Resources

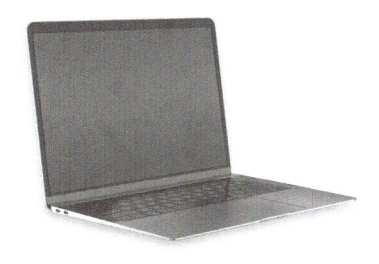

Open Discussion Boards

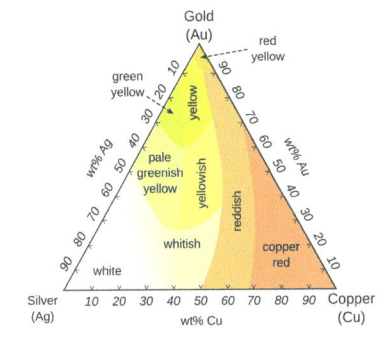

Special Guest

GAMSAT-Prep.com
GOLD STANDARD MATHS

3.0 GAMSAT Has a *Need for Speed*!

As you have done before, answer any or all of the questions/exercises in the table now. Or, after completing this chapter, return to the table below to ensure that you can complete all entries. Subsequently, you can proceed to answer the additional multiple-choice questions at the end of this chapter. Good luck!

High-level Importance

Section Number	Chapter Practice Questions: Your GAMSAT Maths' *Need for Speed* Exercises
3.1.1C	Solve for x: $2x + 3 = 5$
	Solve for x: $2x + 2/3 = 3x - 2$
3.2.1	Simplify: $3x + 4xy - 2 = xy + 1$
3.2.2	Simplify: $\dfrac{3}{2x} + 5x = 4$
	Simplify: $\dfrac{5}{(x+3)} = \dfrac{2}{x} - \dfrac{1}{3x}$
3.2.3	Factor the following: $2x^3 - 4x^2 + 4x$
3.3.2A	Solve for y: $4y - 3x = 2y + x - 6$
3.3.2B	Solve the following system of equations for x and y: $4y - 3x = 2y + x - 6$ $3x + y = 12$
	Use equation addition or subtraction to solve the following for x and y: $2x - 2y = 1$ $4x + 5y = 11$
3.4.1	Rewrite $3y - 2x = 6$ as a function of x
3.4.3	Graph the line using the grid to the right defined by the equation: $2x + y = 3$

GM-74 CHAPTER 3: ALGEBRA AND GRAPH ANALYSIS

3.4.4	Rewrite the following equation in slope-intercept form: $2y + 5x = 8$
	Find the equation for the line passing through (1, 1) and (2, 3)
3.7.1	$\log_5 (125) =$
	Table 1: Common values for the log base 10
		x	Exponential form	$\log_{10}(x)$
	|---|---|---
		0.0001		
		0.001		
		0.01		
		0.1		
		1		
		10		
		100		
		1000		
		10000		
	$\log 10^0 =$ $\qquad$ $\log 10^2 =$ $\log 10^1 =$ $\qquad$ $\log 10^3 =$
	Simplify or expand based on log rules: 1) $\log_a a =$ $\qquad$ 4) $\log_a(M/N) =$ 2) $\log_a M^k =$ $\qquad$ 5) $10^{\log_{10} M} =$ 3) $\log_a(MN) =$ $\qquad$ 6) $\log_a(1) =$
	$\log (1\,000\,000) =$
	$\log (1/100) =$
	Given that $\ln 2 = 0.69$, what is $\ln 2e^3$?
	Approximate $\log(200) =$
3.8	Circle the correct response: On the axis of a graph using a log scale, halfway between the numbers 100 and 1000 would yield a number most consistent with which of the following? **A.** Between 300 and 400 **B.** Between 400 and 500 **C.** 500 **D.** Above 500
	$2^{10} =$

High-level Importance

GAMSAT-Prep.com
GOLD STANDARD MATHS

3.1 Equation Solving and Functions

3.1.1 Algebraic Equations

High-level Importance

Before we jump into more complicated algebra, let's review the basics.

A. Terms

Variable: A variable is a symbol - usually in the form of a small letter - that represents a number. It can take on any range of values.

Most problems that are strictly algebraic in nature will provide you with an equation (or equations) containing one or more unknown variables. Based on the information given, the values of the variables will most likely be fixed. Your job is to solve for those values.

Constant: A constant is a fixed value. A constant can be a number on its own, or sometimes it is represented by a letter such as a, b, k, π, e, etc. In the chapters to come, you will discover that there are many constants in nature.

Polynomial: A polynomial is an expression (usually part of a function or an equation) that is composed of the sum or difference of some number of terms. Please note that some of the terms can be negative. The **order** of a polynomial is equal to the largest exponent to which a variable is raised in one of the terms.

EXAMPLE $3x^2 + x + 5$

This expression is a polynomial. The variable here is x, and the order of the polynomial is 2 ("2nd order") because that is the largest exponent to which x is raised.

B. Preserving Equality

The #1 Rule of Algebra: Whatever you do to one side of an equation, you *must* do to the other side also!

The equals sign implies equality between two different expressions. When you are given an equation, the equality established must be considered to be always true for that problem (unless you are told otherwise). So if you change one side of the equation and you do not also change the other side in the same way, you fundamentally alter the terms of the equation. The equation will no longer be true.

EXAMPLE

Consider this equation:

$$2x + 3 = 5$$

The following manipulation violates the above rule:

$$(2x + 3) - 3 = 5$$

Here, we have subtracted three from one side but not the other, so the equality no longer holds.

This manipulation, however, does not violate the rule:

$$(2x + 3) - 3 = 5 - 3$$

Here, we have subtracted three from both sides, so the equality still holds true.

C. Solving Basic Equations

We can use the rule of algebra described in Part B to help solve algebraic equations for an unknown variable. Keep in mind that addition and subtraction, along with multiplication and division, are inverse operations: They undo each other. First decide the operation that has been applied and then use the inverse operation to undo this (make sure to apply the operation to both sides of the equation). The idea is to isolate the variable on one side of the equation. Then, whatever is left on the other side of the equation is the value of the variable.

EXAMPLE

Solve: $2x + 3 = 5$

$2x + 3 - 3 = 5 - 3$
$2x = 2$

Subtracting 3, however, has not isolated the variable x. Hence, we need to continue undoing by dividing 2 on both sides.

$2x \div 2 = 2 \div 2$
$x = 1$

Here's a little more complicated equation for you to try: $2x + 2/3 = 3x - 2$

Objective: isolate the variable in order to provide a solution to the equation. When you have an equation with the variable on both sides, choose whichever you think will be easier to focus on. In this case, we will isolate x on the right. First, subtract $2x$ from both sides.

$$(2x + 2/3) - 2x = (3x - 2) - 2x$$

> **NOTE**
>
> If two sides of an equation are equal, you can add or subtract the same amount to/from both sides, and they will still be equal.
>
> **EXAMPLE**
> $a = b$
> $a + c = b + c$
> $a - c = b - c$
>
> The same rule applies to multiplication and division.
>
> **EXAMPLE**
> $a = b$
> $ac = bc$
> $a \div c = b \div c$

GAMSAT-Prep.com
GOLD STANDARD MATHS

$\Rightarrow 2/3 = x - 2$

Next, add 2 to both sides to isolate x.

$(2/3) + 2 = (x - 2) + 2$
$\Rightarrow 8/3 = x$

3.1.2 Addition and Subtraction of Polynomials

When adding or subtracting polynomials, the general rules for exponents are applied and like terms are grouped together. You can think of it as similar to collecting the same things together.

EXAMPLE

$4x^3y + 5z^2 + 5xy^4 + 3z^2$

$= 4x^3y + 5xy^4 + (5+3)z^2$
$= 4x^3y + 5xy^4 + 8z^2$

By grouping the similar terms, seeing which terms may be added or subtracted becomes easier.

3.1.3 Simplifying Algebraic Expressions

Algebraic expressions can be factored or simplified using standard formulae:

$$a(b + c) = ab + ac$$
$$(a + b)(a - b) = a^2 - b^2$$
$$(a + b)(a + b) = (a + b)^2 = a^2 + 2ab + b^2$$
$$(a - b)(a - b) = (a - b)^2 = a^2 - 2ab + b^2$$
$$(a + b)(c + d) = ac + ad + bc + bd$$

3.2 Simplifying Equations

In order to make solving algebraic equations easy and quick, you should simplify terms whenever possible. The following are the most common and important ways of doing so.

3.2.1 Combining Terms

This is the most basic thing you can do to simplify an equation. If there are multiple terms being added or subtracted in your equation that contain the same variables, you can combine them.

EXAMPLE

Simplify the equation: $3x + 4xy - 2 = xy + 1$

Notice that there are two terms we can combine that contain xy and two terms we can combine that are just constants.

$(3x + 4xy - 2) - xy = (xy + 1) - xy$
$\Rightarrow 3x + 3xy - 2 = 1$

$(3x + 3xy - 2) + 2 = 1 + 2$
$\Rightarrow 3x + 3xy = 3$

$\Rightarrow \left(\dfrac{3x + 3xy}{3}\right) = \dfrac{3}{3}$
$\Rightarrow x + xy = 1$

Always make sure to look for like terms to combine when you are solving an algebra problem.

3.2.2 Variables in Denominators

When you are trying to manipulate an equation, having variables in the denominators of fractions can make things difficult. In order to get rid of such denominators entirely, simply multiply the entire equation by the quantity in the denominator. This will probably cause other terms to become more complicated, but you will no longer have the problem of a variable denominator.

EXAMPLE

Simplify the expression: $\dfrac{3}{2x} + 5x = 4$.

The problem denominator is $2x$, so we multiply both sides by $2x$.

$(\dfrac{3}{2x} + 5x)2x = (4)2x$
$\Rightarrow 3 + 10x^2 = 8x$

When there are different denominators containing variables, cross multiply the denominator to cancel out. Try the following example.

EXAMPLE

$\dfrac{5}{(x+3)} = \dfrac{2}{x} - \dfrac{1}{3x}$

High-level Importance

Multiply 3x on both sides:

$$\frac{5}{(x+3)}(3x) = \frac{2}{x} - \frac{1}{3x}(3x)$$

$$\frac{15x}{(x+3)} = 6 - 1$$

Multiply (x+3) on both sides:

$$\frac{15x}{(x+3)}(x+3) = 5(x+3)$$

$$15x = 5x + 15$$

$$15x - 5x = 5x + 15 - 5x$$

$$10x = 15$$

$$x = \frac{15}{10} = \frac{3}{2}$$

3.2.3 Factoring

If every term of a polynomial is divisible by the same quantity, that quantity can be factored out. This means that we can express the polynomial as the product of that quantity times a new, smaller polynomial.

EXAMPLE

Factor the following expression:

$$2x^3 - 4x^2 + 4x$$

Every term in this polynomial is divisible by 2x, so we can factor it out of each term. The simplified expression, then, is

$$2x(x^2 - 2x + 2).$$

To verify that you have properly factored an expression, multiply out your solution. If you get back to where you started, you've done it correctly.

3.3 Linear Equations

3.3.1 Linearity

Linear equation is an equation between two (or three) variables that gives a straight line when plotted on a graph (GM 3.5.1). In a linear equation, there can neither be variables raised to exponents nor variables multiplied together.

(a) $3x + 2y = z + 5$

This equation is linear.

(b) $3x^2 - 2xy = 1$

This equation is not linear. The terms $3x^2$ and $2xy$ cannot appear in a linear equation.

The reason such equations are called "linear" is that they can be represented on a Cartesian graph as a straight line. "Cartesian" is the basic coordinate system composed of an x-axis and a y-axis (and sometimes z-axis as well) which we will review shortly.

3.3.2 Solving Linear Equations with Multiple Variables

In the previous sections we have only considered equations with single variables. In some cases though, GAMSAT problems will require you to deal with a second variable.

A. Isolating a Variable

When you have a single equation with two variables, you will not be able to solve for specific values. What you can do is solve for one variable in terms of the other. To do this, pick a variable to isolate on one side of the equation and move all other terms to the other side.

EXAMPLE

Solve the following for y: $4y - 3x = 2y + x - 6$.

Let's isolate y on the left side:
$$(4y - 3x) + 3x - 2y = (2y + x - 6) + 3x - 2y$$
$$\frac{(2y)}{2} = \frac{(4x - 6)}{2}$$
$$y = 2x - 3$$

Now we know the value of y, but only in relation to the value of x. If we are now given some value for x, we can simply plug it in to our solution and obtain y. For example, if $x = 1$ then $y = 2 - 3 = -1$.

B. Solving Systems of Equations

How do you know if you will be able to solve for specific values in an equation or not? The general rule is that if you have the same number of unique equations as variables (or more equations), you will be able find a specific value for every variable. So for the example in Part A, since we have two variables and only one equation, in order to solve for the variables, we would need one more unique equation.

In order for an equation to be unique, it must not be algebraically derived from another equation.

EXAMPLE

$$300 = 30x - 10y$$
$$30 = 3x - y$$

From the above example, the two equations describe the same line and therefore are not unique since they are scalar multiples of each other.

There are two strategies you should know for solving a system of equations (AKA, *simultaneous equations*):

I. **Substitution.** This strategy can be used every time, although, it will not always be the fastest way to come up with a solution. You begin with one equation and isolate a variable as in Part A. Next, wherever the isolated variable appears in the second equation, replace it with the expression this variable is equal to. This effectively eliminates that variable from the second equation.

If you only have two equations, all you need are two steps. Once you have followed the procedure above, you can solve for the second variable in the second equation and substitute that value back into the first equation to find the value of the first variable. If you have more than two variables and equations, you will need to continue this process of isolation and substitution until you reach the last equation.

EXAMPLE

Solve the following system of equations for x and y.

$$4y - 3x = 2y + x - 6$$
$$3x + y = 12$$

We have already isolated y in the first equation, so the first step is done. The new system is as follows:

$$y = 2x - 3$$
$$3x + y = 12$$

Next, we substitute $2x - 3$ for y in the second equation.

$$3x + (2x - 3) = 12$$
$$\Rightarrow 5x - 3 = 12$$
$$\Rightarrow 5x = 15$$
$$\Rightarrow x = 3$$

Now, we have a value for x, but we still need a value for y. Substitute 3 for x in the y-isolated equation.

$$y = 2(3) - 3$$
$$y = 3$$

So our solution to this system of equations is $x = 3$, $y = 3$.

II. **Equation Addition or Subtraction.** You will not always be able to apply this strategy, but in some cases, it will save you from having to do all of the time-consuming substitutions of Strategy I. The basic idea of equation addition or subtraction is exactly what you would expect: Addition or subtraction of equations directly to each other.

Say you have two equations, A and B. Because both sides of any equation are by definition equal, you can add, say, the left side of equation A to the left side of equation B and the right side of equation A to the right side of equation B without changing anything. In performing this addition, you are doing the same thing to both sides of equation B.

The purpose of performing such an addition is to try and get a variable to cancel out completely. If you can accomplish this, you can solve for the other variable easily (assuming you only have two variables, of course). Before adding the equations together, you can manipulate either of them however you like (as long as you maintain equality) in order to set up the cancellation of a variable.

If the only way to cancel out a variable is by subtracting the equation, this may be done as well.

EXAMPLE

Use equation addition or subtraction to solve the following for x and y.

$$2x - 2y = 1$$
$$4x + 5y = 11$$

If we multiply the first equation by two, we will have $4x$ present in each equation. Then if we subtract, the $4x$ in each equation will cancel.

$$\begin{array}{r} 4x - 4y = 2 \\ -(4x + 5y = 11) \\ \hline 0x - 9y = -9 \end{array}$$
$$\Rightarrow y = 1$$

Now, we can substitute this value of y into whichever equation looks simpler to solve for x (either one will work though).

$$2x - 2(1) = 1$$
$$\Rightarrow 2x = 3$$
$$\Rightarrow x = \frac{3}{2}$$

So our solution to this system of equations is $y = 1$, $x = \frac{3}{2}$.

> **NOTE**
>
> A 'classic' GAMSAT-style question requires an understanding of Strategy II to solve Hess' Law problems (CHM 8.3). We will also apply Strategy II to solve simultaneous equations for a pulley system (PHY 3.4).

High-level Importance

GAMSAT-Prep.com
GOLD STANDARD MATHS

3.4 Graphing Linear Functions

3.4.1 Linear Equations and Functions

Every linear equation can be rewritten as a linear function. To do so, simply isolate one of the variables as in GM 3.1.1C. This variable is now a function of the variables on the other side of the equation.

EXAMPLE

Rewrite the equation $3y - 2x = 6$ as a function of x.

$$3y - 2x = 6$$
$$\Rightarrow 3y = 2x + 6$$
$$\Rightarrow y = \frac{2}{3}x + 2$$

Now that we have isolated y, it is actually dependent on, or a *function* of, x. For every input of x, we get a unique output of y. If you like, you can rewrite y as $f(x)$.

$$f(x) = \frac{2}{3}x + 2$$

3.4.2 Cartesian Coordinates in 2D

The Cartesian coordinate system is the most commonly used system for graphing. A Cartesian graph in two dimensions has two axes: The *x*-axis is the horizontal one, and the *y*-axis is the vertical one. The independent variable is always along the *x*-axis and the dependent variable is along the *y*-axis. The independent variable is controlled and the output depends on the independent variable.

The further right you go on the *x*-axis, the larger the numbers get; and on the *y*-axis, the numbers get larger the further up you go. A point on the graph is specified as an ordered pair of an *x* value and a *y* value like this: (x, y). This point exists *x* units from the origin (the point $(0, 0)$ where the axes cross) along the *x*-axis, and *y* units from the origin along the *y*-axis.

EXAMPLE

A *grid* is a network of lines that cross each other to form a series of squares or rectangles. Find the point $(3, -1)$ on the 8x8-grid Cartesian graph shown. To plot this point, simply count three units to the right along the *x*-axis and one unit down along the *y*-axis.

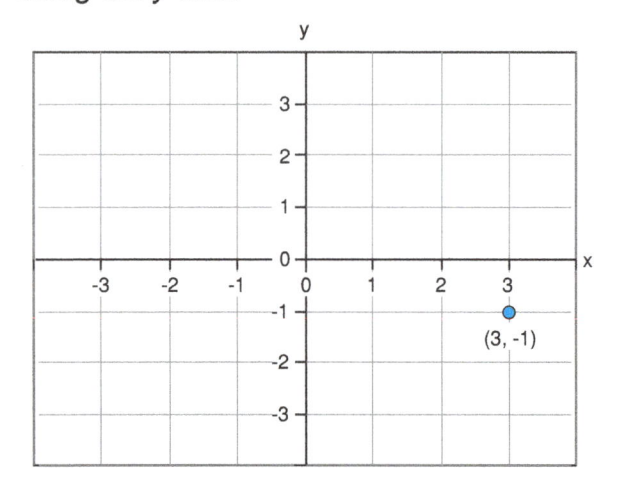

High-level Importance

3.4.3 Graphing Linear Equations

In order to graph a straight line in Cartesian coordinates, all you need to know is two points. Every set of two points has only one unique line that passes through both of them.

To find two points from a linear equation, simply choose two values to plug in for one of the variables. It is best to pick values that will make your calculations easier, such as 0 and 1. Plugging in each of these values, we can solve for y and obtain two points.

EXAMPLE

Graph the line defined by $2x + y = 3$.

First, let's plug in $x = 0$ and $x = 1$ to find two points on the line.

$2(0) + y = 3$ $2(1) + y = 3$
$\Rightarrow y = 3$ $\Rightarrow y = 1$

Now, we have two points: (0, 3) and (1, 1). To graph the line, all we have to do is plot these points on a graph and draw a straight line between them.

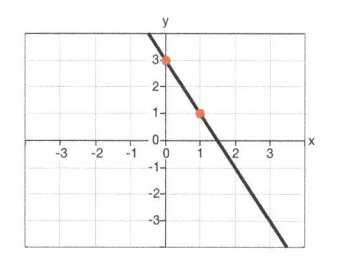

3.4.4 Slope-Intercept Form

There are two pieces of information that are very useful in the graphing of a linear equation: The slope (*gradient*) of the line and its *y*-intercept.

Slope refers to the steepness of a line. It is the ratio (slope = rise/run) of the number of units along the y-axis to the number of units along the x-axis between two points.

EXAMPLE

$y = 5x + 3$ and $y = 5x + 10$

The preceding 2 equations would be parallel to each other since both slopes (m) = 5.

$y = 3x + 6$ and $y = -\dfrac{1}{3x} + 3$

These two equations are perpendicular. The line of the first equation has a positive slope and the perpendicular line has a decreasing slope and therefore both slopes have opposite signs. In fact, the general rule is that when slopes are negative reciprocals of each other, the 2 lines in question must be perpendicular to each other.

The *y*-**intercept** of a line is the *y*-coordinate of the point at which the line crosses the *y*-axis. The value of x where the line intersects, is always zero and its coordinates will be (0, *y*).

One of the standard forms of a linear equation is the slope-intercept form, from which the slope and the *y*-intercept of the line are immediately obvious. This form resembles $y = mx + b$. Here m and b are constants such that m is the slope of the line and b is the y-intercept.

EXAMPLE

Rewrite the following equation in slope-intercept form: $2y + 5x = 8$.

$$\Rightarrow 2y = -5x + 8$$
$$\Rightarrow y = -\frac{5}{2}x + 4$$

This is now in slope-intercept form. In this case, the slope m is $-5/2$ and the y-intercept is 4.

Slope-intercept form is also useful for constructing the equation of a line from other information. If you are given the slope and the intercept, obviously you can simply plug them in to $y = mx + b$ to get the equation. It is also very simple to obtain the slope and intercept if you know two points on the line, (x_1, y_1) and (x_2, y_2). The slope can be obtained directly from this information:

Slope = rise/run = $(y_2 - y_1)/(x_2 - x_1)$

Once the slope m is obtained, you only need to solve for b. To do so, plug in one of the points as well as m into the slope-intercept equation. You can then solve for b.

EXAMPLE

Find the equation for the line passing through (1, 1) and (2, 3).

First, determine the slope.

$$m = \frac{(3-1)}{(2-1)} = 2$$

Now plug m and a point into the slope-intercept equation to find b.

$$y = mx + b$$
$$\Rightarrow 1 = 2(1) + b$$
$$\Rightarrow -1 = b$$

Plugging in all of this information, we now have a complete equation.

$$y = 2x - 1$$

3.5 Basic Graphs

3.5.1 The Graph of a Linear Equation

Given any two points (x_1, y_1) and (x_2, y_2) on the line, we have:

$$y_1 = ax_1 + b$$

and

$$y_2 = ax_2 + b.$$

Subtracting the upper equation from the lower one and dividing through by $x_2 - x_1$ gives the value of the slope,

$$a = (y_2 - y_1)/(x_2 - x_1)$$
$$= \Delta y/\Delta x = \text{rise/run}$$

GAMSAT MASTERS SERIES

> **NOTE**
> Often on the real GAMSAT, you will need to either calculate the slope of a line or the area under a graph or line, or both.

Lines that have positive slopes slant "up hill" (as viewed from left to right), like the graph on this page. Lines that have negative slopes slant "down hill" (as viewed from left to right). Lines that are horizontal have no slope (= a slope of zero; *see* PHY 1.4.1).

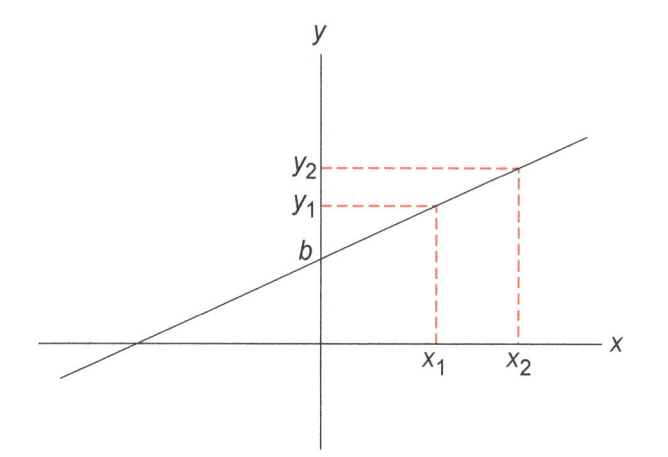

> **NOTE**
> Don't get attached to variables in equations. Only focus on the meaning of the equation. Among and within different textbooks and exams, different variables may be used in the same equations (*a* or *m* for slope; *S* or *d* or *x* for displacement, and many others). Some exam questions are designed to catch students who try to memorise without understanding equations.

3.5.2 Illustrations of Common Graphs

For the graphs in this section (GM 3.5.2), please consider replacing *x* by 0, 1 and 2 (or other values) to ensure that the graph behaves in a way that makes sense to you. In the following graph, note that the red and blue lines have the same slope (gradient); the red and green lines have the same *y*-intercept:

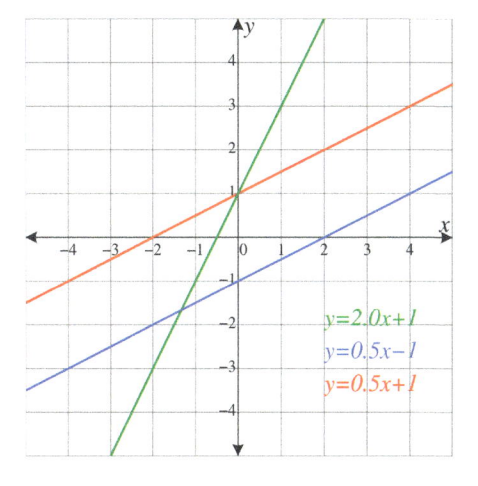

$y = 2.0x + 1$
$y = 0.5x - 1$
$y = 0.5x + 1$

For any real number *x*, there exists a unique real number called the multiplicative inverse or *reciprocal* of *x* denoted $1/x$ or x^{-1} such that $x(1/x) = 1$. The graph of the reciprocal $1/x$ for any *x* is:

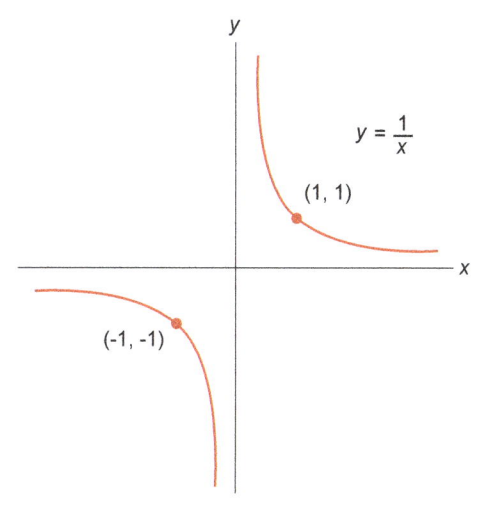

$y = \frac{1}{x}$

(1, 1)

(-1, -1)

GAMSAT MATHS   GM-87

A quadratic equation (e.g. CHM 6.6.1) is a polynomial (GM 3.1.1) in which the highest-order term is 'to the power of 2'. For example, $y = ax^2$. A quadratic equation describes a parabola which is approximately U-shaped:

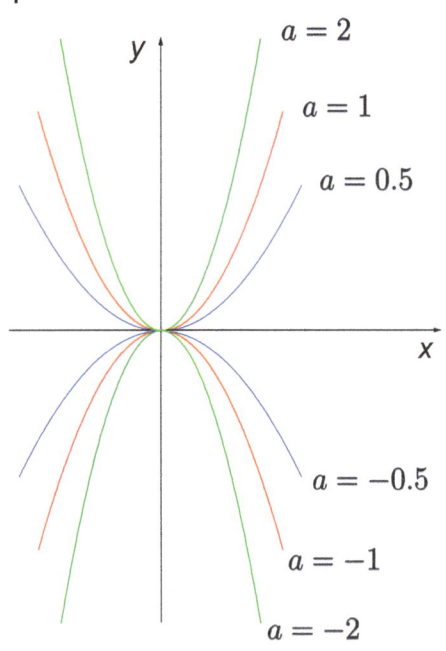

Interestingly, there are important graphs and shapes, including a parabola, that can be obtained by taking a simple cone and cutting it at various angles. This only requires a bit of imagination:

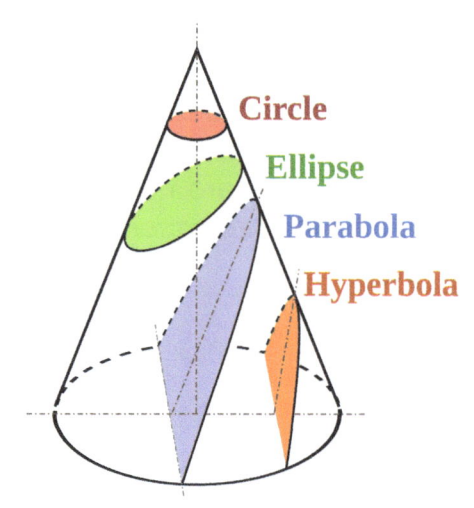

For GAMSAT purposes, it would not be helpful to commit the equation of any graph to memory – aside, of course, for the equation that describes a straight line.

3.5.3 Common Graphs Found in Other Sections or Chapters

There are classic curves which are represented or approximated in the science text as follows: Sigmoidal curve (CHM 6.9.1, BIO 7.5.1), sinusoidal curve (GM 5.2.3, PHY 7.1), hyperbolic curves (CHM 9.7 Fig III.A.9.3, BIO 1.1.2), exponential rise (GM 3.8, CHM 9.8.1) and decay (PHY 10.4, CHM 9.2). Another type of graph that you will likely see during the real GAMSAT is where one or both axes are logarithmic (so called semi-log and log-log graphs, respectively; GM 3.8 + CHM 4.3.3, CHM 6.9.1/2).

If you were to plot a set of experimental data, often one can draw a line or curve which can "best fit" the data. The preceding defines a *regression* line or curve (GM 6.3.1).

One purpose of the regression graph is to predict what would likely occur outside of the experimental data. The skill to extend a graph by inferring unknown values from trends in the known data is *extrapolation* (e.g., BIO 14, Q7).

3.5.4 Tangential Slope and Area under a Curve

During the real GAMSAT, you will very likely need to calculate a slope based on a curve (i.e. the slope of the straight line must just glance the curve at a specific point = *tangential*), and/or you will need to calculate the area under a curve (depending on the presentation, you would estimate the answer by either counting boxes below the graph or by multiplying some part of the x-axis by some part of the y-axis; the question could be in Physics, Chemistry or Biology). In neither instance will you be told which you should calculate, but rather you must learn, as part of basic graph analysis performed in this chapter, when one or the other applies (usually dimensional analysis is the key; GM 2.2).

As long as you pay attention to the units (dimensional analysis), then you do not have to memorise these common facts: velocity is the slope of a displacement vs. time graph (PHY 1.3); acceleration is the slope and displacement is the area under the curve of a velocity vs. time graph (PHY 1.4.1); the change in momentum (= impulse) is the area under a force vs. time graph (PHY 4.3); work is the area under the force vs. displacement graph (PHY 7.2.1).

Do not worry about the Physics for now. Just focus on the maths. Let's examine a velocity vs. time graph of a bullet fired from a gun (side note: notice that the curve resembles ½ of an upside-down parabola). The y-axis is velocity which is in the SI units of metres/second (m/s). The x-axis is time in the SI units of seconds (s). Here are 2 questions that you can try to work out before looking at the solutions:

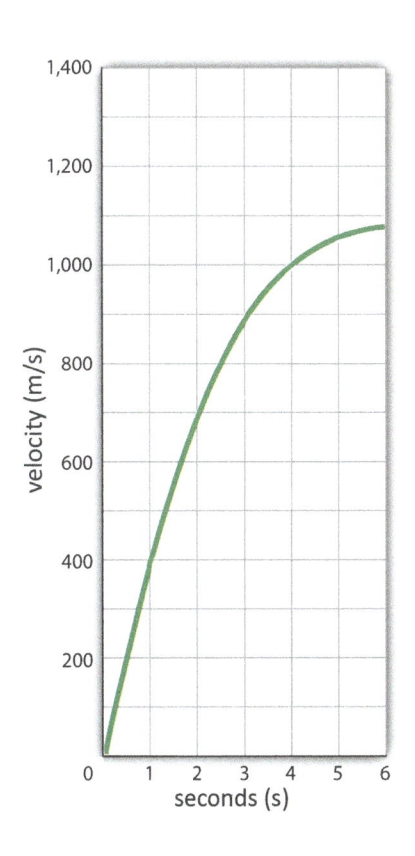

EXAMPLES

(1) Given that acceleration is in units of m/s^2, calculate the instantaneous acceleration at time = 3 seconds.

(2) Given that displacement is in the units of metres (m), calculate the displacement of the bullet in the first 2 seconds of being fired.

GAMSAT-Prep.com
GOLD STANDARD MATHS

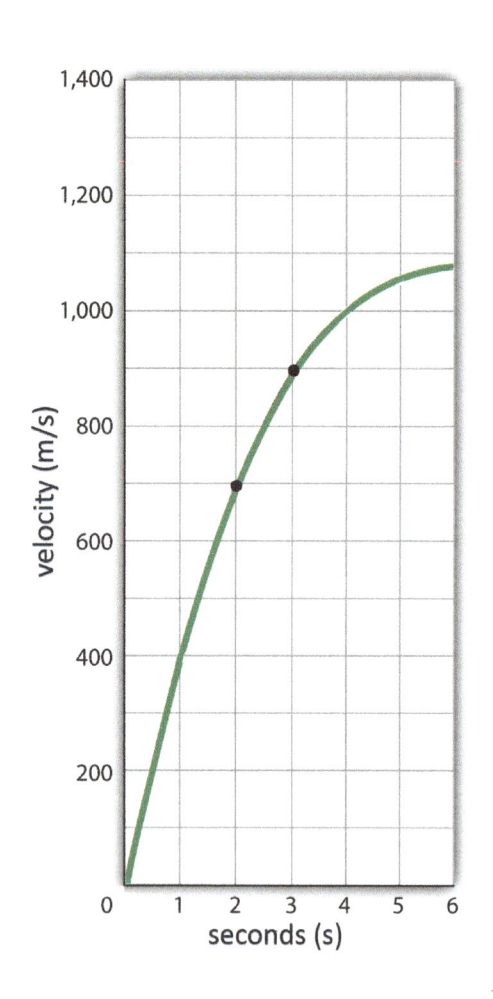

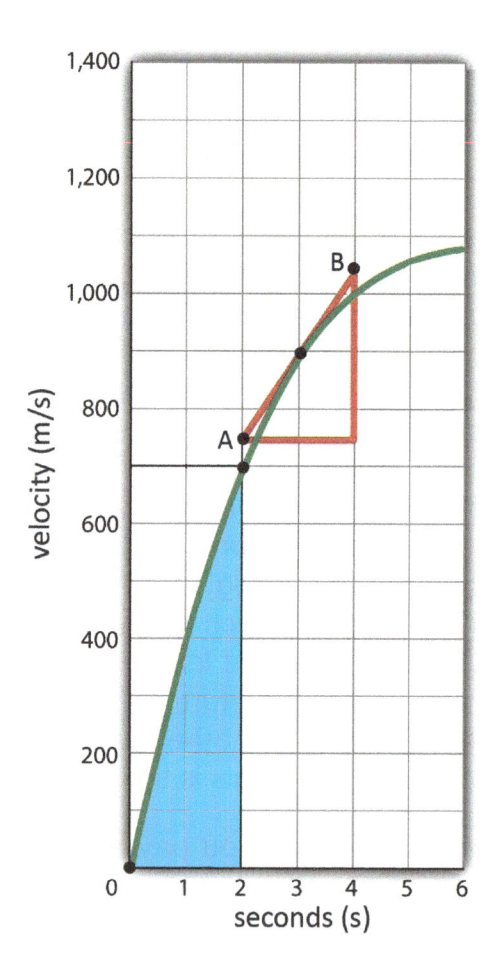

High-level Importance

Hints if required:

(1) **Hint:** try to calculate the slope of a straight line off the curve at 3 seconds. Why does the slope solve the problem? Take a look at the units. A slope is the change of y divided by the change of x. In terms of units, this would make m/s/s = m/s^2 = acceleration.

(2) **Hint:** determine the area of the curve below that segment of the graph (i.e. the first 2 seconds). One way to do so is to calculate the area of one box and then estimate how many boxes are below the curve. Why the area? Again, the units: the area of a square or rectangle is one side times the other side. For a graph, it is x times y. So here is what happens to the units: m/s x s = m = metres which is displacement.

GM-90   CHAPTER 3: ALGEBRA AND GRAPH ANALYSIS

ANSWERS

(1) To calculate the slope at a point, the line that you draw needs to be tangential to the curve as described previously (*see* the preceding graphs). The line can be as long or as short as you want (basically, you choose the length to make the calculation as easy as possible).

We chose a change in x (i.e. from points A to B as seen from the x-axis) which is easy to calculate = 2 seconds (i.e. 4 − 2 = 2). The change in y (i.e. from points A to B as seen from the y-axis) is also easy = 300 m/s (1050 − 750 = 300). The slope is the change in y divided by the change in x so: (300 m/s)/(2 s) = 150 m/s^2.

Notice that point A in the graph is our point (x_1, y_1) and point B is (x_2, y_2); *see* GM 3.5.1. While sitting the GAMSAT, you may need to assess a slope by holding your writing implement up against the computer monitor, or by laying it down on your scratch paper if you have sketched the graph, followed by a reasonable estimate of the data points.

(2) As explained in the "hint", we are trying to calculate the area under the curve in the first 2 seconds. If you put your pen in the line (0, 0) to (2, 700), you will notice that your pen approximates the green line (do not use a ruler because they are not permitted during the GAMSAT!).

In other words, if we were to imagine a rectangle that includes the points (0, 0) to (2, 700), then the area under the curve seems to be about ½ that value. Because a rectangle is simply one side times the other, we can multiply 2 seconds x 700 m/s = 1400 metres. The area below the green graph is about ½ that or 700 metres, which is thus the displacement.

Of course, it depends on the multiple choice answers. Careful observation will show you that the area under the curve is slightly more than 700 m.

An alternative way to calculate the area in blue would be to calculate the area of one single small box from the graph: 100 m/s times 1 s = 100 metres. If you carefully count the boxes in the blue shaded area (which you can see better from the graph on the left), you will be able to count about 7 complete boxes (i.e. approx. 700 m; of course, sometimes you need to add 2 incomplete boxes to make one full box).

Yet another alternative may have been the first choice of those with a science background: estimate the area in blue as a triangle (which we will discuss in GM 4.2.2) which is 1/2(base)(height) = 1/2(2)(700) = 700 m.

GAMSAT-Prep.com
GOLD STANDARD MATHS

3.5.5 Breaking Axes and Error Bars

Among the many reasons that an axis could be broken would be if the missing part of the graph is not key to understanding the trend, and/or when the trend is obvious which allows more data to be shown in a smaller graph.

The following represents 3 different symbols for a broken axis.

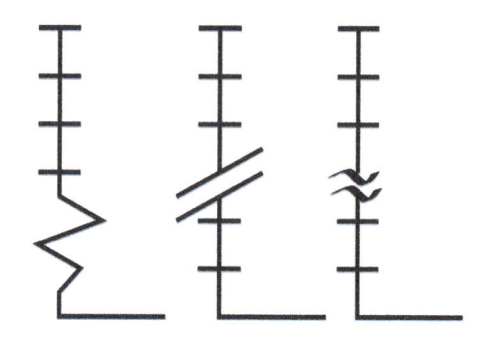

EXAMPLE 1

Consider the following diagram. The break in the *x*-axis does not change the scale; however, the break in the *y*-axis clearly permits the scale to jump from 0 to 0.5 in a way that is remarkably different from the rest of the *y*-axis.

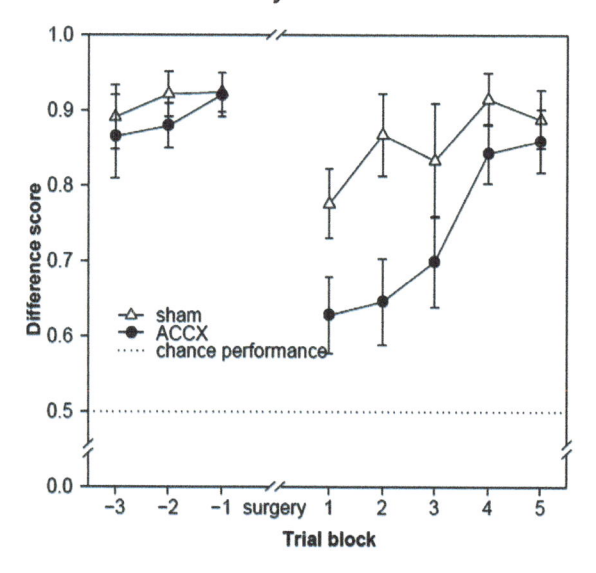

Error bars show the variability of data and indicate the error or *uncertainty* in a measurement. Error bars often represent one standard deviation of uncertainty (GM 6.3.2), or a particular confidence interval (e.g., a 95% chance that the actual data point falls within the extremes of the error bar). From the preceding graph, it can be seen that the error bars for the measurements for Trial block 3 are longer than for Trial block 1, meaning the latter has an average (*mean*) value that is more representative of the data (= more reliable). Also notice that only 2 trials (Trial block 1 and 2) have non-overlapping error bars. This means that in all of the other trials, because of the overlap, the difference between the data points of the sham versus ACCX trials may not be statistically significant.

Thus, even though you are not provided any details, the graph informs us that ACCX (whatever that means) has a statistically significant post-surgical 'difference score' within the first two trial blocks as compared to the sham group. Of course, 'sham' implies 'fake' and in science that implies a group (= *control* group; BIO 2.5) that is exposed to the same conditions as the experimental group, except that the control group does not receive the treatment (e.g. no ACCX).

Mathematically, we can describe a data point's error as 'plus or minus' the point seen in the graph. For example, for ACCX trial block 3, the data point is approximately 0.7 with a range given by the error bar of about 0.64 to 0.76. Thus the point can be described as 0.7 plus or minus 0.06 (i.e. 0.7 ± 0.06).

Let us consider another example of a broken axis but in this case the data is presented using rectangular bars of different heights (= a *histogram*, AKA bar graph or chart). Please note that the following histogram is presented with error bars and is using a linear scale (i.e. it is not logarithmic which we will explore in GM 3.7).

EXAMPLE 2

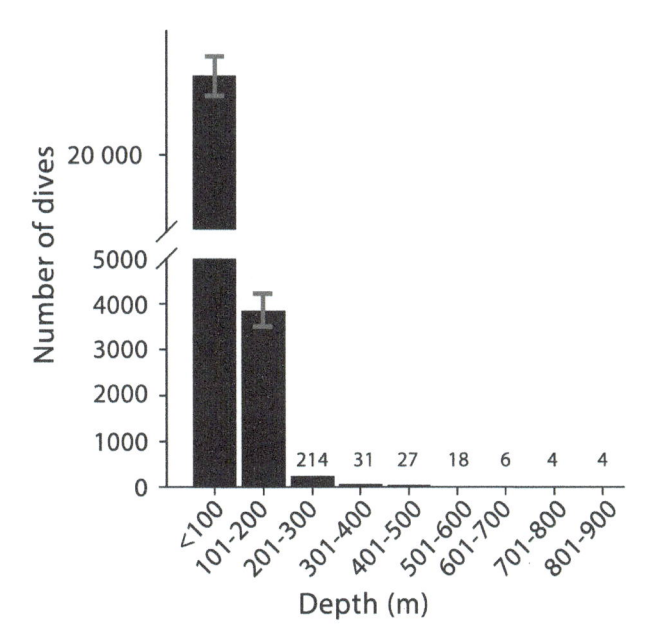

Figure 1 Depth ranges with respective number of dives of leatherback turtles under investigation. Adapted from Hays, Journal of Experimental Biology 2008 211: 2566-2575; doi: 10.1242/jeb.020065.

According to Figure 1, as compared to dives between 100 and 200 metres, dives below 100 metres occur:

A. more than twice as often but less than three times as often.
B. less than 15 000 dives more often.
C. between 15 000 and 20 000 dives more often.
D. over 20 000 dives more often.

Note that glancing at the histogram, without taking into account the broken y-axis, could lead one to be misled into thinking that answer choice A is correct.

Using the distance on the y-axis from 0 to 2000 as a guide, we can see that the first bar diagram seems to end approximately 2000 dives above 20 000 (i.e. 22 000; we can only make this conclusion because the increments are linear).

During the real exam, students sometimes use their ID card (for example, driver's license) to 'measure' distances since rulers are not permitted. We suggest having a long, straight pencil (NOT ergodynamic) which could be helpful for this purpose among others (e.g. slopes off of curves).

The second bar diagram seems to be between 3500 and 4000, which we can approximate as 3750. Thus we can estimate the difference as 22 000 − 3750 = 18 250 dives, thus answer choice C is correct.

The error bars are just an added distraction since they do not come into play here (i.e. they do not overlap). Had they overlapped, we could have no confidence that any difference between the 2 dives exists — even if there appeared to be a difference in the heights of the histograms.

GAMSAT-Prep.com
GOLD STANDARD MATHS

3.6 Cartesian Coordinates in 3D

High-level Importance

The GAMSAT will sometimes present 3D (3-dimensional) graphs to see if you are capable of a basic analysis.

EXAMPLE 1

Consider the following illustration of a 3D Cartesian coordinate system. Notice the origin *O* and the 3 axis lines *X*, *Y* and *Z*, oriented as shown by the arrows. The tick marks on the axes are one length unit apart. Look carefully at the black dot. What coordinate (x, y, z) would you give to identify the position of that dot? (2,2,3)? (3,2,4)? (4,3,2)? (2,4,3)? (2,3,4)? The black dot represents a point with coordinates x = 2, y = 3, and z = 4, or (2,3,4).

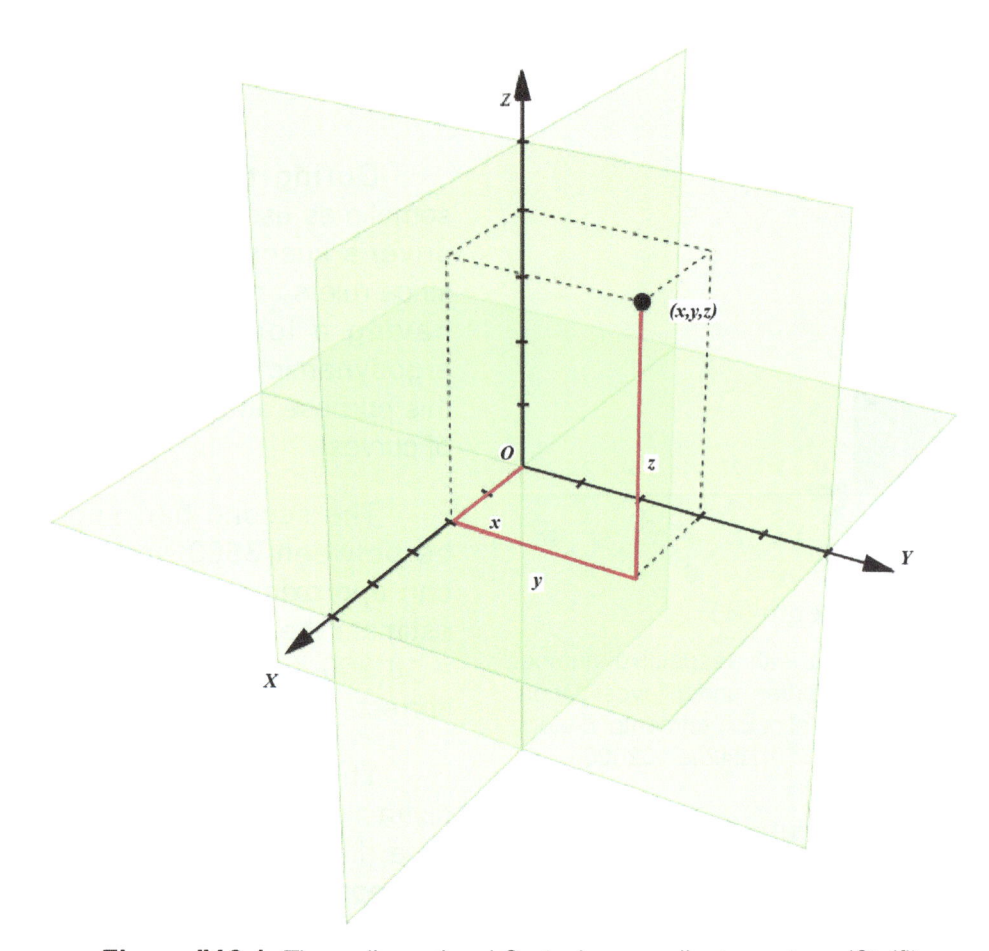

Figure IV.3.1: Three-dimensional Cartesian coordinate system. (Stolfi)

EXAMPLE 2

We will be looking at phase diagrams in General Chemistry Chapter 4. For now, we'll ignore the chemistry and just focus on graph analysis. So as an exercise to read 3D graphs, comment on the relative magnitudes of temperature and pressure for the SOLID (only) portion of the curve in Figure IV.3.2.

First, you must see the graph as a 3-dimensional object. This particular graph looks like a wooden block with parts of 4 sides gouged out, as well as part of the middle. The 3 arrows in the graph indicate increasing magnitudes in the directions of the arrows. Notice that the pressure for solids could be either high or low. However, the specific volume is always relatively low as is the temperature in the region where the graph shows only solid (of course, it makes sense that something that is solid takes up less volume than the gaseous state; also, because of our experience with water - for example, ice and steam - we expect solids to be at low temperatures and gas to be at high temperatures with liquid somewhere in between).

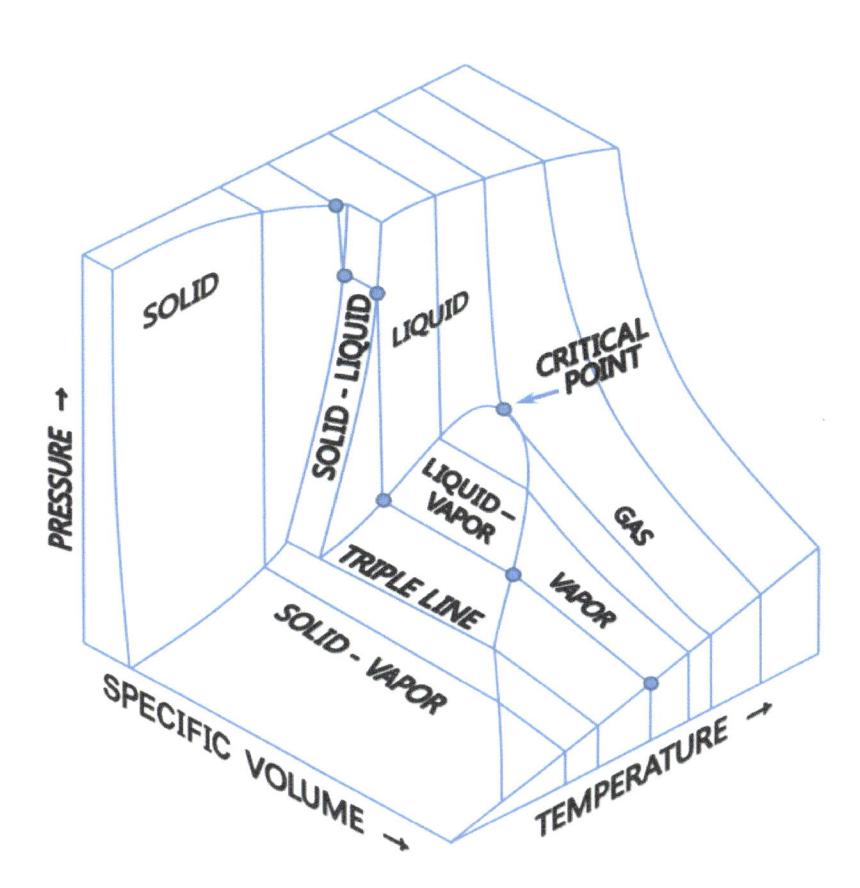

Figure IV.3.2: Pressure-volume-temperature diagram for a pure substance. (Lee/Padleckas)

In conclusion, the relative magnitude of the temperature for the SOLID (only) portion of the curve is low while the pressure can range from high to low.

EXAMPLE 3

In Figure IV.3.2, which of the following can be relatively high at the solid-vapor equilibrium: pressure, temperature or specific volume?

Notice the pressure is always low at the solid-vapor equilibrium (i.e. the part of the graph that says SOLID-VAPOR near the bottom). Temperature also seems to be relatively low at the SOLID-VAPOR part of the graph. However, the volume can be either high or low and thus the volume would be the correct answer.

Just as an aside, the line on the surface called a **triple line** is where solid, liquid and vapor can all coexist in equilibrium.

EXAMPLE 4

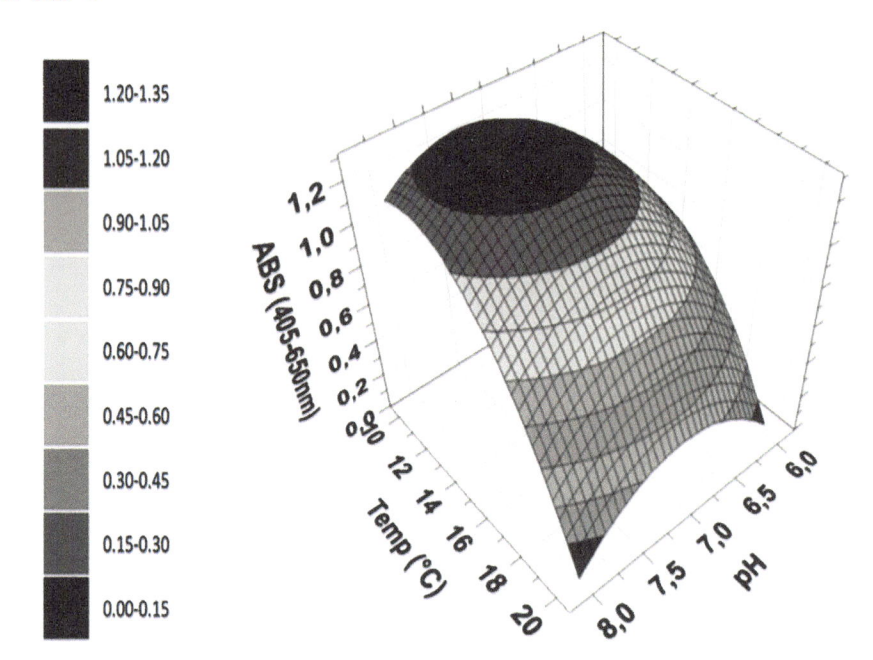

Figure IV.3.2b 3D surface plot demonstrating the effect of temperature and pH on the expression of the TS1-218 protein; the latter is positively correlated with spectrophotometric absorbance (ABS); in yeast cells monitored by ELISA. Jafari R., *Microb. Cell Fact.*, 2011.

GAMSAT MASTERS SERIES

We will continue to try many GAMSAT-level practice questions. As for the real exam, as long as your focus remains 'understanding, reasoning and data interpretation', you can answer the questions without a science background (of course, assuming that you have reviewed all previous GAMSAT Maths sections and chapters). However, you must become accustomed to reading scientific material that is beyond the assumed knowledge for GAMSAT but with the confidence that the actual questions will be founded on basic, introductory-level concepts.

QUESTION 1

According to the data presented in Figure IV.3.2b, approximately what pH and temperature is best for TS1-218 expression?

- A. 7.5, 9.5 °C
- B. 7.5, 14 °C
- C. 6.5, 11 °C
- D. 7.0, 11 °C

QUESTION 2

Which of the following is most consistent with the peak absorbance in Figure IV.3.2b?

- A. Less than 1.2
- B. Exactly 1.2
- C. Above 1.2
- D. None of the above

EXPLANATION

You should develop a standard way to approach all GAMSAT graphs. Here is our Gold Standard 5-step Graph Analysis Technique which you can modify to your liking (we also use this technique during our YouTube videos providing the worked solutions to ACER's GAMSAT practice materials). With experience, it should take you about 30 seconds:

Step 1) Quickly read the labels for all axes (i.e. ABS, Temp, pH) and, most importantly, the caption below the graph, if present. "3D surface plot" suggests that although it is a 3D diagram, we only need to be concerned with the surface of the graph (e.g. it seems to be shaped like a segment of an egg but we only need to be concerned with the eggshell); the rest of the caption can be reasonably interpreted to mean that pH and temperature affects TS1-218 expression which increases with increasing ABS. Thus high ABS = high TS1-218 expression (though the preceding could be inferred, for more about positive correlation: GM 6.3.1). {Note: Sometimes ACER will not have a caption for a diagram, if there is none, make one up! Taking 5-10 seconds to consider your own description of a diagram can focus your mind on the 'big picture'.}

As part of your routine for reading the labels for a graph, you must consider any *key* if present. A key or *legend* is an explanatory list of symbols and/or categories used in a graph, map or table. The key for Figure IV.3.2b is to the left of the graph and clearly shows that the darkest shading at the top refers to values of 1.20-1.35 which means that for the second question, answer choice C is correct. Had you chosen otherwise, it is likely because you did not identify the key and/or fully appreciate the 3D aspect of the diagram. You can tell by the 3 axes that we must be looking at the "top of the eggshell" from the top down, and at an angle.

GAMSAT-Prep.com
GOLD STANDARD MATHS

In other words, you can't just read the ABS value (1.2) from the top of the curve because we are not looking at the graph head-on.

Step 2) Always double check the units (e.g. nm, °C, pH) and the graph's intervals. The latter can be the source of many trick questions, so always check the regularity of the actual distance between the lines on each axis; the unit distance between those lines; as well as the point of origin for each axis to identify cases where the axis begins at a number other than zero.

The intervals for our particular 3D graph are linear (we will later see that pH is logarithmic and so trick questions are still possible but we will not explore that issue for now). Notice that from pH 6 to 8, each major interval is regular at 0.5 pH units. Also note that the surface graph has a grid (GM 3.4.2), and although you do not have to be too precise, you can count - more or less - 30 lines by 30 lines for the grid. That means that to correspond to a pH of 7 (half way between 6 and 8), you would follow a line at approximately 15 on the grid (half of 30, which is due to the graph's visual symmetry; note: you could be off by 3 grid lines - higher or lower - and you would still get the correct answer which is D).

We have placed red asterisks on the 3D graph for you to follow a line from pH 7.0 to the imaginary (approx.) apex of the diagram.

Thus pH has determined that the answer for the first question must be D. The temperature does not need to be precisely calculated but it appears that the Temp axis ranges from about 9 to 21, or about 12 degrees; 30 lines/12 degrees, about 2.5 lines per degree so 11 degrees is about 5 3D-grid lines from the back of the graph, counting along the axis for Temp (side note: we discuss this graph in the Gold Standard Graph Analysis, Part 2 video).

We have already answered both questions, but we will continue with the GS 5-step Graph Analysis Technique which you may need for other types of questions.

Step 3) Recheck the axes to ensure there is not a second labelling system (note that the second graph in GM 3.9 has 2 different labels for the same x-axis), nor any broken axes (i.e. GM 3.5.5).

Step 4) Double check for logarithmic or exponential changes (GM 3.7; yes, it's that important!).

Step 5) Depending on the question type (i.e. GM 3.5.4), assess what the slope or area under the curve would give. This stage may require the equation of a line (GM 3.5.1) and/or dimensional analysis (GM 2.2).

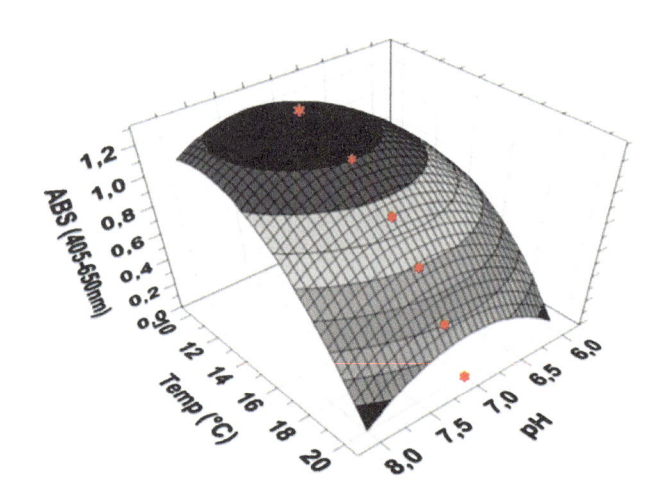

GM-98   CHAPTER 3: ALGEBRA AND GRAPH ANALYSIS

3.7 Logarithms

3.7.1 Log Rules and Logarithmic Scales

A logarithm (i.e. log) is simply the opposite of expressing exponents (GM 1.5). Using a logarithm answers the question: "How many of one number do we multiply to get another number?"

For example: How many 5s must we multiply to get 125? Answer: $5 \times 5 \times 5 = 125$ (GM 1.5.6), so we had to multiply 3 of the 5s to get 125. Now we can say that the log of 125 with base 5 is 3: $\log_5(125) = 3$.

Just as we have already reviewed various rules for exponents (GM 1.5.1-1.5.5), we will shortly learn basic log rules which will permit manipulations for more complex logs, and we will see that the rules can also be applied to the preceding example thus: $\log_5(125) = \log_5(5)^3 = 3\log_5(5) = 3$.

Like many aspects of maths, riding a bike is a good analogy: familiarity will have you applying log rules effortlessly. Logarithmic and exponential scales are found widely in medicine as well as, of course, the basic sciences that we are studying for the GAMSAT.

The rules of logarithms are also discussed in context, for example, Acids and Bases in General Chemistry (CHM 6.5.1). These basic log rules also apply to the "natural logarithm" which is the logarithm to the base e, where "e" is an irrational constant approximately equal to 2.71... (GM 1.1.2). The natural logarithm is usually written as $\ln x$ or $\log_e x$.

Table 1: Common values for the log base 10 (note the trends)

x	Exponential form	$\log_{10}(x)$
0.0001	10^{-4}	-4
0.001	10^{-3}	-3
0.01	10^{-2}	-2
0.1	10^{-1}	-1
1	10^{0}	0
10	10^{1}	1
100	10^{2}	2
1000	10^{3}	3
10000	10^{4}	4

GAMSAT-Prep.com
GOLD STANDARD MATHS

High-level Importance

In general, the power of logarithms is to reduce wide-ranging numbers to quantities with a far smaller range. For example, the graphs commonly seen in this text, including the preceding 2-dimensional graphs, are drawn to a unit or *arithmetic scale*. In other words, each unit on the *x* and *y*-axes represents exactly *one* unit. This scale can be adjusted to accommodate rapidly changing curves. For example, in a unit scale the numbers 1 (= 10^0), 10 (= 10^1), 100 (= 10^2), and 1000 (= 10^3), are all far apart with varying intervals. Using a logarithmic scale, the sparse values suddenly become separated by one unit: Log 10^0 = 0, log 10^1 = 1, log 10^2 = 2, log 10^3 = 3, and so on.

In practice, logarithmic scales are often used to convert a rapidly changing curve (e.g. an exponential curve) into a straight line (see Fig IV.3.4 in GM 3.8). It is called a *semi-log* scale when either the *x*-axis *or* the *y*-axis is logarithmic. It is called a *log-log* scale when both the *x*-axis *and* the *y*-axis are logarithmic. Note: if not specified otherwise, when you just see "log" with no base, then it is considered to be the "common log" which means log base 10.

Here are the rules you must know:

1) $\log_a a = 1$
2) $\log_a M^k = k \log_a M$
3) $\log_a(MN) = \log_a M + \log_a N$
4) $\log_a(M/N) = \log_a M - \log_a N$
5) $10^{\log_{10} M} = M$
6) $\log_a(1) = 0$, given "a" is greater than zero.

EXAMPLE 1

Given:

$$pH = -\log_{10}[H^+]$$

Let us calculate the pH of 0.001 H^+ (for now, ignore the chemistry, focus only on the maths):

[H^+] = 0.001
using the #1 Rule of Algebra (GM 3.1.1):
-log[H^+] = -log (0.001)
pH = -log(10^{-3})
pH = 3 log 10   (log rule #2)
pH = 3   (rule #1, a = 10)

EXAMPLE 2

What is log (1 000 000)?
log (1 000 000) = log 10^6 = 6

EXAMPLE 3

What is log (1/100)?
log (1/100) = log 10^{-2} = -2

EXAMPLE 4

Given that ln2 = 0.69, what is ln2e^3?

Try to solve the problem while keeping in mind: (1) ln is the natural logarithm, meaning that it is log to the base e; (2) our 3rd rule of logarithms permits you separate factors.

ln2e^3 = ln2 + lne^3 = 0.69 + 3 = 3.69

Notice that if you have the base of the log and the base of the number with the exponent the same, then the answer is simply the exponent. Thus

Log(1000) = log10^3 = lne^3 = 3.

> **NOTE**
>
> GAMSAT log problems come in the form of pH, pKa, pKb, rate law, Nernst equation, semi-log graphs, log-log graphs, decibels/sound intensity (PHY 8.3), Gibbs free energy (CHM 9.10), just to name a few! The relevant equations are usually provided. In other words, the 'science' reduces to a basic maths problem.

EXAMPLE 5

Approximate log(200).

Because the number 200 is between 100 and 1000 (but clearly closer to 100), and since log(100) = 2 and log(1000) = 3, log(200) must be a number between 2 and 3 but closer to the number 2. Such an approximation is sufficient for a multiple choice exam. {Incidentally, log(200) happens to be approximately 2.3.}

3.8 Exponential and Logarithmic Curves

The exponential and logarithmic functions are *inverse functions*. That is, their graphs can be reflected about the $y = x$ line which you can see in Figure IV.3.3.

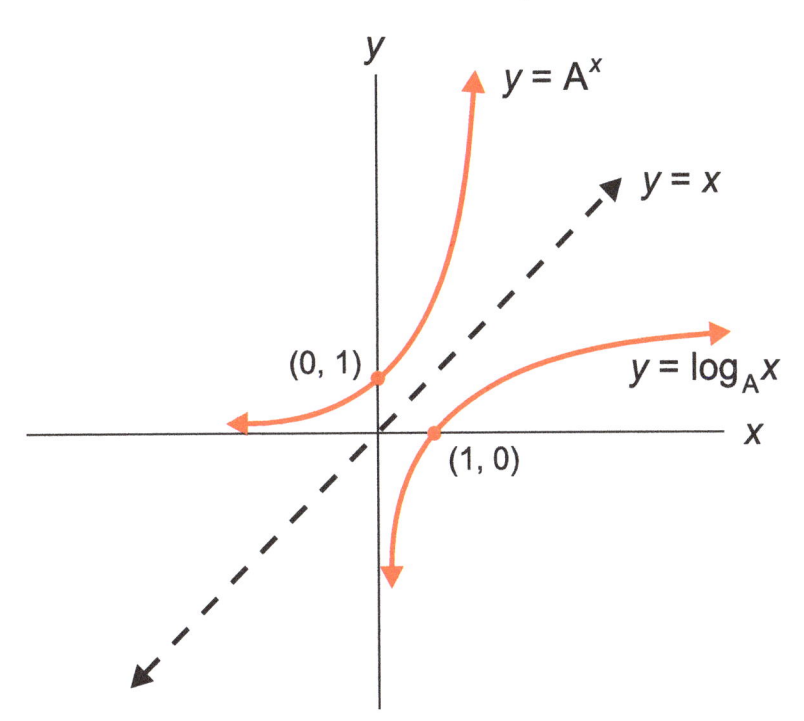

Figure IV.3.3: Exponential and Logarithmic Graphs, A > 1. Notice that when a positive number is raised to the power of 0, then the result is 1 [i.e. the point (0, 1); see also GM 1.5.4, 1.5.5 for rules of exponents]. Also note that log(1) = ln (1) = 0 [i.e. the point (1, 0) on the generic logarithmic curve].

GAMSAT-Prep.com
GOLD STANDARD MATHS

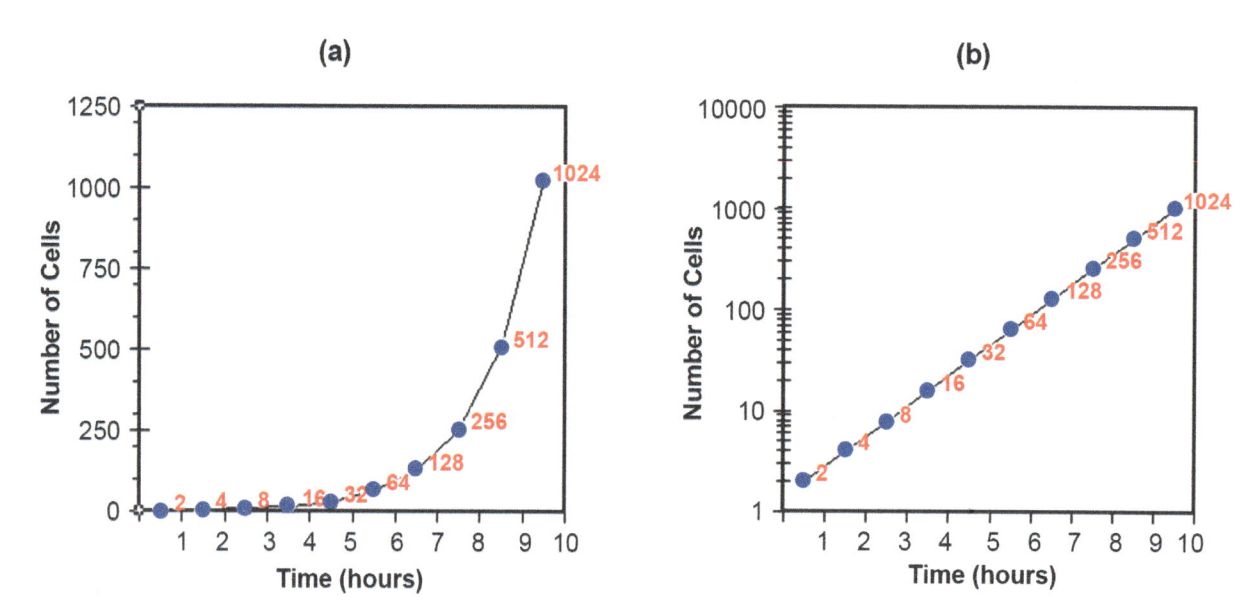

Figure IV.3.4: Growth curves of cells dividing mitotically. (a) An exponential curve with a linear scale for the x and y-axis. (b) A logarithmic scale on the y-axis converts the data rising exponentially into a linear graph. This is referred to as a semi-log graph or semi-log plot (GM 3.7.1). Notice that it is observation or analysis that leads to the conclusion as to what type of graph is being assessed as neither graph is labelled "exponential" nor "logarithm" anywhere. Also, carefully count the notches along the y-axis of the log scale (b), and notice that halfway between 1 and 10, is a number between 3 and 4, halfway between 10 and 100 is 30-40, halfway between 100 and 1000 is 300-400 (answer A in GM 3.0 *Need for Speed*), and so on.

Let's revisit one of the key reasons for using logarithms: when the data points vary from low numbers to very high numbers, sometimes a log helps to better demonstrate all the data points on one graph. Consider Figure IV.3.4: two growth curves that both represent the same data of bacteria doubling over time (2^n = 2, 2^2, 2^3, 2^4, 2^5, 2^6, 2^7, 2^8, 2^9, 2^{10} which is 1024; BIO 2.2).

Notice that in the first graph, the y-axis increases in a linear fashion: the difference between each major marking is 250 cells and it starts at zero. The problem however is that the first 4 or 5 points on the exponential curve are not really distinguishable. They are all such small relative numbers making the first ½ of the curve quite flat before it increases rapidly. It is that rapid rise that we recognise visually as an exponential increase (even though, of course, it is the entire curve which is exponential, being 2 to the power of n).

On the other hand, the second graph uses a logarithmic scale on the *y*-axis (i.e. each number is 10 times the preceding number and equally spaced; the 4th number does not represent 4 times some number, rather, it represents 10 to the power of 4 times which is 10 000 times larger); suddenly the exponential curve is converted to a manageable, more clear, linear relationship where small and large data points are

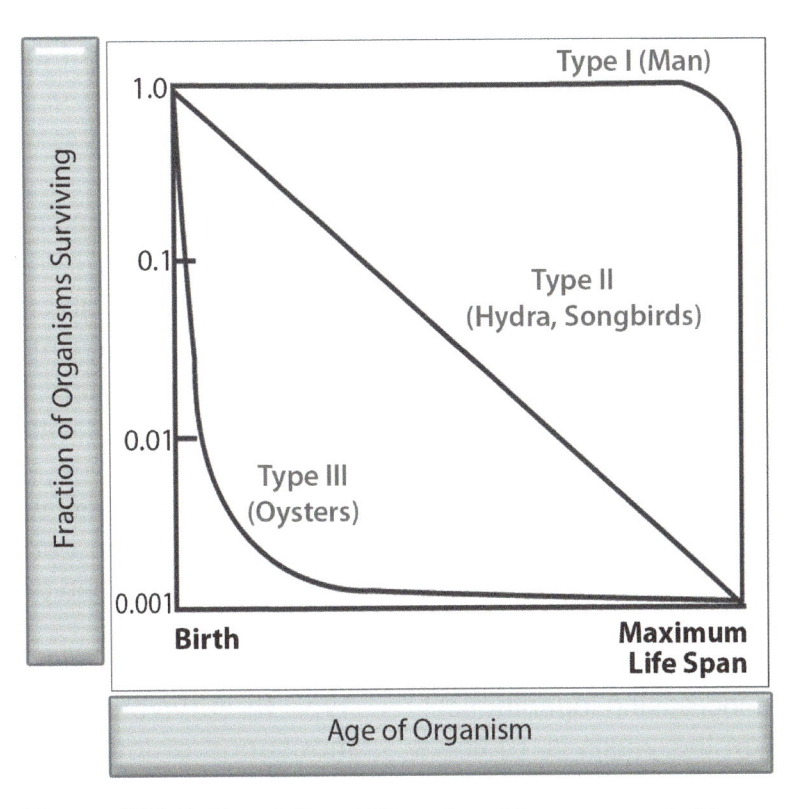

Figure IV.3.5: Type I, II and III survivorship curves scaled to a maximum life span for each species.

easily visible on one graph. Notice that if you took the log of the 5 numbers along the y-axis, you would get the quite regular result of 0, 1, 2, 3 and 4 (recall that log 10 000 = log10^4 = 4). Incidentally, because the x-axis increases in a linear fashion, the preceding is a semi-log graph.

Thus a graph that has a scale that is logarithmic on one axis but is linear on the other axis is semi-log. The term for the graph is unimportant for the GAMSAT but recognising that you are dealing with such a graph is often critical to answering the questions properly. We will now explore another semi-log graph (Figure IV.3.5).

Spend a few moments considering Figure IV.3.5.

QUESTION 1

Based on the diagram provided, is it true that approximately ½ of songbirds would be expected to survive ½ of their maximum lifespan? {Please consider your answer before turning the page.}

QUESTION 2

One perspective regarding the biological success of a species would be to equate success with the absolute number of individual organisms belonging to the species in question. Given this perspective, if oysters, songbirds and humans are all equally successful, based on the diagram, which of the three likely produces the least number of organisms (i.e. the least number of offspring per organism)?

EXPLANATION 1

NO! Not even close!! First, let's get a sense of the scales. We must assume that the *x*-axis is linear because no other information is provided. However, the *y*-axis is clearly logarithmic. It looks like it is regular (in a linear sense) but when you look at the numbers, they are increasing logarithmically. Each marking on the *y*-axis is 10 times the previous marking. After 3 markings, 1000 times or 10^3. If you take the log of the 4 numbers on the *y*-axis, you would get the very regular numbers of -3, -2, -1 and 0.

Now let's look at ½ of the maximum life span (so ½ of the length of the *x*-axis). When you look at the Type II line at that point (signifying songbirds and hydra; it's not important that you know what hydra means) and look across to the *y*-axis, you get a point ½ way between 0.01 and 0.1. Even if we imagine the higher of the 2 numbers, 0.1, that is only 1/10th of the surviving organisms (0.1 = 1/10 = 10%). And because the lower number is 1/100th (= 1%) of the surviving organisms, the actual result is between the two which is far lower than ½ of surviving organisms (i.e. 50%). This is a common question type that can appear in any of the GAMSAT science subtopics. If you do not understand the scale, you will get the wrong answer.

EXPLANATION 2

Presumably, for the next generation to exist, the current generation must survive long enough to reproduce. The survivorship curve with the most extreme change between birth and a presumed age of reproductive ability would be the Type III survivorship curve. Let's see what we can infer from the shapes of that curve.

Most individuals in populations with Type III survivorship must produce many thousands of individuals, most of whom, according to the diagram, die right away. Once this initial period is over, survivorship is relatively constant. Examples of this would likely include fish, marine larvae, and of course oysters. Relatively little effort or parental care is likely invested in each individual.

> **NOTE**
>
> Notice that neither Figure IV.3.4 (b) nor Figure IV.3.5 had a clear origin of (0, 0). Though not important here, sometimes questions are designed to test whether you observed that the origin was other than (0, 0) and that you took it into account when necessary. We will see some questions like that in Biology.

Type I survivorship includes humans, likely, we could reason, in developed countries. As a result of environment and the resources invested in each individual, there is a high survivorship throughout the life cycle. Most individuals, according to the graph, die of old age. If Type III must produce a lot of individuals to survive the 'die off' and still be successful, then Type I requires relatively few offspring to be successful because the survivorship is better than the other two groups. Thus the answer is: humans.

EXAMPLE

Consider the following diagram.

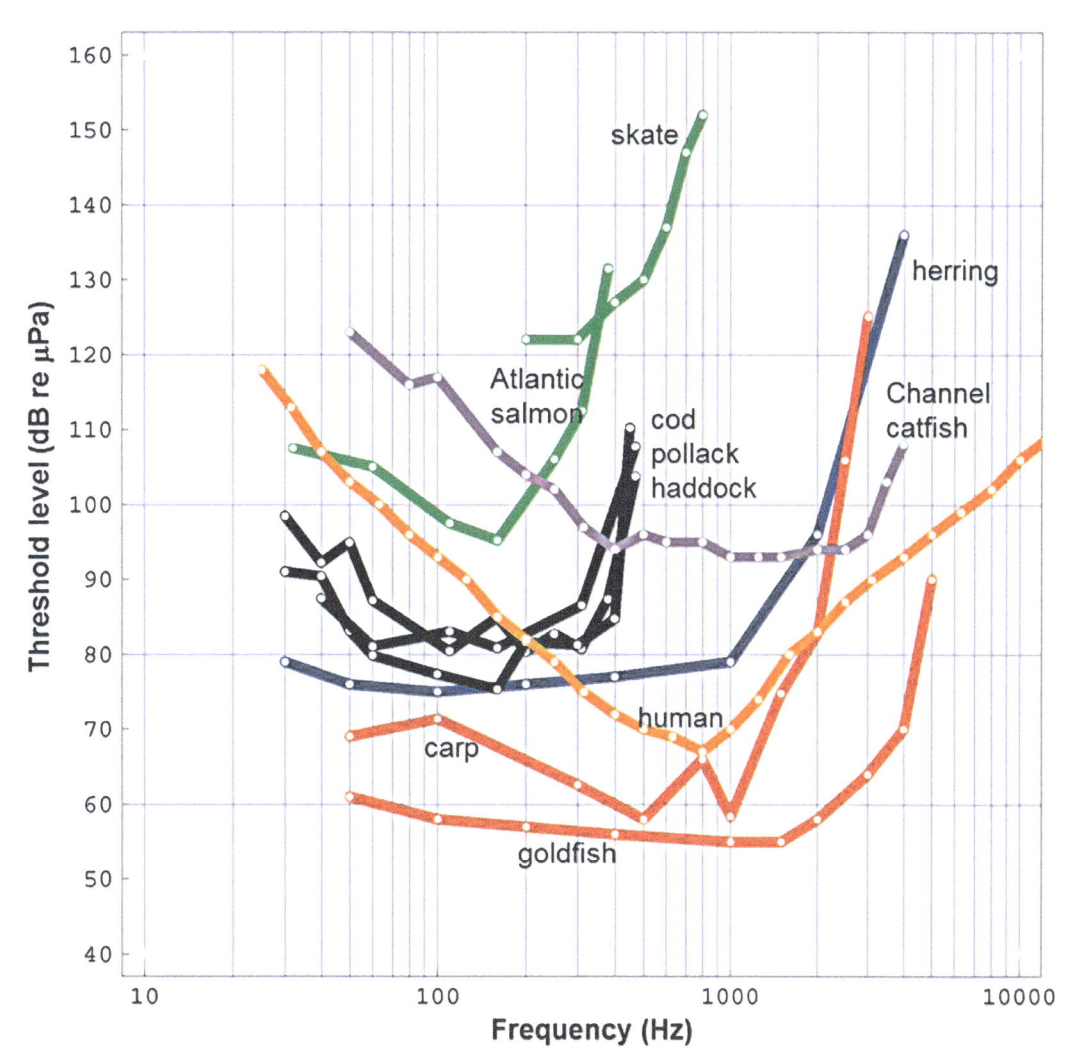

Figure IV.3.6 Audiogram curves showing the faintest sounds – as sound pressure recorded as decibels (dB) – that can be heard at each frequency, underwater. Amundsen and Landrø, GEOexPro Vol. 8, No. 3; 2011.

GAMSAT-Prep.com
GOLD STANDARD MATHS

We will now proceed with some GAMSAT-level multiple-choice questions based on the logarithmic scale (Fig. IV.3.6).

QUESTION 1

According to the diagram, which of the following best approximates the human underwater minimum sound pressure and corresponding frequency, respectively?

- A. 67 dB, 0.8 kHz
- B. 67 dB, 1000 Hz
- C. 66 dB, 9.8 x 10^2 Hz
- D. 66 dB, 9.9 x 10^2 Hz

QUESTION 2

Hearing range describes the range of frequencies, from lowest to highest, that can be heard by humans or other animals. According to the diagram, which of the following has the greatest hearing range?

- A. Herring
- B. Carp
- C. Channel catfish
- D. Goldfish

QUESTION 3

According to the diagram, how many species are likely to hear a sound of 90 dB and 3000 Hz?

- A. 1
- B. 2
- C. 3
- D. More than 3

EXPLANATION

The caption links the expression "sound pressure" to dBs which can be read along the y-axis.

The minimum sound pressure value for the 'human' graph seems to be between 65 and 70 dB, though it is not possible to be overly accurate (yes, ambiguity is embedded in the question). However, we can be very precise about the frequency at that sound pressure: It is clearly and exactly 800 Hz [if you are unsure as to how to read the logarithmic scale, go back to the beginning of this section, GM 3.8, and examine the y-axis of Figure IV.3.4, graph (b); also re-examine our discussion for Figure IV.3.5; and finally, consider labelling Figure IV.3.6 yourself so that between 100 and 1000 along the x-axis, you add the following numbers below the vertical lines: 200, 300, 400, 500, 600, 700, 800, 900]. It is very important for GAMSAT purposes that you also remember your SI unit prefixes (GM 2.1.2, 2.1.3). 800 Hz = 0.8 kiloHz = 0.8 kHz, thus A is the correct answer for the first question. The other 3 answer choices are all above 900 Hz which is clearly incorrect.

For Question 2, as defined, the expression 'range' is generally understood to mean the difference between the highest and lowest number (side note: we will discuss statistical measures for the GAMSAT in Maths Chapter 6).

If the scale were linear, then the easiest way to determine the widest frequency range would simply be to inspect each curve to see which is the widest (from left to right), and then 'herring' would be the winner! However, the x-axis is logarithmic so such simplifications do not apply. By far, 'goldfish' has the greatest range (answer choice D is correct)

High-level Importance

GM-106   CHAPTER 3: ALGEBRA AND GRAPH ANALYSIS

because it begins at a number far higher than the rest:

A. Herring: 4000 − 30 = 3970 Hz
B. Carp: 3000 − 50 = 2950 Hz
C. Channel catfish: 4000 − 50 = 3950 Hz
D. Goldfish: 5000 − 50 = 4950 Hz

For Question 3, label the graph in increments of 1000 between labels 1000 Hz and 10000 Hz so you have no doubt as to where the vertical line for 3000 Hz lies. To meet this line, using a straight pencil from 90 dB, you should intersect a point which is just above (or at) the 'human' graph. Thus the sound in question (90 dB and 3000 Hz) is at - or above - the threshold for human, and far above the threshold for 'goldfish'. The answer is B.

3.9 Nomograms: The Art of Unusual Graphs

A **nomogram** is a diagram representing the relations between three or more changing variables using several scales. Each scale is arranged so that the value of one variable can be found by simple geometry, for example, by drawing a straight line intersecting the other scales at the appropriate values.

Most students, with or without a science background, have little to no experience with nomograms which is exactly why ACER loves them! In addition, there is such a wide variety of what may be loosely called 'nomograms' that it assures ACER that in the long run, almost all students will be confronted with a nomogram which they would see for the first time in the exam room.

EXAMPLE 1

Consider the following nomogram. Using a straight pencil as a guide, you can join a point from the water temperature on the upper scale to the dissolved oxygen reading (ppm) on the bottom scale. You can then read the percentage oxygen saturation from the point at which your pencil crosses the middle scale. For example, at 7 °C and 12 ppm of dissolved oxygen, the result is approximately 100% saturation (note: ACER typically provides an example to get you oriented).

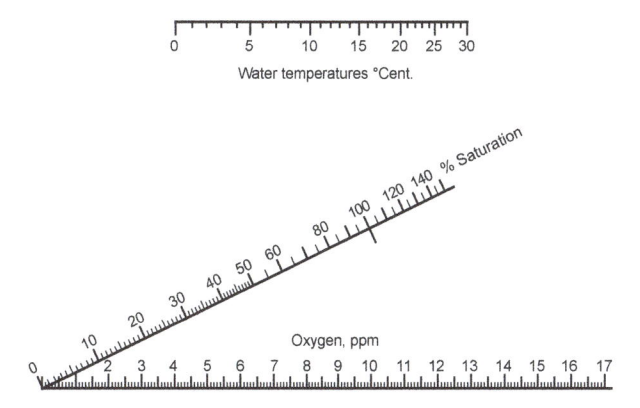

Nomogram for dissolved oxygen saturation.
Ref. Environments in Profile, an aquatic perspective, W Kaill and J Frey, Canfield Press, 1973.

What is the % saturation for 1.5 ppm of dissolved oxygen at a water temperature of 18 °C?

A. Less than 10%   C. 20%
B. 15%   D. More than 20%

GAMSAT-Prep.com
GOLD STANDARD MATHS

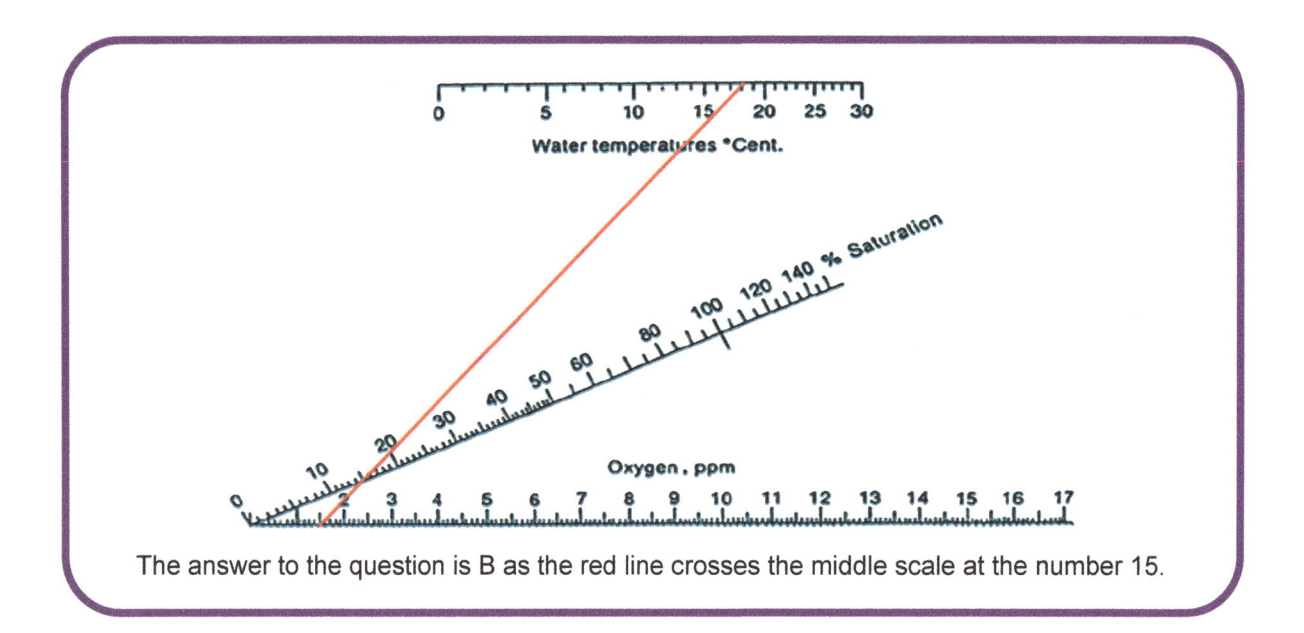

High-level Importance

The answer to the question is B as the red line crosses the middle scale at the number 15.

Side note: Although there is no assumed knowledge for the preceding question, the nomogram teaches an important point about gases dissolved in water which comes up frequently on the real exam. Hopefully, after you study General Chemistry, you will understand why the same concentration of oxygen (in this case, ppm) results in lower saturation in water at lower temperatures. Consequently, more gas can "fit" in water when the temperature is low (like a can of Coke or champagne, the gas bubbles are lost faster at higher temperatures).

EXAMPLE 2

Nomograms can appear to be more complex than the preceding straight lines as will be illustrated next. The many graphs to follow will have associated GAMSAT-level practice questions which do not have any assumed science knowledge (as is often the case with real GAMSAT Section 3 graph-analysis questions).

The following represents normal values for arterial blood in humans: pH 7.4, bicarbonate 24 mmol/L, pCO_2 40 mmHg.

Consider Figure IV.3.7.

> **NOTE**
>
> Please avoid trying to think: 'I will memorise this or that graph for the exam'. The better long-term strategy would be: 'I need to have a reliable method to approach novel graphs so when I see one, I will have the confidence to break it down (and hopefully have some fun along the way!)'. You can try the Gold Standard 5-step Graph Analysis Technique (GM 3.6), or develop your own approach, but do not let graphs intimidate you!

GM-108 CHAPTER 3: ALGEBRA AND GRAPH ANALYSIS

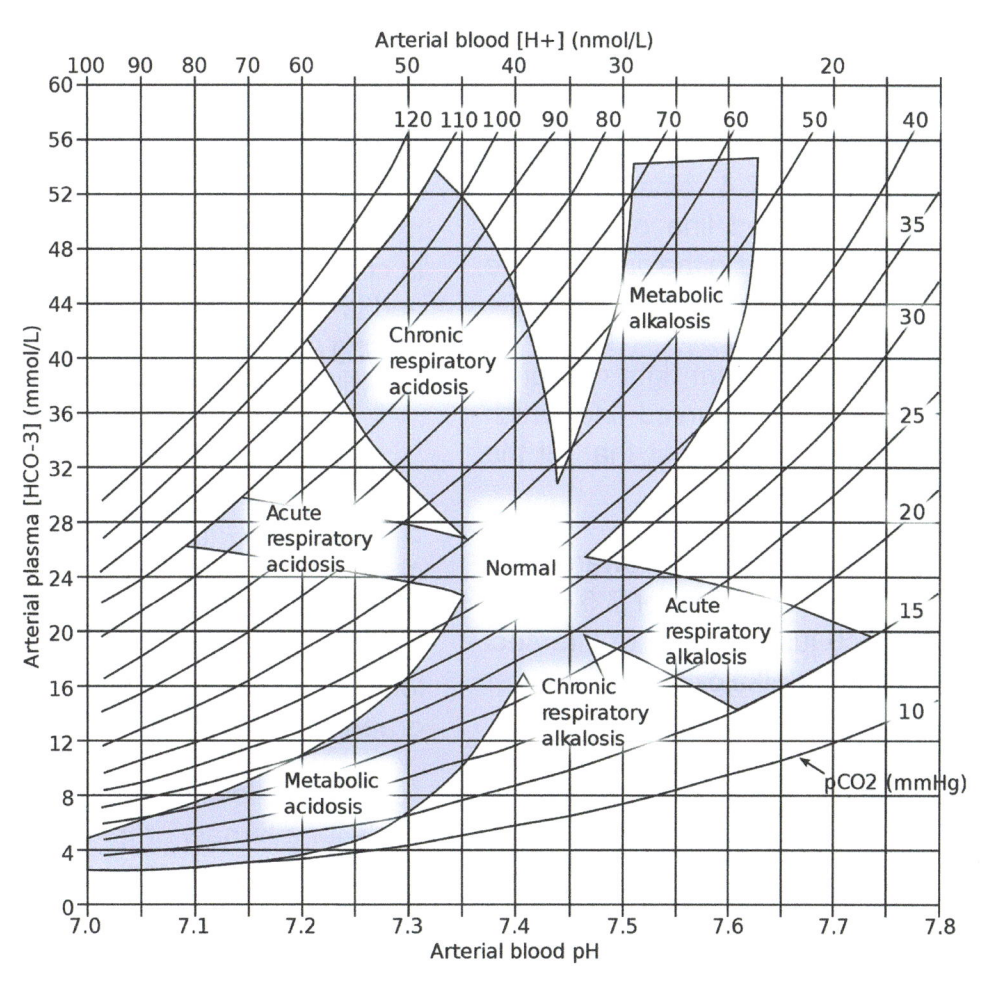

Figure IV.3.7 Human arterial blood acid-base balance and disorders

QUESTION 1

According to Figure IV.3.7, an arterial blood pH of 7.5 with a pCO₂ of 25, corresponds best with which of the following?

A. Metabolic alkalosis
B. Acute respiratory alkalosis
C. Chronic respiratory alkalosis
D. Chronic respiratory acidosis

QUESTION 2

Consider a patient with metabolic alkalosis. Based on Figure IV.3.7, which of the following would be most consistent with returning the patient back to normal?

A. Increase in arterial [H⁺], decrease arterial bicarbonate
B. Increase arterial pH, increase arterial bicarbonate
C. Decrease pCO₂, decrease arterial [H⁺]
D. Increase pCO₂, decrease arterial bicarbonate

GAMSAT-Prep.com
GOLD STANDARD MATHS

EXPLANATION

For Question 1, you must begin with the example provided in the preamble and trace the lines of pH 7.4, bicarbonate 24 mmol/L, and the curved line of pCO_2 40 mmHg which all intersect in the graph at one point – basically, in the middle of 'Normal'.

Notice that the bottom right corner of the diagram points to a curved line which says pCO_2 (mmHg) to suggest that all the curved lines represent pCO_2.

Now our attention turns towards the two lines in the question: pH of 7.5 with a pCO_2 of 25 which just manage to intersect at 'Acute respiratory alkalosis'. The answer is B for Question 1.

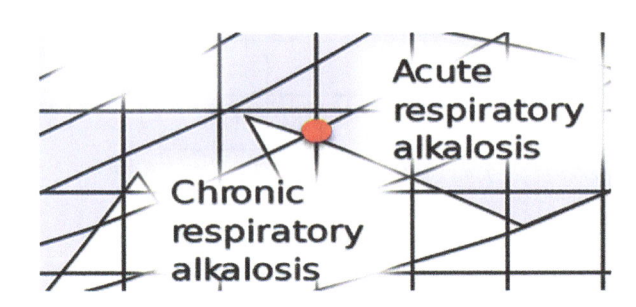

For Question 2, note that 'metabolic alkalosis' is in the top right portion of the graph. 'Normal' is, comparatively, down and to the left of 'metabolic alkalosis'. Looking at the y-axis to the left, we can see that going down means that we would have a decrease in arterial bicarbonate. Now be careful to notice that the x-axis at the top of the graph has arterial [H⁺] decreasing from left to right, which means that moving to the left results in an increase in arterial [H⁺]. The answer is A for Question 2.

Even though we have not formally reviewed General Chemistry, having already seen the equation for pH (GM 3.7.1; pH = $-\log_{10}$[H⁺]), because of the negative sign, when pH rises, you can deduce that [H⁺] must decrease, and vice versa. This point is confirmed by the nomogram (Fig. IV.3.7) and is the source of over a dozen questions among ACER's GAMSAT practice materials. We will review the pH scale next in CHM 6.5.

EXAMPLE 3

Ternary (AKA trilinear, triangular) graphs or plots, tephigrams (commonly used in weather analysis and forecasting), and some thermodynamic diagrams can be loosely defined as nomograms. The ternary graph is encountered the most frequently.

The following is the most widely-used scale for a ternary graph. From time to time, return to this common scale to confirm your understanding.

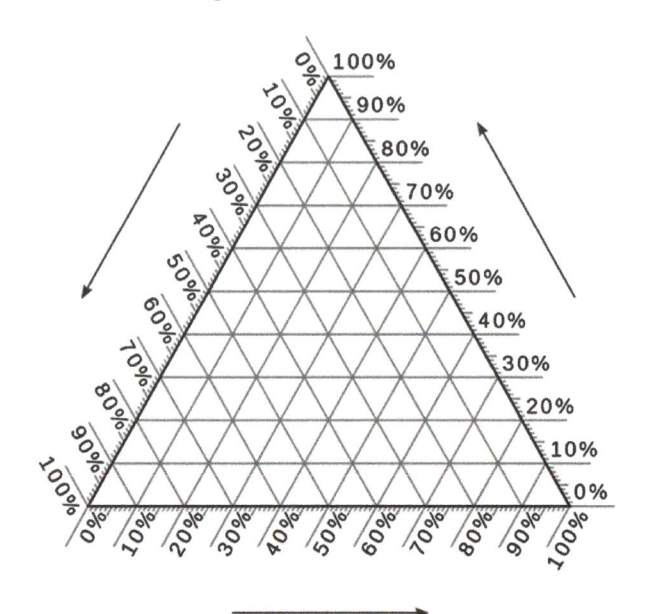

Now we will learn how to read a ternary graph with the following 3 variables: organic matter, clay and sand.

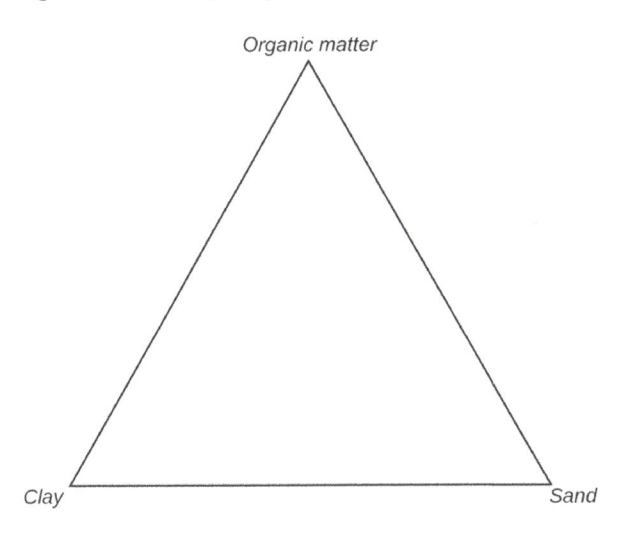

As a general rule, the percentage of one component is given by a line that is parallel with the line between the other 2 components. For example, consider the diagram below. Notice that the percentage of 'Organic matter' is represented by a line that is parallel to the Clay-Sand line.

Notice that the percentage of 'Clay' in the following diagram is represented by a line that is parallel to the Organic matter-Sand line. The caption in the diagram reads: "One coordinate only tells us the one proportion: at any point along these lines, the proportion of Clay is the percentage given, but we don't know the proportions of Organic matter or Sand."

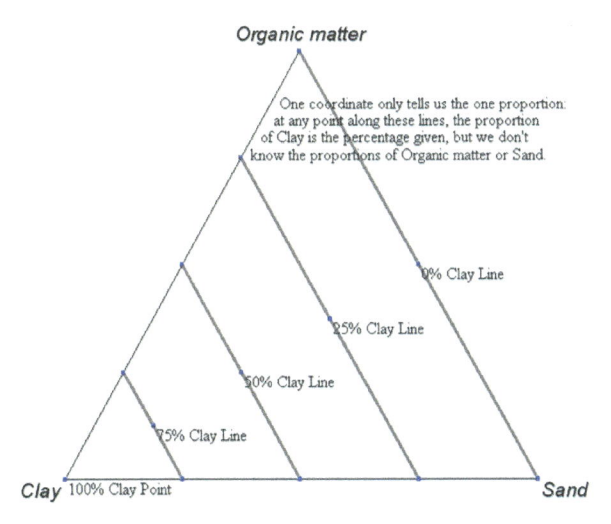

Notice in the following diagram that the percentage of 'Sand' is represented by a line that is parallel to the Clay-Organic matter line.

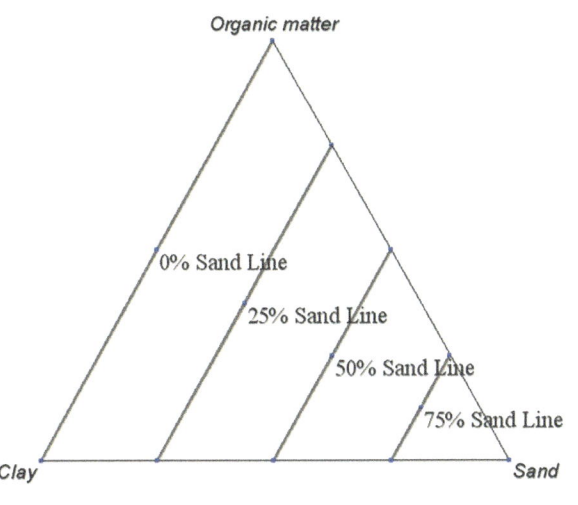

Ref.: Wikipedia Commons Statistics, Smith609

GAMSAT-Prep.com
GOLD STANDARD MATHS

High-level Importance

As long as you know that a ternary graph is based on 100%, you should be able to read it without any percentages showing (this will ensure that you will not fall for any tricks like leaving out key numbers on any or all 3 axes).

As you progress through this section on nomograms, you will likely find some challenging questions. Please take the time that you need to solve the problem.

EXAMPLE 4

Consider the following ternary graph. Note: similar to the previous ternary graphs, the maximum possible for any single component is 100%.

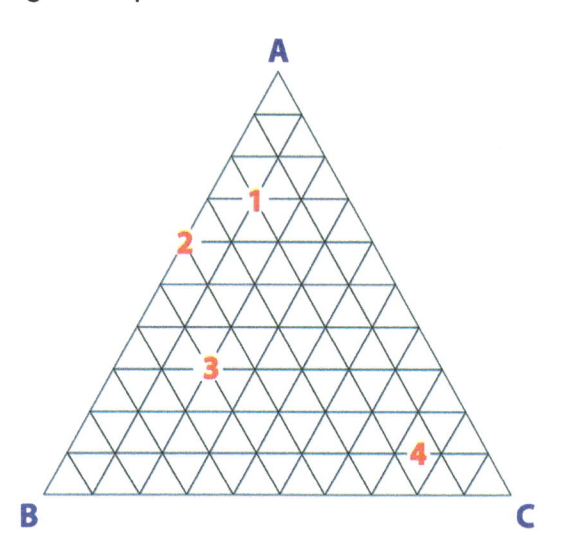

Which of the following correctly corresponds to the label provided in the preceding ternary diagram?

- **A.** 1. 80% A | 10% B | 10% C
- **B.** 2. 60% A | 30% B | 10% C
- **C.** 3. 20% A | 60% B | 20% C
- **D.** 4. 10% A | 15% B | 75% C

Notice that the 3 components can always be added up to a sum total of 100% since that is the scale provided in the question (i.e. A + B + C = 100%). If you are unsure, go back to the first diagram which we described as the "most widely-used scale for a ternary graph." If it is still not clear, you may login to your gamsat-prep.com account, click on Videos, and look for GAMSAT Graph Analysis Recorded Webinar Part 3, and of course we also have the gamsat-prep.com/forum.

Here are the actual percentages which reveal that only answer choice D is correct:

1. 70% A | 20% B | 10% C
2. 60% A | 40% B | 0% C
3. 30% A | 50% B | 20% C
4. 10% A | 15% B | 75% C

EXAMPLE 5

Coloured gold metal may include silver and copper in various proportions, producing white, yellow, green and red golds. Pure 100% gold is 24 karat (K) by definition, so all coloured golds are less than this, with the common ones being 18K (75%), 14K (58%), and 9K (38%).

Consider the following ternary plot showing different colours of Ag-Au-Cu alloys.

We suggest using a pencil to determine your answers – as you would do for the real exam – since you may change your mind and wish to erase and restart.

GM-112   CHAPTER 3: ALGEBRA AND GRAPH ANALYSIS

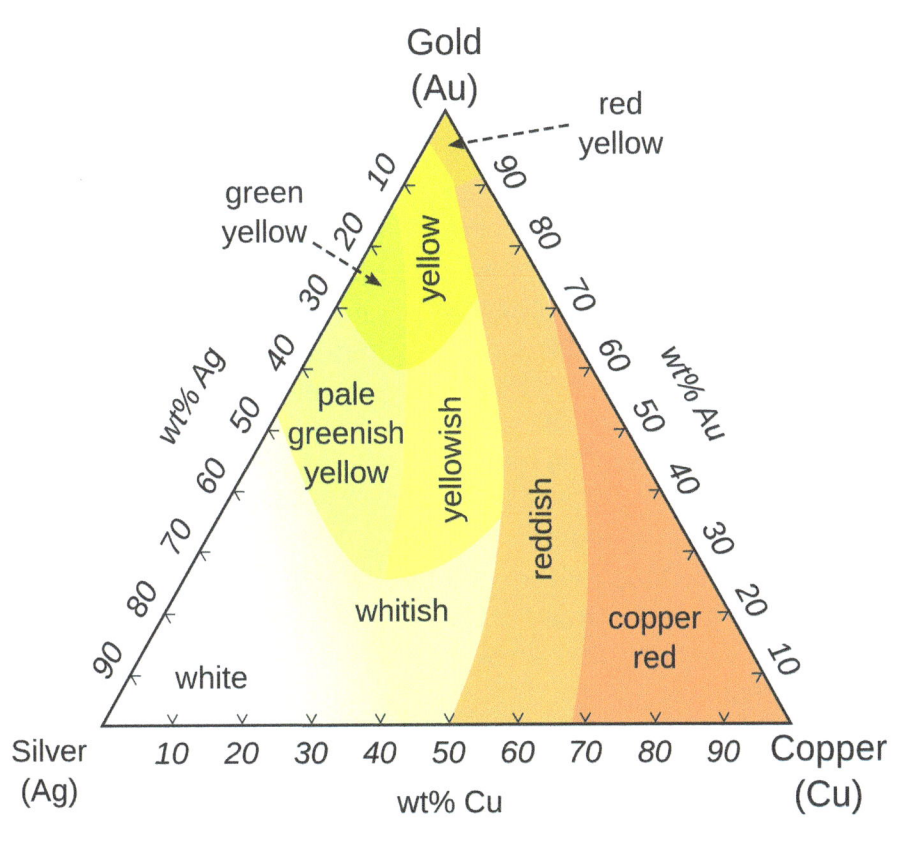

Figure IV.3.8 Trilinear diagram representing the percent by weight of 3 different metals and the resultant appearance of the mixture (= *metal alloy*). en.wikipedia.org/wiki/Colored_gold Ref: Metallos

QUESTION 1

Based on the information provided, choose the correct statement.

A. Pure gold is 'yellow' gold.
B. Increasing copper in the alloy increases the chance of a possible greenish appearance.
C. "Yellowish" gold is present when ½ of the mixture is gold, while silver and copper are equal.
D. Pure silver added to 'pale greenish yellow' gold can produce 'yellow' gold.

QUESTION 2

Equal amounts by weight of 14K and 9K gold are mixed together. According to Figure IV.3.8, which of the following is the likely result of the appearance of the mixture if it contains 10% copper?

A. Pale greenish yellow
B. Yellow
C Yellowish
D. Whitish

GAMSAT-Prep.com
GOLD STANDARD MATHS

EXPLANATION 1

For the first question:

A. Pure gold, according to the preamble before the diagram, is 100% gold which is clearly labelled 'red yellow' in the diagram as opposed to simply 'yellow'.

B. Increasing copper increases the chance of a red appearance (in fact, the corner where copper is highest is labelled "copper red". The 'pale greenish yellow' appearance is possible only when copper is 0-30%.

C. Converting the words to maths: gold must be 50%, and thus silver and copper must be 25% each. Drawing the appropriate lines confirms that answer choice C is correct.

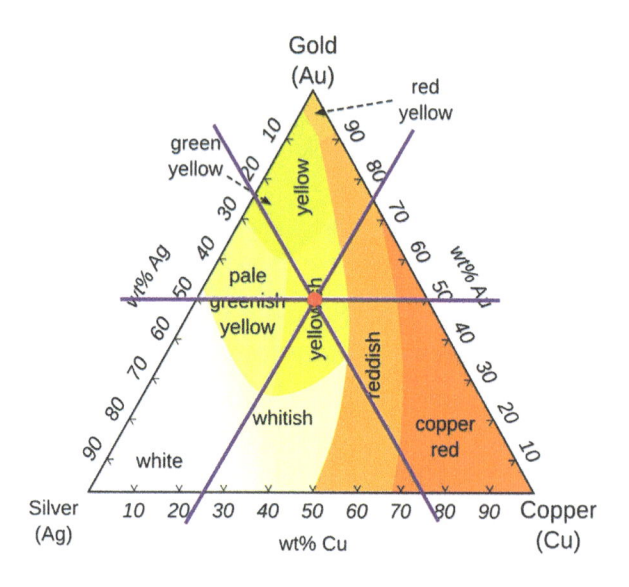

D. To add pure silver is to increase the silver % which means to go from 'pale greenish yellow' to 'whitish' or 'white' rather than the opposite direction to 'yellow'.

EXPLANATION 2

For the second question:

14K (58% gold according to the preamble) and 9K (38% gold) are combined thus we have (58 + 38)/2 = 48% gold (combining percentages: GM 1.4.3C). We can use the 2 lines (48% gold and 10% copper) to determine that the answer is 'pale greenish yellow' and to confirm the concentration of the 3rd component (100 – 48 – 10 = 42% silver). Answer choice A is correct.

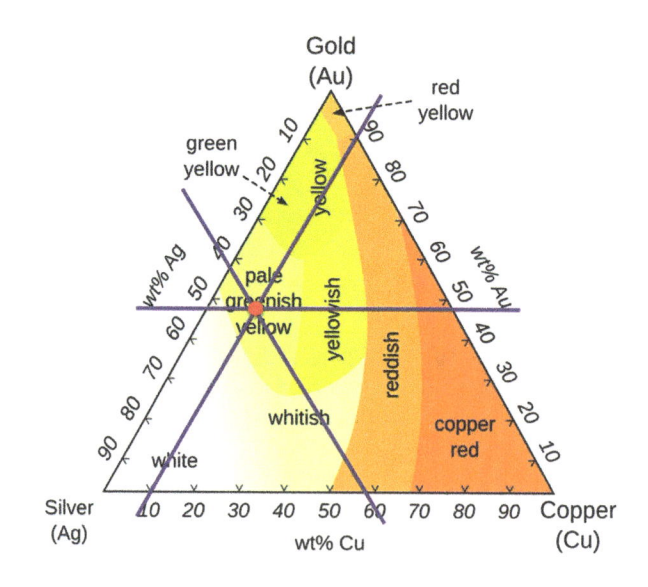

EXAMPLE 6

A piper plot is often used to visualise the chemistry of a rock, soil, or water sample. There are 3 components: a ternary (or triangular) diagram in the lower left representing cations, a ternary diagram in the lower right representing anions, and a diamond plot (or 'rhomboid') in the middle representing a combination of the two. Note that following a line parallel to the outer axis of each ternary diagram, and projecting

GM-114   CHAPTER 3: ALGEBRA AND GRAPH ANALYSIS

each point in the ternary diagrams upward until they intersect will create one associated point in the diamond plot. These three points represent one sample. For example, for potable groundwater, the sample labelled 'A' in Figure IV.3.9, we can make the following approximations from the combined (diamond) plot: Ca + Mg = 23%; SO$_4$ + Cl = 98%.

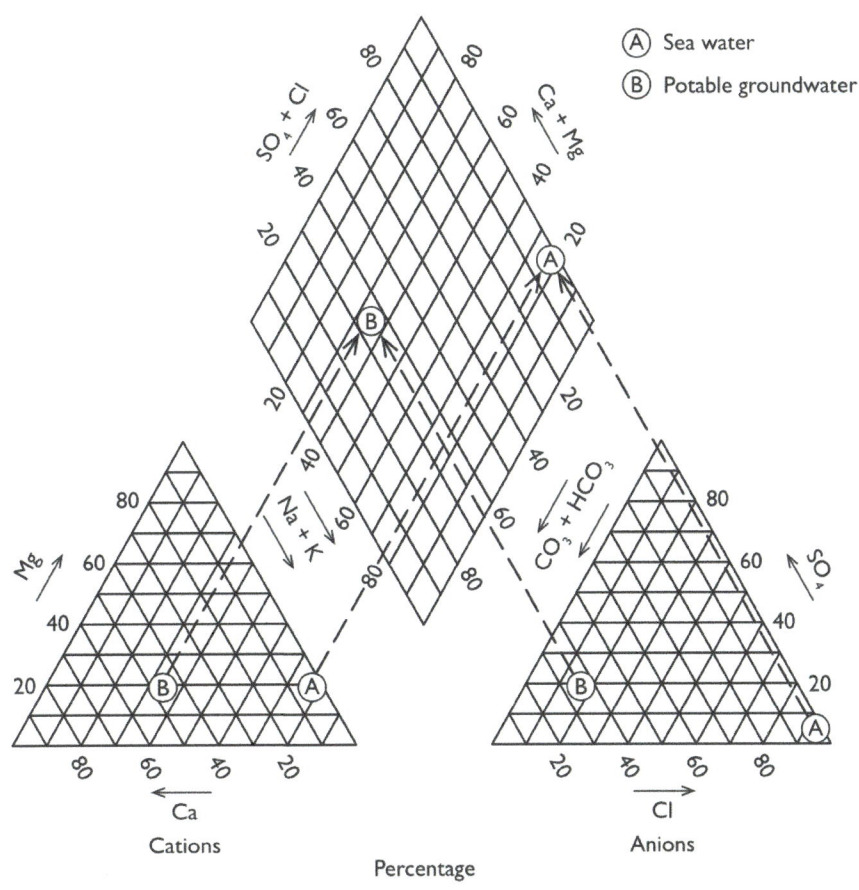

Figure IV.3.9 Chemical analyses of water represented as percentages of total equivalents per litre on the diagram developed by Hill (1940) and Piper (1944).

QUESTION 1

According to Figure IV.3.9, the percent concentration of which of the following is most consistent with the percent concentration of K?

A. Na
B. Mg + Ca
C. 100 − (Mg + Ca + Na)
D. Cannot be determined by the information provided.

QUESTION 2

There are 4 general categories of groundwater based on the dominant ions: 1) Ca-SO$_4$; 2) Ca-HCO$_3$; 3) Na-HCO$_3$; 4) Na-Cl. Using these 4 numbered categories, which of the following is most consistent with sea water and potable groundwater in Figure IV.3.9, respectively?

A. 4, 2
B. 2, 3
C. 1, 1
D. 3, 4

GAMSAT-Prep.com
GOLD STANDARD MATHS

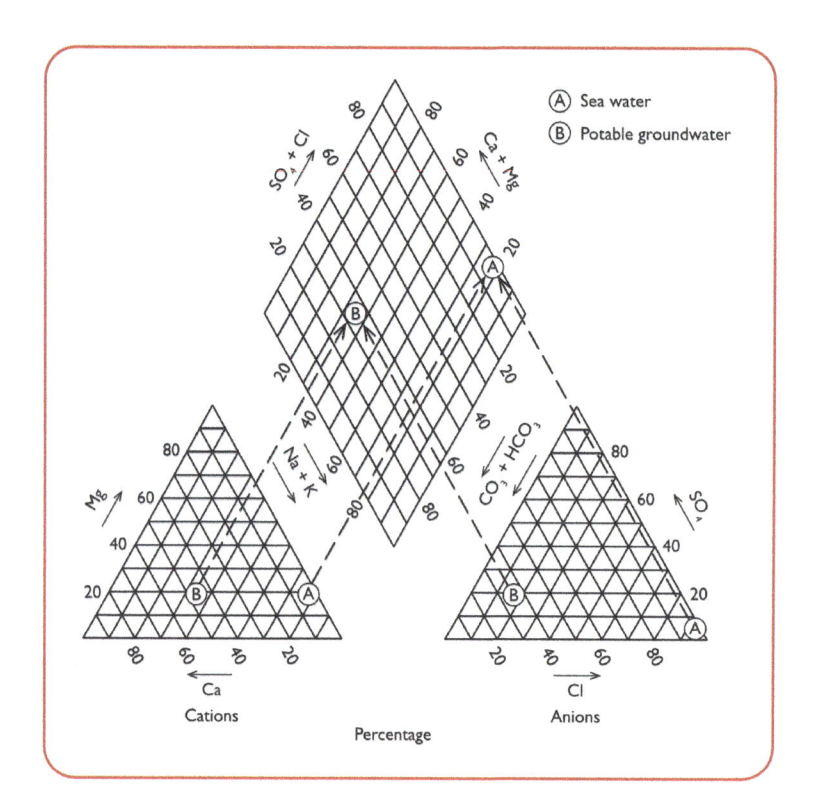

High-level Importance

EXPLANATION 1

If you had trouble reading the ternary graph, consider going back to the scale and examples that we have already seen. Then consider completing the labelling of the diagrams: for example, in the ternary graph in the bottom left of Fig. IV.3.9, write '100% Mg' at the top (that is where it is 100%), write '100% Ca' in the bottom left of the triangle and '100% Na + K' in the bottom right, this may help orient you (of course, additional labelling may not occur on the real exam so you should do it manually if needed).

Side note: notice that the samples labelled A and B have the same concentration of one of the ions! Which one? Consider looking back at the diagram.

We have established a couple of times that the components of the trilinear diagram must add to the maximum value – which is 100% – according to the diagram and caption. So, for the cations we have:

Mg + Ca + Na + K = 100
K = 100 – Mg – Ca – Na
 = 100 – (Mg + Ca + Na)

Thus the correct answer for the first question is C.

For our "Side note" question, samples A and B both have 20% Mg.

EXPLANATION 2

For the second question, the diagram's key indicates that the samples labelled A and B represent sea water and potable

GM-116   CHAPTER 3: ALGEBRA AND GRAPH ANALYSIS

GAMSAT MASTERS SERIES

groundwater, respectively. The diamond plot's dashed lines provide a clear statement: Each sample is composed of both cations and anions. There is no assumed science knowledge.

We are told in the question stem that the categories are based on dominant ions. So, let us determine the balance of ions in each sample and then choose the dominant (foremost) cations and anions.

Using the technique we have practiced:

- From the ternary graph in the bottom left corner, approx. (± 3%): A = Mg: 20%, Ca: 5%, Na + K: 75%; B = Mg: 20%, Ca: 45%, Na + K: 35%.
- From the ternary graph in the bottom right corner, approx. (± 3%): A = SO_4: 5%, Cl: 90%, CO_3 + HCO_3: 5%; B = SO_4: 20%, Cl: 15%, CO_3 + HCO_3: 65%.

Dominant (highest percentage) for A: Na + K and Cl, which resembles category 4 (notice that K – alone – is never dominant among the categories). Dominant (highest percentage) for B: Ca and CO_3 + HCO_3, which resembles category 2 (notice that CO_3 – alone – is never dominant among the categories). Thus the correct answer is A and the other 3 answer choices present at least one of the samples with an ion with minimum concentration thus the process of elimination would also confirm that only one answer is possible.

The following image shows the names of the various ions which we will learn in GS GAMSAT General Chemistry Chapter 5, Solution Chemistry. At that time, you can return to Fig. IV.3.9 and insert the missing superscripts (i.e. the charges for each species) since each component in the diagram is either a positively-charged cation or a negatively-charged anion.

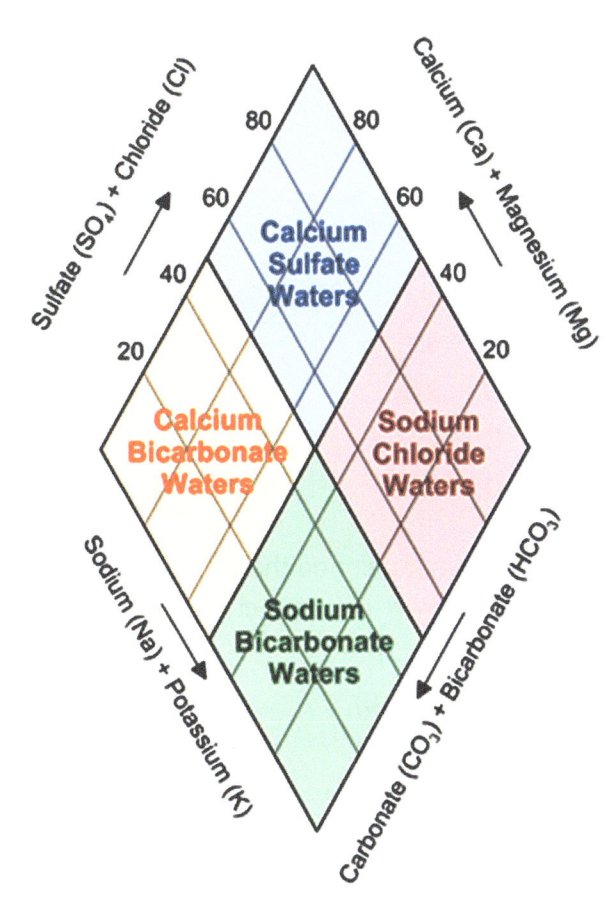

Golden Software LLC Interpretation of the diamond plot (modified from inside.mines.edu/~epoeter/_GW/18WaterChem2/WaterChem2pdf.pdf).

If it is still not clear, you may login to your gamsat-prep.com account, click on Lessons, General Chemistry, Chapter 5: Solution Chemistry, GAMSAT Section 3 PBL: Ions and The Piper Plot; of course, we also have gamsat-prep.com/forum.

GOLD STANDARD WARM-UP EXERCISES

CHAPTER 3: Algebra and Graph Analysis

1. If $y = \dfrac{12}{4x^3 - 6x + 5}$, then if $x = 2$ then y equals:
   A. 12/17
   B. 12/49
   C. 12/9
   D. 12/25

2. $13xy^2z$ is to $39y$ as $9xyz^6$ is to:
   A. $3z^5$
   B. $27z$
   C. $9y$
   D. $27z^5$

3. At what point do the lines $y = 2x - 1$ and $6x - 5y = -3$ intersect?
   A. (2, 3)
   B. (0.5, 0)
   C. (−1,−3)
   D. (−0.5, −2)

4. Loubha has a total of $.85. If she has two less dimes than nickels, how many dimes and nickels does she have? {Note that: One dollar ($1) is composed of 100 cents; a dime is a 10-cent piece and a nickel is a 5-cent piece.}
   A. 5 nickels, 7 dimes
   B. 6 nickels, 4 dimes
   C. 4 nickels, 2 dimes
   D. 7 nickels, 5 dimes

5. If $2.5 \times 10^3 (3 \times 10^x) = 0.075$, then x equals:
   A. −3
   B. −5
   C. 0
   D. −4

6. A plank of wood is leaning against the left side of a house with vertical walls. Both are on level ground. If the plank touches the ground 7 feet away from the base of the house, and touches the house at a point 5 feet above the ground, at what slope is the plank lying?
   A. −5/7
   B. 7/5
   C. −7/5
   D. 5/7

7. If $n + n = k + k + k$ and $n + k = 5$, then $n = ?$
   A. 9
   B. 6
   C. 5
   D. 3

8. Let $x = 4$ and $y = 8$. Evaluate the expression: $((y^{-2/3})^{1/2}) / (x^{-1/2})$.
   A. 8
   B. 4
   C. 1
   D. 1/2

9. Evaluate the expression: $\log_6(24) + \log_6(9)$.
   A. 3
   B. 2
   C. 1
   D. 1/2

10. Solve for x: $\log_{10}(70) = x + \log_{10}(7)$.
    A. 0
    B. 1
    C. 2
    D. 3

11. Simplify the expression: $x(\log_b(y)) + y(\log_b(y))$.

- A. $\log_b(y^{x-y})$
- B. $\log_b(y^{x+y})$
- C. $\log_b(y^{xy})$
- D. $\log_b(xy^{xy})$

12. Evaluate the expression: $\ln(e^3)\log_3(27) + \ln(1)\ln(e)$.

- A. e
- B. 3
- C. 6
- D. 9

13. Which of the following GAMSAT Physics equations would not be expected to represent the graph of a straight line? (note: you do not need to understand any of the equations in order to answer the question)

- A. $F = ma$
- B. $M = mv$
- C. $W = Fd$
- D. $E = \frac{1}{2}mv^2$

14. pH is measured on a logarithmic scale given by the equation $pH = -\log_{10}(H)$. Given that H is positive but less than 1, as H decreases, the slope of the graph of pH vs H:

- A. decreases.
- B. increases.
- C. remains constant.
- D. sometimes decreases, sometimes increases.

15. Consider the following reaction:

$$2A \longrightarrow B$$

The integrated rate law for the preceding reaction is given below, where the rate constant is k_1, the concentration of A at any time t is $[A]$ and at time 0 is $[A]_0$:

$$k_1 t = \ln\frac{[A]_0}{[A]}$$

The following graph illustrates the relationship between the change in concentration and time for the preceding reaction.

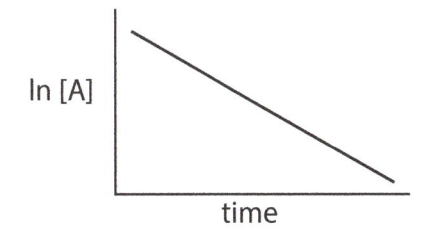

The slope of the line is equal to which of the following?

- A. $-1/k_1$
- B. $-k_1$
- C. $-\ln[A]$
- D. k_1

HINT (upside down if you need it):

Use your log rules for division (GM 3.7.1; as though ln, which is the natural logarithm, is simply any log) then rearrange the equation to look like y = mx + b (notice that ln[A] is y in the graph, and time is x). Why? Because we are given a straight line so we must mold the equation that we are provided into the format of a straight line. If you have not considered this yet, please try the question before looking at the worked solution.

GAMSAT-Prep.com
GOLD STANDARD MATHS

Questions 16–17

In microbiology, a colony-forming unit (CFU) is a unit used to estimate the number of viable bacterial cells in a sample. Consider Figure 1.

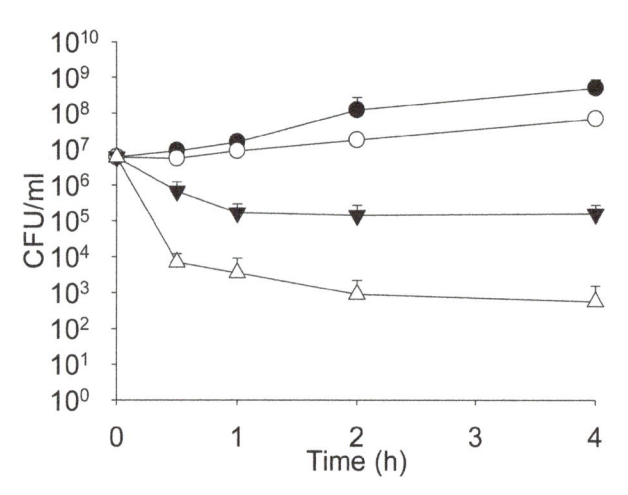

Figure 1: Effect of the control (filled circles), 4 µg imipenem (IMI)/mL (open circles), 8 µg AMP38/mL (filled triangles), and 8 µg AMP38/mL + 4 µg IMI/mL (open triangles) on the bacterium *Pseudomonas aeruginosa* (open source: AIMS Microbiology; doi: 10.3934/microbiol.2018.3.522)

16. According to Figure 1, the largest drop in the number of viable bacterial cells per mL, between 30 minutes into the trial and hour 4, occurs with which of the following trials?

- A. Control
- B. 4 µg IMI/mL
- C. 8 µg AMP38/mL
- D. 8 µg AMP38/mL + 4 µg IMI/mL

17. At hour 4 in Figure 1, the difference in viable bacterial cell numbers per mL between the control trial and the trial with only 8 µg AMP38/mL would be expected to be a number between which of the following ranges?

- A. 1000 – 10 000
- B. 100 000 – 1 000 000
- C. 10 000 000 – 100 000 000
- D. 100 000 000 – 1 000 000 000

18. Consider Figure 1.

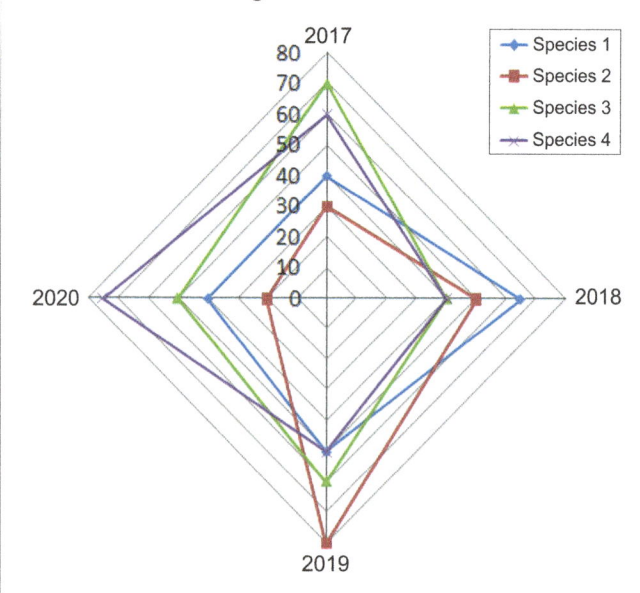

Figure 1: Radar chart displaying the population of 4 bird species in thousands of individuals on an isolated island during a 4-year period. As an example, Species 2 had a population of 40 000 in 2018.

Which bird species shows the maximum change in population numbers from 2017 to 2020?

- A. Species 1
- B. Species 2
- C. Species 3
- D. Species 4

GM-120   CHAPTER 3: ALGEBRA AND GRAPH ANALYSIS

Questions 19–20

19. Sandstone is a classic sedimentary rock composed mainly of sand-sized mineral particles or rock fragments. In Figure 1, the region for sandstone is indicated by shaded areas which demonstrate 5 different forms of sandstone (Fm).

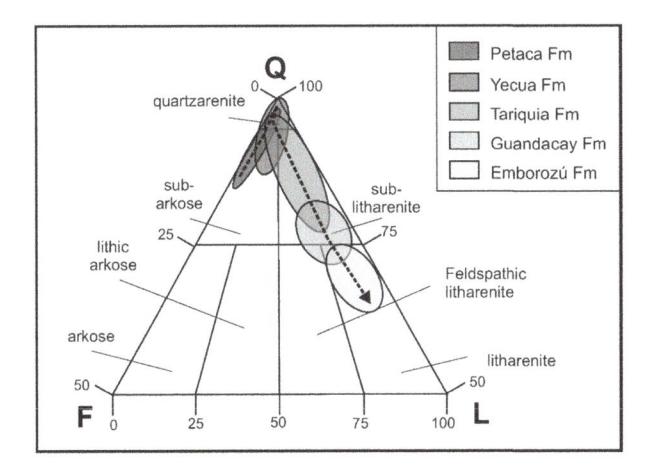

Figure 1: Ternary graph of sandstone showing the percent composition
(Hulka, Uba, Heubeck; Sandstone petrology; 228821091; 2020)

Note that: Q = quartz; F = feldspar; L = lithic.

According to Figure 1, of the 3 components of sandstone, which is least significant?

A. Quartz
B. Feldspar
C. Lithic
D. All of the above are equally present in sandstone.

20. The region indicated in Figure 1 as 'lithic arkose' is what percent lithic?

A. Less than 50%
B. 50-60%
C. 60-70%
D. More than 70%

21. Consider Figure 1.

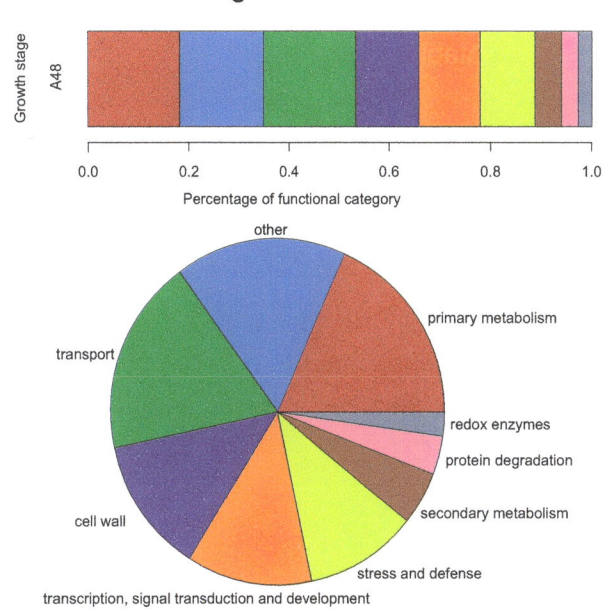

Figure 1: Percentage of major biological processes within differentiated genes (adapted from Horn F. et al, Front. Genet., 2014)

Which biological processes combine to produce the largest percentage of major biological processes for the organism presented in Figure 1?

A. Primary metabolism and protein degradation
B. Redox enzymes and transport
C. Stress, defense and 'other' processes
D. Cell wall and stress and defense

GAMSAT-Prep.com
GOLD STANDARD MATHS

Questions 22–24

To answer the following 3 questions, go back to the last nomogram in section GM 3.9, **Figure IV.3.9: The Piper Plot**.

22. According to Figure IV.3.9, which of the following best approximates the percent concentration of the combination of sodium (Na) and potassium (K) ions in potable groundwater?
    A. 35%
    B. 50%
    C. 65%
    D. 80%

23. According to Figure IV.3.9, which of the following ions is in equal concentration in both sea water and potable groundwater?
    A. Cl
    B. SO$_4$
    C. Na + K
    D. Neither **A**, nor **B**, nor **C**

24. An unknown Sample C was taken that is not shown in Figure IV.3.9 with the following results... Ca: 38%, Cl: 32%, SO$_4$: 59%, Na and K: 35%. Only using information gleaned from this unit, determine the concentration of Mg.
    A. 35%
    B. 27%
    C. 21%
    D. 11%

25. A tephigram is a type of nomogram used for weather analysis and forecasting. Temperatures (Celcius, C, and Absolute, A) are marked on the x-axes, while entropy and potential temperatures (pot temp) are marked along the y-axes. Other features such as pressure are marked as shown.

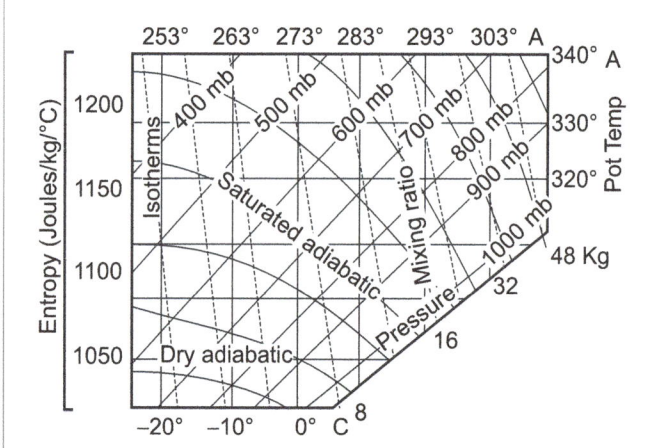

Figure 1: Tephigram. Note that temperature along the bottom x-axis is in degrees Celcius (C) and corresponds precisely and vertically with the absolute temperature (A; these are isothermal lines). For example, 0 °C corresponds to 273 on the absolute (A) temperature scale. Entropy, along the left-most y-axis, runs horizontally. (Redrawn from aviation_dictionary.enacademic.com/6690/tephigram)

According to Figure 1, if the entropy is 1150 Joules/kg/°C and the pressure is 800 mb, the expected temperature in degrees Celcius would be in the range of which of the following?
    A. 0-10
    B. 10-20
    C. 20-30
    D. 30-40

High-level Importance

Chapter 3 Worked Solutions

Question 1   D
See: GM 3.1.4
Substitute 2 for *x* in the function:

$$y = \frac{12}{4(2)^3 - 6(2) + 5}$$
$$= \frac{12}{4(8) - 12 + 5}$$
$$= \frac{12}{32 - 12 + 5} = \frac{12}{25}$$

Question 2   D
See: GM 3.3.2, 3.3.3
Create a ratio with the first two values and simplify:

$$\frac{13xy^2z}{39y} = \frac{xyz}{3}$$

The unknown ratio must also be equal to this value. Let *k* represent the variable and cross-multiply:

$$\frac{9xyz^6}{k} = \frac{xyz}{3}$$
$$3(9xyz^6) = (xyz)k$$
$$\frac{27xyz^6}{xyz} = k$$
$$27z^5 = k$$

Question 3   A
See: GM 3.4.2A, 3.4.2B
Substitute the first equation into the second, replacing *y*:

$$6x - 5y = -3$$
$$6x - 5(2x - 1) = -3$$
$$6x - 10x + 5 = -3$$
$$-4x + 5 = -3$$
$$-4x = -8$$
$$x = 2$$

Substitute this value back into either equation to find y:

$$y = 2x - 1$$
$$y = 2(2) - 1$$
$$y = 3$$

Question 4   D
See: GM 3.4.2B
We will need to write equations that correspond to the sentences. Let *d* represent the number of dimes, and *n* represent the number of nickels. Since there are two less dimes than nickels,

$$d = n - 2.$$

The amount of money a group of coins is worth is equal to the value of the coins times the number of coins. The total value of Loubha's nickels is $0.05n$ and the total value of her dimes is $0.10d$. These add up to all of the money she has:

$$\$0.05n + \$0.10d = \$0.85.$$

Substitute the first equation into the second for *n*:

$$\$0.05n + \$0.10(n - 2) = \$0.85$$
$$\$0.05n + \$0.10n - \$0.20 = \$0.85$$
$$\$0.15n = \$0.85 + \$0.20$$
$$\$0.15n = \$1.05$$

$$n = \$1.05 / \$0.15$$
$$n = 7$$

There are 7 nickels. We can plug this into either of the two original equations, but the first is easiest to use:

$$d = n - 2$$
$$d = 7 - 2$$
$$d = 5$$

NOTE: In this particular problem, the fastest way is to just try the different answers until one fits the requirements. We have shown the work in case it was a different question type then you would still know the approach.

GAMSAT-Prep.com
GOLD STANDARD MATHS

Question 5   B
See: GM 3.3.1
Simplify the expression:

$$(2.5 \times 10^3)(3 \times 10^x) = 0.075$$
$$(2.5 \times 3)(10^3 \times 10^x) = 0.075$$
$$(7.5)(10^{3+x}) = 0.075$$

Divide both sides of the equation 7.5, or simply note that 0.075 is one–hundredth $\left(\frac{1}{100}\right) = 10^{-2}$ of 7.5:

$$10^{3+x} = 10^{-2}$$
$$3 + x = -2$$
$$x = -5$$

Question 6   D
See: GM 3.5.4
If we think of the plank as a straight line in a coordinate system, we can use the points at which its ends are located to find its slope. The origin can be anywhere we choose, and the base of the house's left wall is a good choice. This point of the house must be located at (0, 0), and so the base of the plank, 7 feet to the left, is located at (−7, 0). The point at which the plank touches the left wall is 5 feet above the origin, at (0, 5). The slope of the plank is therefore

$$m = \frac{0-5}{-7-0} = \frac{-5}{-7} = \frac{5}{7}$$

Question 7   D
See: GM 3.3.1, 3.4.2A, 3.4.2B
It is given that $2n = 3k$, which implies that $\frac{2}{3}n = k$. $n + k = 5$ can therefore be rewritten:

$$n + \frac{2}{3}n = 5$$
$$\frac{5}{3}n = 5$$
$$n = 3$$

Question 8   C
See: GM 1.5
First combine the exponents where possible, and rearrange so they are all positive:

$$((y^{-2/3})^{1/2}) / (x^{-1/2})$$
$$= (y^{-1/3}) / (x^{-1/2})$$
$$= (x^{1/2}) / (y^{1/3})$$

Now plug in x=4 and y=8. Notice that $4=2^2$ and $8=2^3$.

$$= (4^{1/2}) / (8^{1/3})$$
$$= (2^{(2)1/2}) / (2^{(3)1/3})$$
$$= 2^1/2^1$$
$$= 1.$$

Question 9   A
See: GM 3.7
When adding logarithms of the same base, combine them by multiplying the numbers in parentheses (note: an asterisk - or dot • - can be used as a multiplication symbol). In this case:

$$\log_6(24) + \log_6(9)$$
$$= \log_6(24*9)$$
$$= \log_6(216)$$
$$= \log_6(6^3)$$

Now remember, a logarithm is an exponent. The question it poses is, "the base raised to what power is equal to the number in the parentheses?" So 6 raised to what power is equal to 6^3? The answer is, of course, 3.

Question 10   B
See: GM 3.7
First isolate the x terms on one side and all other terms on the other side of the equation.

$$\log_{10}(70) = x + \log_{10}(7)$$
$$\log_{10}(70) - \log_{10}(7) = x$$

Now combine the logarithms. When subtracting logarithms of the same base, combine them by dividing the numbers in parentheses.

$$\log_{10}(70/7) = x$$
$$\log_{10}(10) = x$$
$$1 = x.$$

Question 11   B

See: GM 1.5, 3.7
A coefficient multiplied by a logarithm can by brought inside the parentheses as an exponent.

$x(\log_b(y)) + y(\log_b(y))$
$= \log_b(y^x) + \log_b(y^y)$
$= \log_b(y^x y^y)$
$= \log_b(y^{x+y})$.

Question 12   D

See: GM 1.5, 3.7
The natural log has base e. Note that a logarithm of 1, no matter what the base, is equal to 0. And a log of its own base is equal to 1. So:

$\ln(e^3)\log_3(27) + \ln(1)\ln(e)$
$= \ln(e^3)\log_3(27) + 0*1$
$= 3\log_3(27)$
$= 3(3)$
$= 9$.

Question 13   D

See: GM 3.3, 3.4
We will learn about all of these equations in the GAMSAT Physics chapters, A: Newton's 2nd Law; B: Momentum; C: Work; D: Kinetic energy. From a maths standpoint, y = mx + b is the equation of a straight line. Notice that b can equal 0, meaning that the line intersects at the point (0, 0), and so y can be equal to mx. Answer choices A, B and C have the same format as y = mx. Answer choice D has a variable raised to the power of 2 which is not consistent with the format: y = mx + b. Identifying whether or not an equation could produce a straight line is an important GAMSAT skill.

Spelling out some examples: A graph of F vs a, has m as a slope. A graph of W vs d, has F as a slope. A graph of E vs v would be an exponential curve (GM 3.8; notice the word 'exponent' in exponential!).

Question 14   B

See: GM 3.7, 3.8
A standard graph is y vs x, so if we are looking for pH vs H, then pH is y and H is x. Given pH = $-\log_{10}(H)$, and H is positive but below 1… well, let's try a couple of numbers that would make our calculation as easy as possible. Of course, the log of 1 is 0 so that would be our first point: (1, 0). Let's say H went down from 1 to 1/10 (10^{-1}), then the pH = $-\log_{10}(10^{-1}) = \log_{10}(10) = 1$ (from GM 3.7.1, log rules 1 and 2). So, pH went from 0 to 1. Let's try decreasing H again: from 1/10 to 1/100, thus pH goes from 1 to 2, thereby the trend of increasing. Now we can see that the smaller H becomes, the larger pH will always become (between 0 and 1).

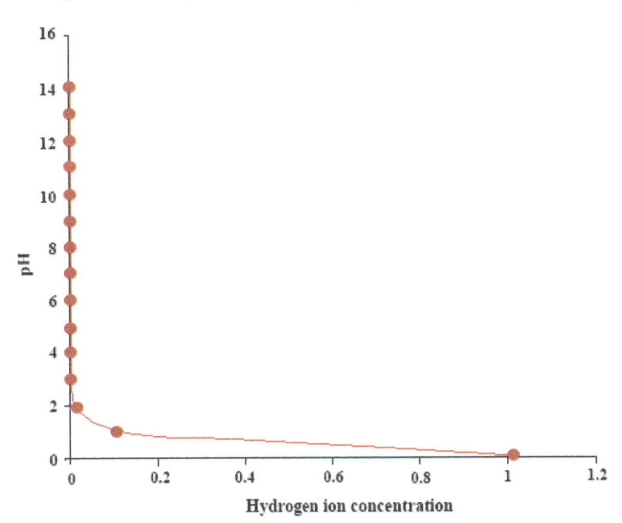

Question 15   B

See: GM 3.3, 3.4, 3.7
We start with the equation that we are given: $k_1 t = \ln[A]_0/[A]$

Apply the rule of logarithms: $\log x/y = \log x - \log y$

$k_1 t = \ln[A]_0 - \ln[A]$

Rearrange so that y, ln [A], is alone on the left and everything else is on the right:

$\ln[A] = -k_1 t + \ln[A]_0$

which is the equation of a straight line:

y = mx + b

where the graph is ln [A] vs *t* with a negative slope (meaning the line is going down from left to right) of constant $-k_1$ and the y-intercept (b) would be $\ln[A]_0$.

Question 16   C

See: GM 3.7
The caption below the figure identifies the symbols with labels. Answer choices A and B are clearly rising during

the time period mentioned in the question so we are really only considering C and D. Visually, it seems that D is decreasing a bit more than C during the period of ½ hour to 4 hours. But, the y-axis scale is clearly not linear, it is exponential. C begins around 1 000 000 and goes to around 100 000, which is a reduction of an incredible 900 000. D (at 30 minutes) starts at a paltry 10 000 and finishes 1000 which is a reduction of just 9 000. Answer choice C wins by an incredible amount. If you did not consider the exponential scale, try answering the next question again before looking at the solution.

Question 17 D

See: GM 1.5, 3.7

The trial with 8 µg AMP38/mL (dark triangles) at hour 4 seems to line up with approximately 100 000 (which is 10 to the power of 5). At hour 4, control (dark circles) seems to line up between 1 000 000 000 and 100 000 000. The answer choices are so incredibly wide apart, it does not matter which of the two you choose. Keep in mind that 100 000, as a difference, does not impact the control which is, literally, orders of magnitude greater:

$$\frac{1\,000\,000\,000 - 100\,000}{}$$

is approximately 1 000 000 000

Don't make the mistake of treating subtraction in the same way that you would division.

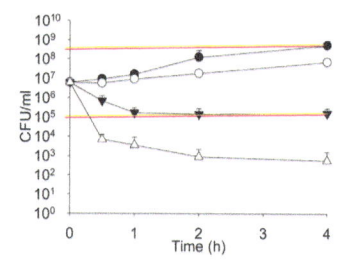

Question 18 C

See: GM 3.9

On the Surface: The increments are linear (0, 10, 20, etc., nothing exponential) and there are 4 axes for the 4 different years. We just need to identify, from 2017 to 2020 (only look at the upper left of Figure 1), which line crosses the most space between lines: Green, Species 3, answer C.

Note that ACER often, but does not always, provide an example as to how to read a graph before asking questions. For this question, you were given a strong hint in the caption. You can see that Species 2 is the small red square on a grey line. Now you need to think: How does that point near 2018 give me 40 000? Now just look for a way to get to 40 and you notice that the increments of 10 are for all directions along the grey lines, and the caption states "in thousands."

Going Deeper: Radar charts (AKA, web chart, spider chart, star plot, polar chart) can show up in Section 1 or Section 3. Just read it as though you have 4 different x-axes. Notice where 0 must be for each direction, then 10 and so on. From 2017 to 2020, write down on your scratch paper the values in thousands for each species: answer choice A: 30 to 30 (notice how 'blue' just stays on the 30 line in the top left of Figure 1); B: 20 to 10; C: 60 to 40; D: 50 to 65. Clearly the biggest change is the 20 000 drop in population for Species 3, answer C.

Other questions that could have been asked? 1) Biggest percent change: B (a whopping 50% decrease!); Largest decrease: C; Largest increase: D.

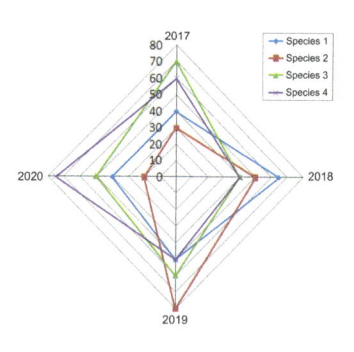

Question 19 B

See: GM 3.9

The top is labelled Q so that is where the maximum Quartz must be, thus 100%, and you must read the downward sloping line on the right ranging from 100 Q to 50 Q. L is maximum at the bottom right thus 100% L going down to 0% L horizontally to the left ("x-axis" for L). F is maximum at the bottom left and its top value is only 50% and goes down to zero with the left uphill axis. F starts lower than the others. Additionally, by looking at the shaded areas, all 5 types of sandstone have significantly less than 15% feldspar which is the lowest percentage of the 3 components.

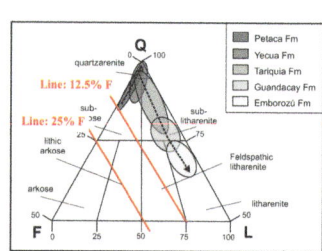

GAMSAT MASTERS SERIES

Question 20   A

See: GM 3.9

Once you are comfortable reading ternary graphs, it is clear that the region described is less than 50%. If not clear, consider revising Chapter 3. You can also watch Dr. Ferdinand read ternary graphs from an older edition of the book by going to the Gold Standard GAMSAT YouTube Channel, Pink Booklet Worked Solutions, Questions 14–17. Note that in the image, from the perspective of L, lithic arkose is completely below 50%.

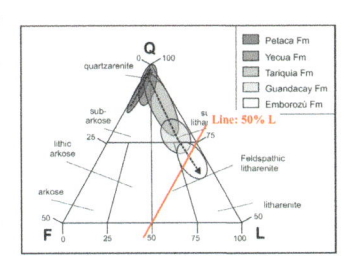

Question 21   C

See: GM 3, deduce

If you are skilled at noticing differences, since there is no log scale, you can find the answer visually. Notice that answer choices C and D both have 'stress and defense' so you only have to compare: other vs cell wall, and other is visually bigger.

If not visually, this question requires discipline and patience. Don't worry if you made +/– 10% approximations, your answers would be the same. Estimate based on the legend (key), keeping in mind that all of the processes, according to the legend, add up to 1 (the components of the pie chart add up to 100%):

primary metabolism: 0.18	A. 0.21
redox enzymes: 0.03 (a little less?)	B. 0.22
protein degradation: 0.03	C. 0.27
secondary metabolism: 0.05	D. 0.23
transport: 0.19	
stress and defense: 0.10	
other processes: 0.17	
cell wall: 0.13	

Question 22   A

See: GM 3.9

This is basically an orientation question to test if you can read a ternary diagram (keep your focus on the triangle in the bottom left because we are asked about Na + K). If you cannot, please go through the step-by-step instructions in GM 3.9, Nomograms. If you trace the dashed line to B to the Na + K axis, it hits approx. 35% (perhaps closer to 33%!).

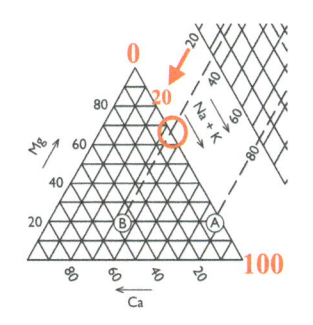

Question 23   D

See: GM 3.9

From Figure 1, both A and B have equal concentrations of Mg and for no other ion(s). A and B sit on the same line for Mg only. Note that in the EXPLANATION 1 for the Piper Plot in GM 3.9, we concluded that samples A and B each have 20% Mg.

Question 24   B

See: GM 3.9

Recognise that the 3 sides of the ternary plot form a triangle that has a maximum of 100%, so this is the total for the 3 components. So, [Mg] = 100% – [Na + K] – [Ca] = 100% – 73% = 27%. There is no need to try to graph the point in this question.

Question 25   C

See: GM 3.9

There is a fair chance that you will see a graph that you had never imagined on the real exam! Let's start with the information we are given in this 'unit': Entropy represents horizontal lines which means that the value of 1150 can be traced horizontally to see what it meets. Next, pressure? We are not told anything specific, but, similar to carbon dioxide in the GM 3.9 nomogram, Fig. IV.3.7, we can see the label for Pressure on the graph which suggests that lines which are oblique (*slanting*) and have a number ending with mb represent the pressure.

OK, so we can make a point with the entropy of 1150 and the pressure of 800 mb (oblique line). We are told that straight vertical lines have the same temperature (isotherms) so we follow that line up and see a number just above 293. Well, let's follow that number straight down and it looks like it is around 16, but we have a problem: the direction and labelling seems to have changed. Before temperature was increasing by 10 and now by 16, at an angle, and ending with 48 Kg, which is NOT temperature!

GAMSAT MATHS   GM-127

GAMSAT-Prep.com
GOLD STANDARD MATHS

High-level Importance

Now we need to reason that from 253 to 273, the absolute temperature clearly followed Celcius by increments of 10 (linear, no logs). If 273 is 0, then 283 must be 10, 293 must be 20, and thus the point represents 20-30 degrees Celcius. You will be seeing many more nomograms across the GS universe of materials.

Side note: The absolute (A) scale actually refers to the (big K) Kelvin scale, and 0 °C is indeed 273 K, but (small k) kelvin is not technically regarded as degrees. We will explore this more in CHM 7.4.

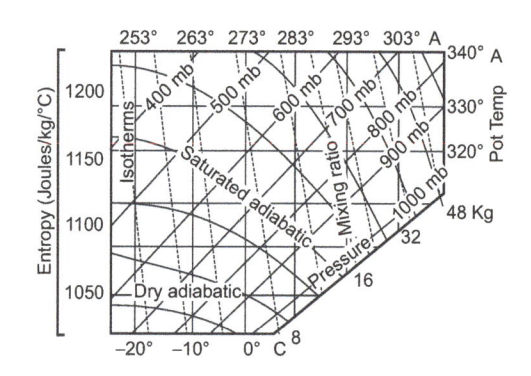

Dear GAMSAT Maths,

Please stop asking me to find your x.

She's not coming back and I don't know y either.

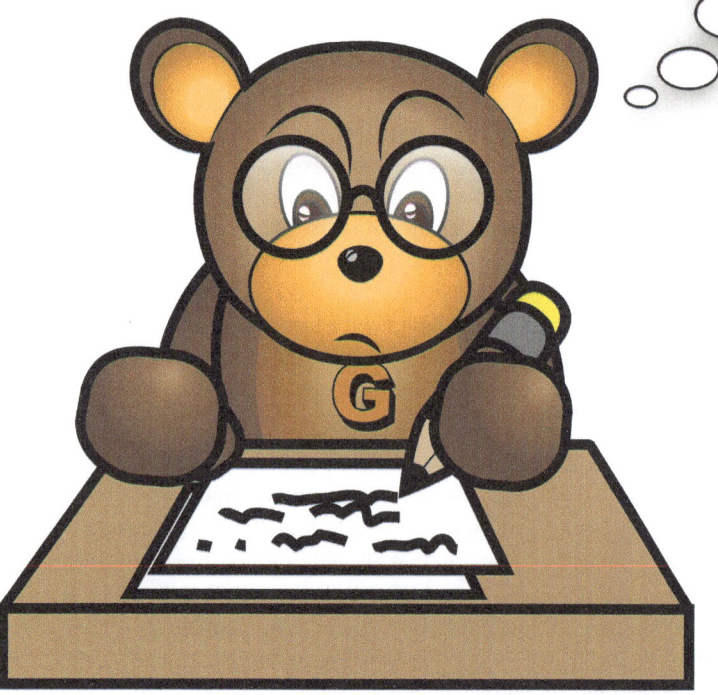

NOTE

As a rule, we do not recommend reading Masters Series chapters multiple times. It is best to read once, take brief notes, and then study using your notes on a regular basis moving forward. However, these first 3 GAMSAT Maths chapters are exceptional. We do suggest the same note-taking process but, also, we think that 1-2 weeks before the real exam, you should come back to briefly revise these chapters.

CHAPTER 3: ALGEBRA AND GRAPH ANALYSIS

GAMSAT MASTERS SERIES

SPOILER ALERT ⚠️

Gold Standard has cross-referenced the content in this chapter to examples from ACER's official GAMSAT practice materials. It is for you to decide when you want to explore these questions since you may want to preserve some of ACER's materials for timed mock-exam practice.

Examples – Area under the curve: Q32-35 of 2; ternary graph: Q14-17 of 5; nomogram: Q67-68 of 5; logs: Q33-34, Q55, Q73-75, Q104-107 of 4, Q8-10 and Q109-110 of 5; histogram: Q1-4 of 2; Q85-88 of 4, Q61-65 of 5. Note that "Q" is followed by the question number, and, for example, "of 1" refers to booklet number 1 which is referenced in the Spoiler Alert table at the end of Chapter 1. The 10 full-length HEAPS GAMSAT practice tests (by Gold Standard and MediRed), exams 1 through 10, contain specific cross-references to this chapter within the worked solutions. Note that there are over a hundred graphs in the HEAPS book and the online portion (which now comes with digital exams with the new GAMSAT formatting). The GAMSAT Physics chapters of the book that you are using has many awesome graphs including the beautiful nomogram at the end of Chapter 3. Physics Chapter 8 has audiogram-based questions along the lines of GM 3.8, Figure IV.3.6. Both Chemistry Chapter 5 and Biology Chapter 11 have multiple questions based on ternary graphs, as do several HEAPS exams. You will find histograms in this chapter and throughout our materials including a 3D histogram in Biology Chapter 14.

High-level Importance

Chapter Checklist

- ☐ Reassess your 'learning objectives' for this chapter: Go back to the first page of this chapter and re-evaluate the top 3 boxes and the Introduction.
    - ☐ Please be sure that you have completed the *Need for Speed* exercises at the beginning of this chapter.
- ☐ Complete a maximum of 1 page of notes using symbols/abbreviations to represent the entire chapter based on your learning objectives. These are your Gold Notes.
- ☐ Consider your multimedia options based on your optimal way of learning:
    - ☐ Download the free Gold Standard GAMSAT app for your Android device or iPhone.
    - ☐ Create your own, tangible study cards or try the free app: Anki.
    - ☐ Record your voice reading your Gold Notes onto your smartphone (MP3s) and listen during exercise, transportation, etc.
    - ☐ Try out the Gold Standard GAMSAT Physics online videos at gamsat-prep.com which have heaps of calculations, or you can try other maths options on YouTube like Khan Academy or Leah4sciMCAT playlist for Maths Without a Calculator (the latter was produced for MCAT preparation but it remains helpful for GAMSAT).
- ☐ Reassess your schedule for your full-length GAMSAT practice tests: ACER and/or HEAPS exams. Ensure that you have scheduled one full day to complete a practice test and 1-2 days for a thorough assessment of worked solutions while adding to your abbreviated Gold Notes.
- ☐ Reassess your progress in scheduling and/or evaluating stress reduction techniques such as regular exercise (sports), yoga, meditation and/or mindfulness exercises (*see* YouTube for suggestions).

High-level Importance

GOLD NOTES

GEOMETRY
Chapter 4

Memorise
* The Pythagorean Theorem
* Perimeter, Area, and Volume Formulas
* Properties of Triangles

Understand
* Points in Cartesian Coordinates
* Parallel and Perpendicular Lines
* Similar Polygons
* Types of Triangles and Angles

Importance
Medium level: 7% of GAMSAT Section 3 maths-based questions released by ACER are related to content in this chapter (in our estimation).
* Note that approximately 90% of such questions are related to just 3 chapters: 1, 2, and 3.

GAMSAT-Prep.com

Introduction

Geometry is a very visual branch of mathematics dealing with lines and shapes and relations in space, so drawing and labelling pictures can be extremely helpful when you are confronted with certain GAMSAT Physics problems. But don't forget about algebra! More often than not, these problems are simply algebraic equations in disguise.

Past questions have shown that ACER expects that you know the area of a triangle and rectangle, the volume of a block, and the Pythagorean Theorem. Anything else that you want to learn/revise in this chapter is because you have a strong background in science and you want to prepare for unlikely questions, or that you want to improve spatial awareness.

Additional Resources

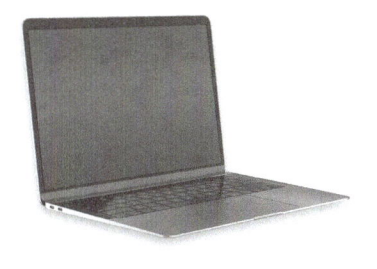

Open Discussion Boards

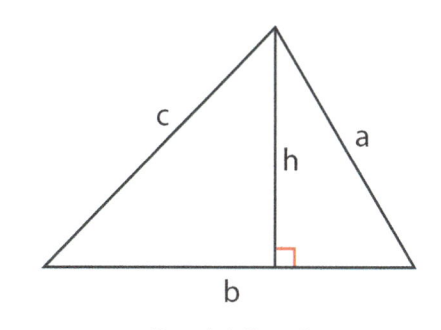

Special Guest

GAMSAT MATHS GM-131

> # GAMSAT-Prep.com
> # GOLD STANDARD MATHS

> **4.1 Points, Lines and Angles**

> **4.1.1 Points and Distance**

Knowing your way around the Cartesian coordinate systems begins with understanding the relationships between simple points. As discussed in section 3.5, points on a graph are represented as an ordered pair of an *x* and *y* coordinate, (x, y).

A. Addition and Subtraction of Points

To add or subtract two points, simply add or subtract the two *x* values to obtain the new *x* value and add or subtract the two *y* values to obtain the new *y* value.

EXAMPLE

Add the points (2, 3) and (1, -5).

$$(2, 3) + (1, -5)$$
$$= (2 + 1, 3 - 5)$$
$$= (3, -2)$$

Graphically, addition of points is easy to visualise. All you are doing when you add two points is treating the first point as the new origin. You then plot the second point in terms of this new origin to find the sum of the two points.

You can add more than two points in the same way. Just add all of the *x* values together, and then add all of the *y* values together.

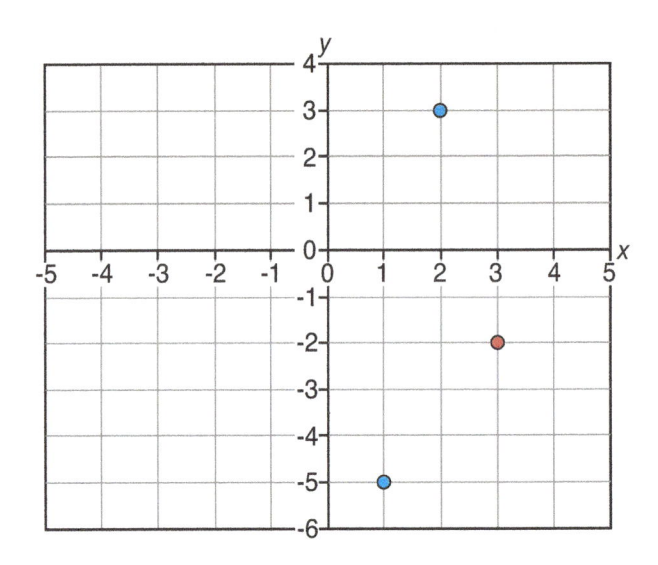

B. Distance between Points

Finding the distance between two points requires the use of the Pythagorean Theorem. This theorem is probably the most important tool you have for solving geometric problems.

> **Pythagorean Theorem:** $x^2 + y^2 = z^2$

This theorem describes the relationship between the lengths of the sides of a right triangle. The lengths *x* and *y* correspond to the two legs of the triangle adjacent to the right angle, and the length *z* corresponds to the hypotenuse of the triangle.

Medium-level Importance

In order to find the distance between two points (x_1, y_1) and (x_2, y_2), consider there to be a line segment connecting them. This line segment (with length z equivalent to the distance between the points) can be thought of as the hypotenuse of a right triangle. The other two sides extend from the points: One is parallel to the x-axis; the other, to the y-axis (with lengths x and y, respectively).

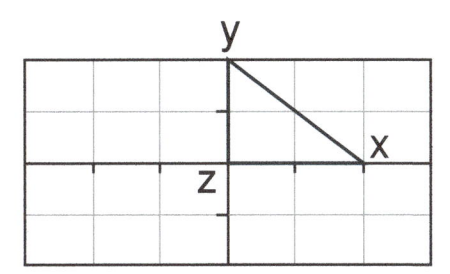

$$x = (x_2 - x_1)$$
$$y = (y_2 - y_1)$$
$$z = \sqrt{(x^2 + y^2)}$$

Plugging in the point coordinates will yield z, the distance between the two points.

EXAMPLE

Find the distance between the points (5, 0) and (2, -4).

$$x = (2 - 5) = -3$$
$$y = (-4 - 0) = -4$$
$$z = \sqrt{(-3^2 + -4^2)}$$
$$= \sqrt{(9 + 16)} = \sqrt{25} = 5$$

So the distance between the points is z = 5.

To find the distance between the two points, simply apply the Pythagorean Theorem.

4.1.2 Line Segments

A. Segmentation Problems

These problems are a kind of geometry-algebra hybrid. You are given a line segment that has been subdivided into smaller segments, and some information is provided. You are then asked to deduce some of the missing information.

In a segmentation problem, some of the information you are given may be geometric, and some may be algebraic. There is not, however, a clear algebraic equation to solve. You will need to logically determine the steps needed to reach a solution.

EXAMPLE

The line segment QT of length $4x + 6$ is shown in the figure that follows. Point S is the midpoint of QT and segment RS has length x – 1. What is the length of line segment QR?

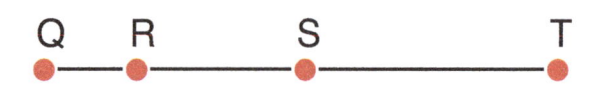

Q   R   S   T

First, determine what information you know. The length of QT and RS are given. Also, since we have a midpoint for QT, the length of QS and ST are simply half of the length of QT.

Now, determine an algebraic relationship regarding the length of QR, which is what we are looking for. We can see that the length of QR is simply QS with the RS segment removed.

$$QR = QS - RS$$

Plugging in our information, we get the following:

$$QR = \frac{(4x+6)}{2} - (x-1)$$
$$= 2x + 3 - x + 1$$
$$= x + 4$$

Before you start working out a solution, it can be extremely helpful to list the information you are given. This will help you understand and organise the problem, both in your own mind and on the page.

B. Segments in the Plane

In segmentation problems, you only have to deal with one dimension. However, line segments can also turn up in problems dealing with a two dimensional Cartesian graph.

To determine the length of a line segment in a plane, simply find the distance between its endpoints using the Pythagorean Theorem (GM 4.1.1).

Any line segment in a plane corresponds to a single linear equation. This can be determined from any two points on the line segment (GM 3.4.3, 3.4.4). Knowing this linear equation can help you find other points on the line segment.

4.1.3 Angles

An **angle** is formed by the intersection of two lines.

In problems that are not trigonometric, angles are almost always measured in degrees. A full circle makes 360°.

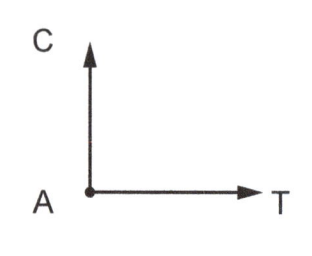

A **right angle** is an angle that is exactly 90° (sometimes symbolised with a small square in the angle: GM 4.2.1, 4.2.2, 4.2.4).

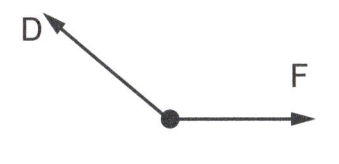

An **obtuse angle** is an angle that is greater than 90°.

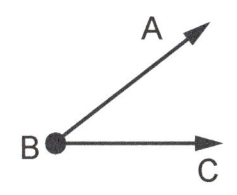

An **acute angle** is an angle that is less than 90°.

A **straight angle** is an angle that is exactly 180°.

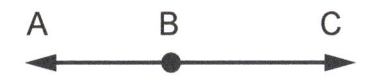

A **vertical angle** is the angle opposite of each other that is formed by two intersecting lines. The two angles across from each other are equal in measure. The following example shows that angles 1 and 3 are vertical angles and equal to each other. Same are angles 2 and 4. At the same time, adjacent vertical angles 1 and 4 or 2 and 3 are also supplementary angles and will form 180°.

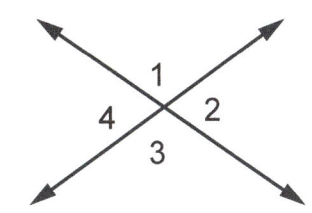

Complementary angles are two angles that add up to 90°. The example that follows shows that angles A and B add up to 90°.

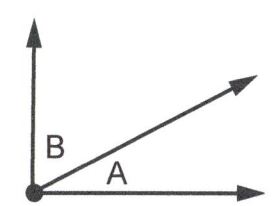

Supplementary angles are two angles that add up to 180°. This example shows that angles A and B add up to 180°.

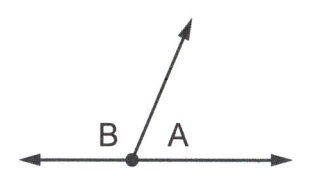

A. Angles and Lines in the Plane

If two lines are **parallel**, they have the same slope. Such lines will never intersect, and so they will never form angles with one another.

If two lines are **perpendicular**, their intersection forms only 90° angles. If the slope of a given line is a/b, then the slope of any perpendicular line is $-b/a$.

EXAMPLE

Consider the line defined by $y = 2x + 3$.

(a) Give the equation for a parallel line:

$$y = 2x + 2.$$

Any line that still has a slope of 2 will suffice. So, in slope-intercept form, any line of the form $y = 2x + a$ will be a parallel line.

GAMSAT-Prep.com
GOLD STANDARD MATHS

(b) Give the equation for the perpendicular line that intersects the given line at the *y*-axis.

In this case, there is only one solution since the line can only intersect the *y*-axis once. The solution will be a line with the same *y*-intercept (which is 3) and the negative reciprocal slope (which is -½): rule from GM 3.4.4.

$$y = -\frac{1}{2}x + 3$$

The standard kind of angle-line problem deals with a setup of two parallel lines that are cut by a transversal, like the one in the following diagram (this type of geometry may present in Physics Chapter 11: Light and Geometric Optics).

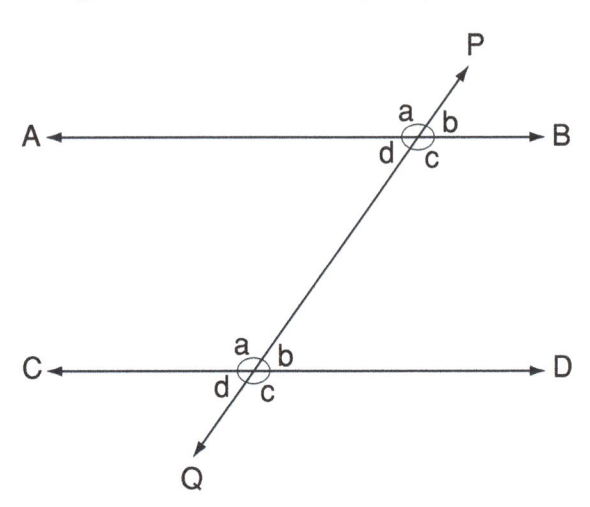

The trick with these problems is to realise that there are only ever two values for the angles.

First, think of the two areas of intersection as exact duplicates of each other.

The upper left angles are equivalent, as are the upper right, the lower left, and the lower right. Using just this information, you automatically know the value of the twin of any angle that is given to you.

Also, angles that are opposite each other are equivalent. So the lower left angle is the same as the upper right and vice versa.

The other fact you can use to determine unknown angles is that the angle along a straight line is 180°. When you are given an angle *a*, you can find supplement *b* by subtracting 180° - *a*.

EXAMPLE

In the figure that follows, if angle *a* is 35°, what is the value of angle *b*?

Angle *b* is the twin of the supplement of *a*, so *b* is equal to 180° - *a*.

$$b = 180° - 35° = 145°$$

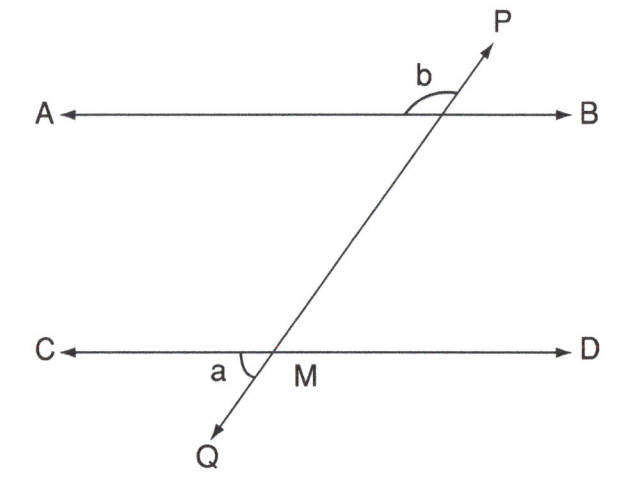

GM-136 CHAPTER 4: GEOMETRY

B. Properties of Parallel Line Angles

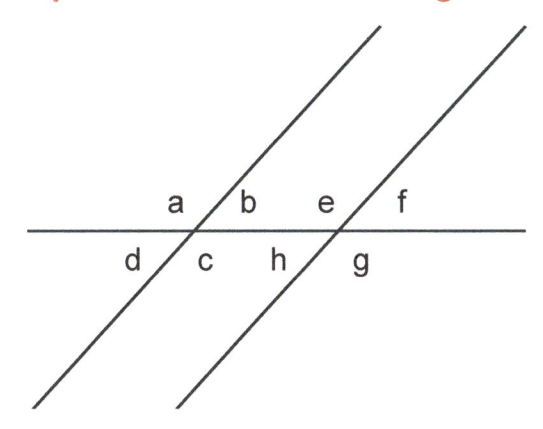

When two parallel lines are cut by a transversal line:

1. both pairs of acute angles as well as obtuse angles are equal: $a = e$, $b = f$, $d = h$, $c = g$.
2. alternate interior angles are equal in measure as well: $c = e$, $b = h$.

C. Interior Angles of a Polygon

Sometimes you may be dealing with a shape that you are not familiar with and that you do not know the total of all interior angles. A polygon is a flat (i.e. plane) figure with at least three straight sides and angles. If the polygon has x sides, the sum, S, is the total of all interior angles for that polygon. For a polygon with x sides, the sum may be calculated by the following formula:

$$S = (x - 2)(180°)$$

EXAMPLE

A triangle has 3 sides, therefore,

$S = (3 - 2) \times 180°$
$S = 180°$

A rectangle has 4 sides,

$S = (4 - 2) \times 180°$
$S = 360°$.

Given the total angles for a polygon, you can determine each interior angle of a polygon by dividing the sum of the polygon by the number of sides.

EXAMPLE

A rectangle has a sum of 360°. Given that $x = 4$, $360° \div 4 = 90°$. Therefore, each angle in a rectangle is 90°.

> **NOTE**
>
> Though not common, these question types are usually related to projectile motion, inclined planes and optics which will be explored in Physics.

GAMSAT MATHS

GAMSAT-Prep.com
GOLD STANDARD MATHS

4.2 2D Figures

Make sure you know how to find the area, perimeter, side lengths, and angles of all the figures in this section. There are all kinds of ways to combine different shapes into the same problem; but if you can deal with them all individually, you'll be able to break down any problem thrown your way!

4.2.1 Rectangles and Squares

A **rectangle** is a figure with four straight sides and four right angles. In rectangles, opposite sides always have the same length, as do the two diagonals that can be drawn from corner to corner.

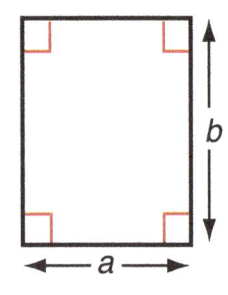

Perimeter: The perimeter of a rectangle is equal to the sum of its sides.

Perimeter = $a + b + a + b = 2a + 2b$

Area: The area of a rectangle is equal to the product of its length and width.

Area = Length × Width = $a \times b$

A **square** is a rectangle with all four sides of the same length, so $a = b$.

The perimeter of a square is

$P = a + a + a + a = 4a$.

The area of a square is

$A = a \times a = a^2$.

4.2.2 Types of Triangles

While there are a wide variety of types of triangles, every one shares these properties:

(i) The sum of the interior angles of a triangle is always equal to 180°. In the following figure, a, b, and c are interior angles.

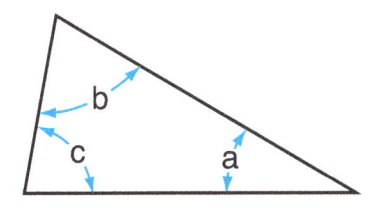

(ii) The sum of the exterior angles of a triangle is always equal to 360°. The following figure shows *d*, *e*, and *f* to be exterior angles.

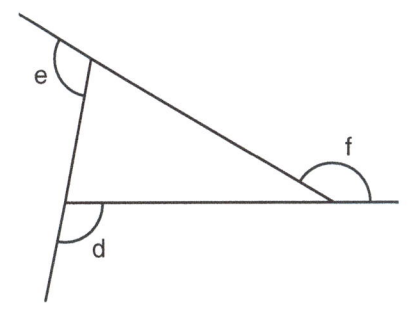

(iii) The value of an exterior angle is equal to the sum of the opposite two interior angles.

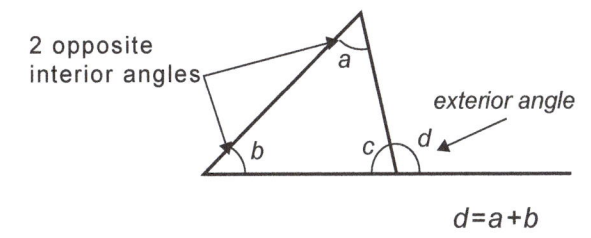

d = a + b

EXAMPLE

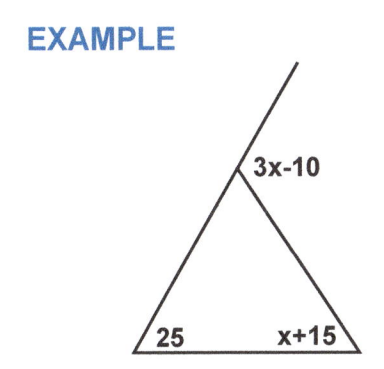

$3x - 10 = 25 + x + 15$
$2x = 10 + 25 + 15$
$2x = 50$
$x = 25$

(iv) The perimeter of a triangle is equal to the sum of its sides.

(v) The area of a triangle is always half the product of the base and the height.

$$\text{Area} = \frac{1}{2} \text{ Base} \times \text{Height}$$

You can pick any side of the triangle to function as the base, and the height will be the line perpendicular to that side that runs between it and the opposite vertex (i.e. highest point).

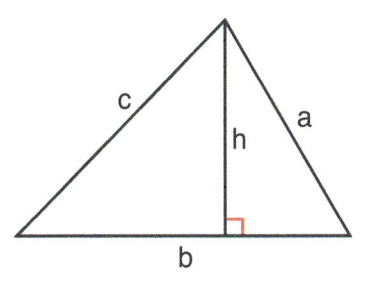

NOTE

If you ever see a triangular shaped graph during the GAMSAT, check the units of one axis multiplied by the other. If the units match the answer choices of any of the questions then you are likely 1/2 way to getting the correct answer without even having read the question yet! As an example, *see* the 2nd question and the 2nd graph (blue shaded area) in GM 3.5.4.

GAMSAT MATHS GM-139

Medium-level Importance

GAMSAT-Prep.com
GOLD STANDARD MATHS

A. Right Triangles

A **right triangle** is a triangle that contains a right angle. The other two angles in a right triangle add up to 90°.

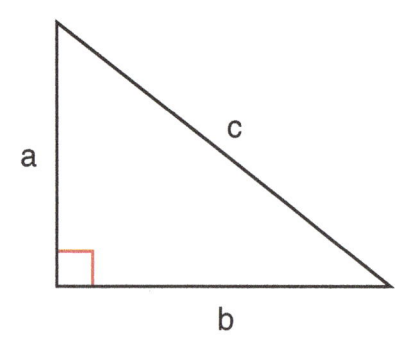

The two short legs of a right triangle (the legs that come together to form the right angle) and the hypotenuse (the side opposite the right angle) are related by the Pythagorean Theorem:

$$a^2 + b^2 = c^2$$

To find a missing side of the triangle, plug the values you have into the Pythagorean Theorem and solve algebraically.

The two legs of a right triangle are its base and height. So to find the area, compute as shown.

NOTE

The area of a triangle, the Pythagorean Theorem and its special ratios appear regularly on the real GAMSAT.

$$\text{Area} = \frac{1}{2}(a \times b)$$

Special Cases: There are a few cases of right triangles you should know. First, the ratios of side lengths 3:4:5 and 5:12:13 are often used. Identifying that a triangle corresponds to one of these cases can save you precious time since you will not have to solve the Pythagorean Theorem.

There are also two special ratios of interior angles for right triangles: 30°-60°-90° and 45°-45°-90°. The sides of a 30°-60°-90° triangle have the ratio $1:\sqrt{3}:2$ and the sides of a 45°-45°-90° triangle have the ratio $1:1:\sqrt{2}$ (ACER would normally provide all of the preceding values if they are needed).

B. Isosceles Triangles

An **isosceles triangle** is a triangle that has two equal sides. The angles that sit opposite the equal sides are also equal.

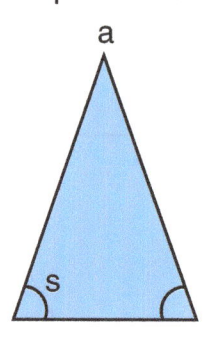

For an isosceles triangle, use the odd side as the base and draw the height line to the odd vertex. This line will bisect the side, so it is simple to determine the height using the Pythagorean Theorem on one of the new right triangles formed.

Medium-level Importance

GM-140   CHAPTER 4: GEOMETRY

> **NOTE**
>
> **Pythagorean Theorem**
>
> Knowing any two sides of a right triangle lets you find the third side by using the Pythagorean formula: $a^2 + b^2 = c^2$.
>
> 3-4-5 triangle: if a right triangle has two legs with a ratio of 3:4, or a leg to a hypotenuse ratio of either 3:5 or 4:5, then it is a 3-4-5 triangle.
>
> 5-12-13 triangle: if a right triangle has two legs with a ratio of 5:12, or a leg to a hypotenuse ratio of either 5:13 or 12:13, then it is a 5-12-13 triangle.
>
> 45°-45°-90° triangle: if a right triangle has two angles that are both 45°, then the ratio of the three legs is $1:1:\sqrt{2}$.
>
> 30°-60°-90° triangle: if a right triangle has two angles of 30° and 60°, then the ratio of the three legs is $1:\sqrt{3}:2$.
>
> Confirm for yourself that the ratio of sides in the 4 preceding triangles actually fulfill the Pythagorean Theorem.

C. Equilateral Triangles

An **equilateral triangle** is a triangle with all three sides equal. All three interior angles are also equal, so they are all 60°.

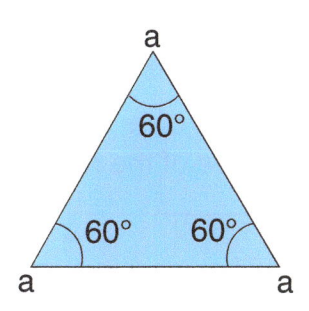

Drawing a height line from any vertex will divide the triangle into two 30°-60°-90° triangles, so you can easily solve for the area.

D. Scalene Triangles

A **scalene triangle** is any triangle that has no equal sides and no equal angles. To find the value for the height of this kind of triangle requires the use of trigonometric functions (*see* Chapter 5).

E. Similar Triangles

Two triangles are **similar** if they have the same values for interior angles. This means that ratios of corresponding sides will be equal. Similar triangles are triangles with the same shape that are scaled to different sizes.

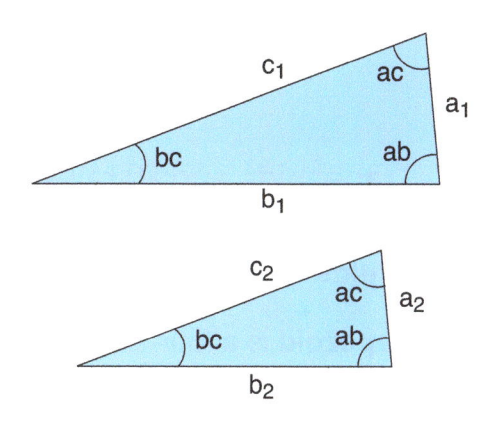

GAMSAT-Prep.com
GOLD STANDARD MATHS

To solve for values in a triangle from information given about a similar triangle, you will need to use ratios. The ratios of corresponding sides are always equal, for example $\frac{a_1}{a_2} = \frac{b_1}{b_2}$. Also, the ratio of two sides in the same triangle is equal to the corresponding ratio in the similar triangle, for example $\frac{a_1}{b_1} = \frac{a_2}{b_2}$.

4.2.3 Circles

A **circle** is a figure in which every point is the same distance from the center. This distance from the center to the edge is known as the **radius** (*r*). The length of any straight line drawn from a point on the circle, through the center, and out to another point on the circle is known as the **diameter** (*d*). The diameter is twice the radius.

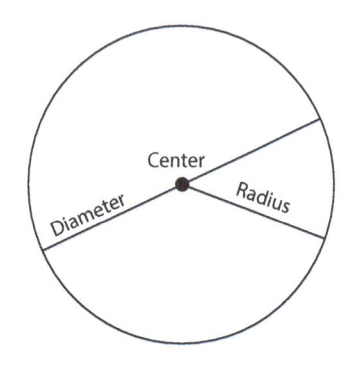

$$d = 2 \times r \quad \text{or} \quad r = \frac{1}{2}d$$

There are no angles in a circle.

Circumference: The circumference of a circle is the total distance around a circle. It is equal to pi times the diameter.

$$\text{Circumference} = \pi \times d = 2\pi \times r$$

Area: The area of a circle is equal to pi times the square of the radius.

$$\text{Area} = \pi \times r^2 = \frac{1}{4}\pi \times d^2$$

4.2.4 Trapezoids and Parallelograms

A. Trapezoids

A **trapezoid** is a four-sided figure with one pair of parallel sides and one pair of non-parallel sides.

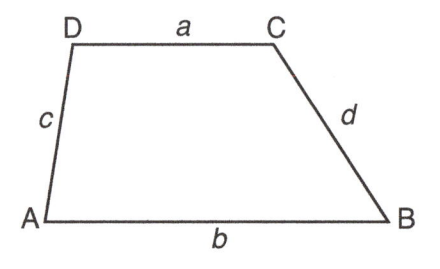

Medium-level Importance

GM-142   CHAPTER 4: GEOMETRY

Usually the easiest way to solve trapezoid problems is to drop vertical lines down from the vertices on the smaller of the two parallel lines. This splits the figure into two right triangles on the ends and a rectangle in the middle. Then, to find information about the trapezoid, you can solve for the information (side length, area, angles, etc.) of these other shapes.

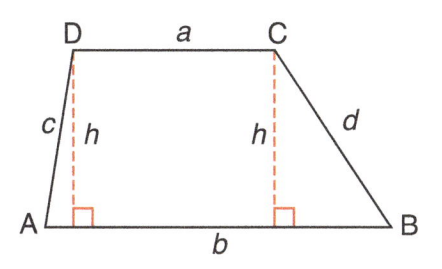

> **NOTE**
>
> "Really, will the GAMSAT ever specifically ask for the area of a trapezoid?" No! But they may occasionally present a graph that is shaped like a trapezoid and the question requires you to calculate the area under the graph or 'curve' (i.e. the area of the trapezoid).

1. The area of a trapezoid is calculated as

$$\frac{a+b}{2}h$$

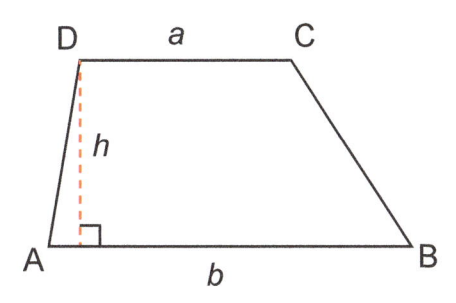

2. The upper and lower base angles are supplementary angles (i.e., they add up to 180°).

   Angle A + Angle D = 180°
   Angle B + Angle C = 180°

Sometimes it can be useful to draw a line from vertex to vertex and construct a triangle that way, but this usually only makes sense if the resulting triangle is special (i.e. isosceles).

Isosceles Trapezoids: Just like isosceles triangles, **isosceles trapezoids** are trapezoids with two equal sides. The sides that are equal are the parallel sides that form angles with the base of the trapezoid. Similarly, if the left and right sides are of the same lengths, these angles are the same as well.

In this isosceles trapezoid, ABCD means that Angle A = Angle B, Angle D = Angle C, and Diagonal AC = Diagonal BD.

The perimeter = $a + b + 2c$

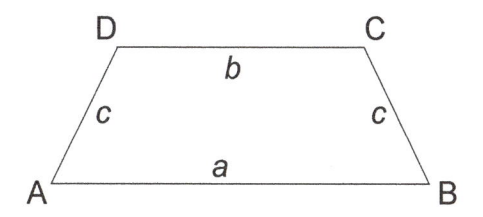

GAMSAT-Prep.com
GOLD STANDARD MATHS

B. Parallelograms

A **parallelogram** is a quadrilateral that has two sets of parallel sides. A square, for example, is a special kind of parallelogram, as is a rhombus (which has four sides of equal length but, unlike a square, has two different pairs of angle values).

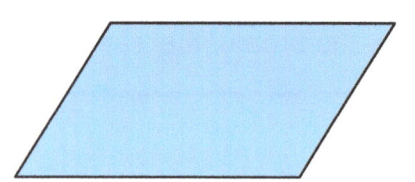

Area: The area of a parallelogram is simply the base times the height.

$$\text{Area} = (\text{Base}) \times (\text{Height})$$

The height of a parallelogram can be found by dropping a vertical from a vertex to the opposite side and evaluating the resulting right triangle.

The sum of all the angles in a parallelogram is 360°. Opposite angles are equivalent, and adjacent angles add up to 180°.

4.3 3D Solids

In three dimensions, it does not always make sense to talk about perimeters. Shapes with defined edges (such as boxes and pyramids) still have them, but rounded shapes (such as spheres) do not. Instead, we are generally concerned with the values of surface area and volume.

4.3.1 Boxes

Boxes are the three-dimensional extension of rectangles. Every angle in a box is 90°, and every box has six rectangular faces, twelve edges, and eight vertices. Opposite (and parallel) faces are always of the same length, height, and width, as are opposite (and parallel) edges. ==None of the equations in these sections (4.3.1, 4.3.2, 4.3.3) should be memorised. Hopefully, most of the equations will make sense to you in some way.==

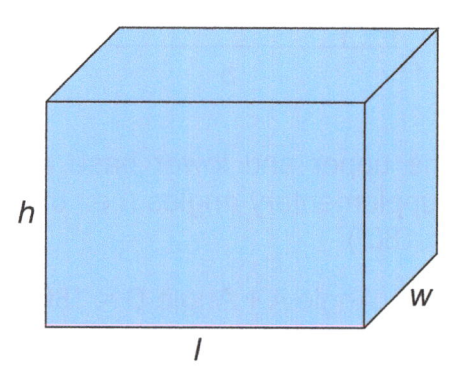

Perimeter: The perimeter of a box is the sum of its edges. There are, however,

GM-144 CHAPTER 4: GEOMETRY

only three different lengths and four edges corresponding to each one. So to find the perimeter, we can simply take the sum of four times each the width, length, and height.

Perimeter = $4l + 4w + 4h = 4(l + w + h)$

Surface Area: The surface area of a box is the sum of the area of each of its faces. Since there is one duplicate of each unique face, we only need to find three products, double them, and add them together.

Surface Area = $2lw + 2wh + 2lh$
            = $2(lw + wh + lh)$

Volume: Calculating the volume of a box can be visualised as taking the surface of any of its rectangular faces and dragging it through space, like you were blowing a box-shaped bubble. So you start with the product of a width times a height, and then you multiply that by a length.

Volume = $l \times w \times h$

4.3.2 Spheres

The definition of a sphere is basically identical to that of a circle, except that it is applied in three dimensions rather than two: It is a collection of points in three dimensions that are all of the same distance from a particular center point. Again, we call this distance the radius, and twice the radius is the diameter. A sphere has no vertices or edges, so it has no circumference.

Surface Area: Surface Area = $4\pi \times r^2$

Volume: Volume = $(4/3)\pi \times r^3$

4.3.3 Cylinders

Spheres may be the 3D equivalent of circles, but if you start with a circle and extend it into the third dimension, you obtain the tube shape known as a cylinder. Cylinders have two parallel circular faces, and their edges are connected by a smooth, edgeless surface.

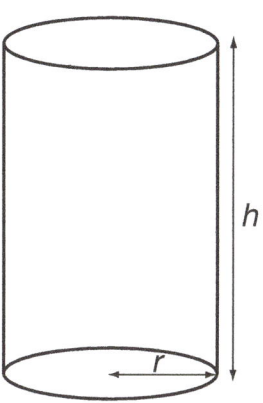

GAMSAT-Prep.com
GOLD STANDARD MATHS

Surface Area: The surface area of a cylinder is composed of three parts: The two circular faces and the connecting portion. To find the total area of a cylinder, add the areas of these two parts. We already know how to calculate area for circles; and for the connecting surface, all we need to do is extend the circumference of one of the circles into three dimensions. So, multiply the circumference by the height of the cylinder.

$$\text{Surface Area} = 2(\pi \times r^2) + (2\pi \times r) \times h$$

Volume: The volume of a cylinder is equal to the area of one of its bases (circle) multiplied by the height.

$$\text{Volume} = (\pi \times r^2) \times h$$

NOTE

Notice that a cylinder approximates a pipe (Physics) or a small part of a blood vessel (Biology).

GOLD STANDARD WARM-UP EXERCISES
CHAPTER 4: Geometry

Medium-level Importance

1. The area of a circle is 144π. What is its circumference?

   A. 6π
   B. 24π
   C. 72π
   D. 12π

2. The points (2,–3) and (2,5) are the endpoints of a diameter of a circle. What is the radius of the circle?

   A. 64
   B. 4π
   C. 8
   D. 4

3. A and B are similar 45°–45°–90° triangles. If B has an area of 12 square metres, and A has three times the area of B, what is the length of A's hypotenuse?

   A. $\sqrt{72}$ m
   B. 36 m
   C. 72 m
   D. 12 m

4. Leslie drives from Highway 1 to the parallel Highway 2 using the road that crosses them, as in the given figure below. Leslie misses the turn onto Highway 1 at point Q and drives 2 km further, to point P. Driving in a straight line from point P to get back to Highway 1, how much further will Leslie travel? (open-book question)

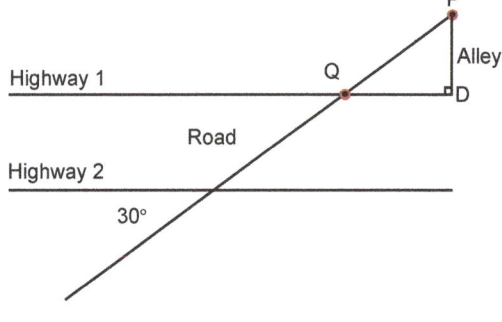

   A. 1/2 km
   B. $\sqrt{3}$ km
   C. 1 km
   D. 2 km

GM-146 CHAPTER 4: GEOMETRY

5. A circle is inscribed in a square with a diagonal of length 5. What is the area of the circle?

A. $\dfrac{25}{8}\pi$ C. $\dfrac{25}{16}\pi$

B. $\dfrac{25}{2}\pi$ D. $\dfrac{25}{4}\pi$

6. A circle is drawn inside a larger circle so that they have the same center. If the smaller circle has 25% the area of the larger circle, which of the following is the ratio of the radius of the small circle to that of the larger circle?

A. $\dfrac{1}{8}$ C. $\dfrac{1}{4}$

B. $\dfrac{3}{4}$ D. $\dfrac{1}{2}$

7. Consider a box with length l, width w and height h, if the thickness of the cardboard is t, how much empty space is inside this cardboard box?

A. $l \times w \times h$
B. $(l - t) \times (w - t) \times (h - t)$
C. $(l + t) \times (w + t) \times (h + t)$
D. $(l - 2t) \times (w - 2t) \times (h - 2t)$

8. What is the measure of the missing length?

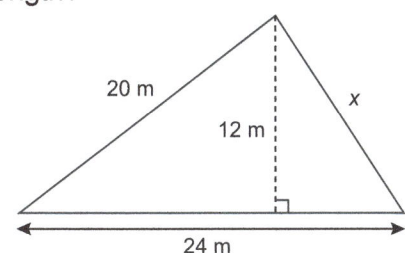

A. 7 m   C. 14 m
B. 10 m   D. 17 m

9. How high is the height h as measured along the wall from the ground to the end of the ladder against the building?

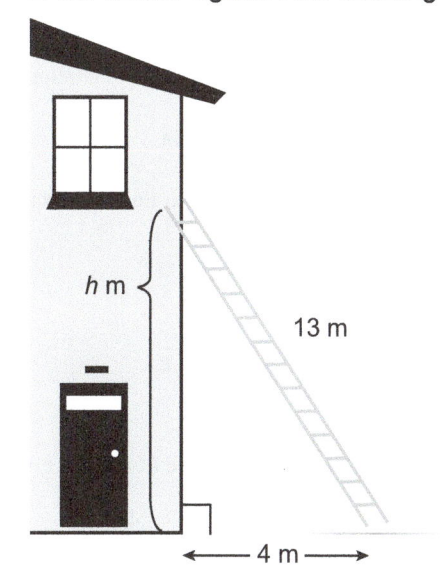

A. $4^2 + h^2 = 13^2$; 12.4 m
B. $4^2 + 13^2 = h^2$; 12.7 m
C. $4^2 + h^2 = 13^2$; 10.6 m
D. $4^2 + h^2 = 13^2$; 14.4 m

10. A square is connected to a triangle below. What is the measure of the hypotenuse of the triangle?

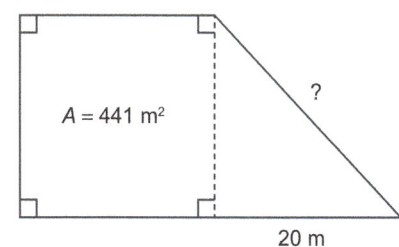

A. 21 m   C. 35 m
B. 29 m   D. 40 m

CHAPTER 4 WORKED SOLUTIONS

Question 1   B
See: GM 4.2, 4.2.3
Using the given information to write an equation, we have:

$$\pi r^2 = 144\pi$$

We need the value of the radius to find the circumference, so we solve for r:

$$r^2 = \frac{144\pi}{\pi}$$
$$r = \sqrt{144}$$
$$r = 12$$

The formula for the circumference of a circle gives us:

$$2\pi r = 2\pi(12) = 24\pi$$

Question 2   D
See: GM 4.2, 4.2.3
The length of the radius is half of the length of the diameter, which is

$$d = \sqrt{(2-2)^2 + (-3-5)^2} = \sqrt{0+64} = 8$$

units long. The radius is therefore equal to 4.

Question 3   D
See: GM 4.2, 4.2.2
Triangle A has an area of $\frac{bh}{2} = 3(12m^2) = 36m^2$ which means that its base times its height is equal to 72 square feet. The base and height of all 45°–45°–90° triangles are the same, so $(b \times h)/2 = (b \times b)/2 = 36$. Solving for b gives us $b = \sqrt{72}$. Using the Pythagorean Theorem, we can solve for the hypotenuse.

$h^2 = (\sqrt{72})^2 + (\sqrt{72})^2 = 144$, therefore $h = \sqrt{144} = 12$.

Question 4   C
See: GM 4.1, 4.1.3

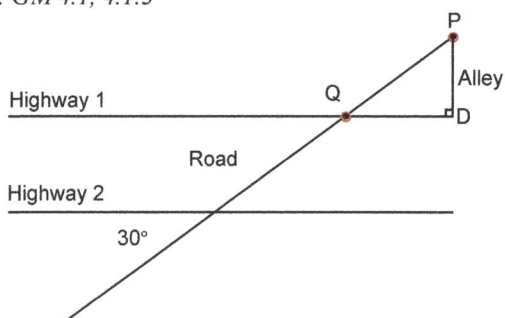

The angle PQD has a measure equal to that of the given angle, 30 degrees, because the highways are parallel and the road forms a transversal across them. The hypotenuse of the right triangle PQD is 2 km long, and the alley, which forms the leg of the triangle that is opposite angle PQD, has a length of

$$(2 \text{ km}) \sin(30°) = 1 \text{ km}$$

Don't worry if you did not know or remember how to solve a problem with the sine function. As long as you understand the set up for the solution, that's fine for now. We will discuss trigonometric functions in the next GAMSAT Maths chapter and again in Physics Chapter 1.

Question 5   A
See: GM 4.2, 4.2.1, 4.2.3
The relationship between the length of a side s and the length of the diagonal d of a square is (i.e. because the diagonal cuts the square into 45–45–90 triangles and remembering the ratio of that triangle's sides):

$$d = s\sqrt{2}$$

The length of a side of the given square is therefore

$$s = \frac{d}{\sqrt{2}} = \frac{5}{\sqrt{2}}$$

This is always the length of the diagonal of the inscribed circle, which has a radius of length $\frac{5}{\sqrt{2}} \div 2 = \frac{5}{2\sqrt{2}}$.

The area of the circle is therefore

$$\pi \left(\frac{5}{2\sqrt{2}}\right)^2 = \frac{25\pi}{8}$$

Question 6   D
See: GM 4.2, 4.2.3

Represent the areas of the large and small circle by πr_L^2 and πr_S^2, respectively. 25% is equivalent to $\frac{1}{4}$, so

$$\pi r_S^2 = \frac{1}{4}(\pi r_L^2)$$

$$r_S^2 = \frac{1}{4} r_L^2$$

$$\sqrt{r_S^2} = \sqrt{\frac{1}{4} r_L^2}$$

$$r_S = \frac{1}{2} r_L$$

and the ratio of the radii is $\frac{r_S}{r_L} = \frac{\frac{1}{2} r_L}{r_L} = \frac{1}{2}$.

Question 7   D
See: GM 4.3.1; deduce

Because it is cube-like, we need to multiply 3 different sides together in order to get the volume. Consider that if you were to just multiply the 3 sides together, you would get a volume which includes the actual cardboard (i.e. calculating the volume that way would get a result which is somewhat greater than the actual volume INSIDE the box). However, if we were to examine the length for example, the space available inside the box would be less than the length of the box because of the thickness at BOTH ends.

Thus the inside measurements are reduced by the thickness of each side:

- The inside length will be l – 2t
- The inside width will be w – 2t
- The inside height will be h – 2t

Thus the space (volume) inside the box = (l – 2t) × (w – 2t) × (h – 2t)

This style of reasoning including the development of an equation (during the exam!) that you have never seen before is a common though infrequent part of the real GAMSAT.

Note: Answer choice A is a reasonable approximation but answer choice D is the best answer among the choice provided. Part of the challenge of multiple choice exams is getting in the habit of identifying the best among options.

Question 8   C
See: GM 4.1.1, 4.2.2

There are several triangles! At the far right, we have the hypotenuse x of a little triangle. We know its height (12 m) but we do not yet know the length of its small base. But, we have the hypotenuse (20 m) of the triangle to the left and its height (12 m). Let's use Pythagoras to calculate the base of the triangle on the left:

$20^2 = 12^2 + b^2$
$400 = 144 + b^2$
$400 - 144 = b^2$
$256 = b^2$
$16 = b$

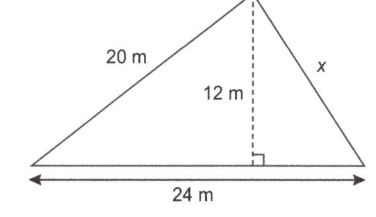

and since the biggest base is 24 m, that means 24 – 16 = the smallest base at 8 m. Now we know 2 sides of the smallest triangle so let's get the hypotenuse x:

$x^2 = 8^2 + 12^2 = 64 + 144 = 208$

The square root of 196 is 14, and the square root of 225 is 15 (GM 1.5.6), so the answer must be just over 14, answer choice C.

GAMSAT-Prep.com
GOLD STANDARD MATHS

Question 9   D

See: GM 4.1.1, 4.2.2

The image is that of a right angle triangle where we know the hypotenuse (the side opposite the right angle, 13) and one side (4) so it is easy to calculate:

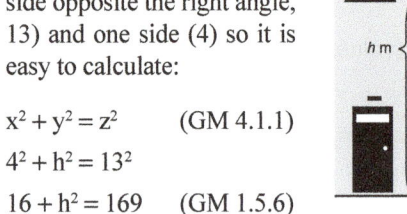

$x^2 + y^2 = z^2$ (GM 4.1.1)

$4^2 + h^2 = 13^2$

$16 + h^2 = 169$ (GM 1.5.6)

$h^2 = 169 - 16 = 153$

So we need the square root of 153 which must be a number between 12 (squared is 144) and 13 (squared is 169), and so the answer is A. Note that you should know the squares of numbers from 1 to 15 (GM 1.5.6).

Question 10   B

See: GM 4.1.1, 4.1.2

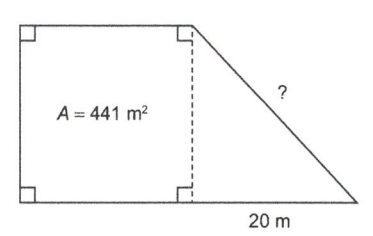

We want the hypotenuse but we only have one side of the triangle (20 m). We can get the height of the triangle by changing the area of the square into length. Area is one side times the other, so we can take the square root of 441 to get length in m. $20 \times 20 = 400$, let's try 21×21 = bingo, 441.

So, we have a triangle with 20 m and 21 m as sides and we need the hypotenuse.

$c^2 = 20^2 + 21^2 = 400 + 441 = 841$

c is equal to a number just below 30 (since $30 \times 30 = 900$), and the closest number is 29 (of course you can double check that 29 x 29 is indeed 841).

Medium-level Importance

GM-150   CHAPTER 4: GEOMETRY

GAMSAT MASTERS SERIES

> **SPOILER ALERT** ⚠️
>
> Gold Standard has cross-referenced the content in this chapter to examples from ACER's official GAMSAT practice materials. It is for you to decide when you want to explore these questions since you may want to preserve some of ACER's materials for timed mock-exam practice.
>
> **Examples** – Triangle: Q32-33 of 2; Q89-90 of 4; Pythagoras and the triangle: Q44-47 of 2; volume of a block Q99 of 3 and Q29-32 of 4. Note that "Q" is followed by the question number, and, for example, "of 1" refers to booklet number 1 which is referenced in the Spoiler Alert table at the end of Chapter 1. The 10 full-length HEAPS GAMSAT practice tests (by Gold Standard and MediRed), exams 1 through 10, contain specific cross-references to this chapter within the worked solutions. Note that the HEAPS exams have geometry in the expected measure for the average, real exam. Note that in this book, we used a triangle for the area under a curve in GM 3.5.4, and we will do it again in Physics Chapter 1; circles in circular motion, Physics Chapter 3; the volume of a block, Physics Chapter 6.

Chapter Checklist

- [ ] Reassess your 'learning objectives' for this chapter: Go back to the first page of this chapter and re-evaluate the top 3 boxes and the Introduction.

- [ ] Complete a maximum of 1 page of notes using symbols/abbreviations to represent the entire chapter based on your learning objectives. These are your Gold Notes.

- [ ] Consider your multimedia options based on your optimal way of learning:
    - [ ] Download the free Gold Standard GAMSAT app for your Android device or iPhone.
    - [ ] Create your own, tangible study cards or try the free app: Anki.
    - [ ] Record your voice reading your Gold Notes onto your smartphone (MP3s) and listen during exercise, transportation, etc.
    - [ ] Try out the Gold Standard GAMSAT Physics online videos at gamsat-prep.com which have heaps of calculations, or you can try other maths options on YouTube like Khan Academy or Leah4sciMCAT playlist for Maths Without a Calculator (the latter was produced for MCAT preparation but it remains helpful for GAMSAT).

- [ ] Reassess your schedule for your full-length GAMSAT practice tests: ACER and/or HEAPS exams. Ensure that you have scheduled one full day to complete a practice test and 1-2 days for a thorough assessment of worked solutions while adding to your abbreviated Gold Notes.

- [ ] Reassess your progress in scheduling and/or evaluating stress reduction techniques such as regular exercise (sports), yoga, meditation and/or mindfulness exercises (*see* YouTube for suggestions).

Medium-level Importance

Medium-level Importance

GOLD NOTES

TRIGONOMETRY
Chapter 5

Memorise
* Formulas for Sine, Cosine, and Tangent

Understand
* Graphing Sine, Cosine, and Tangent
* The Unit Circle
* Inverse Trigonometric Functions

Importance
Low level: **2.5%** of GAMSAT Section 3 maths-based questions released by ACER are related to content in this chapter (in our estimation).
* Note that approximately 90% of such questions are related to just 3 chapters: 1, 2, and 3.

GAMSAT-Prep.com

Introduction

Trigonometry is the most conceptually advanced branch of mathematics with which you will need to be familiar for the GAMSAT test. But don't let that scare you. Basically, everything in this section boils down to right triangles, and after Chapter 5, you will be a triangle pro!

Of the more than 400 official Section 3 practice questions from ACER, very few would benefit from an understanding of the content from this chapter (*see* Spoiler Alert). These concepts will return, in part, in the first 3 chapters of GAMSAT Physics.

Additional Resources

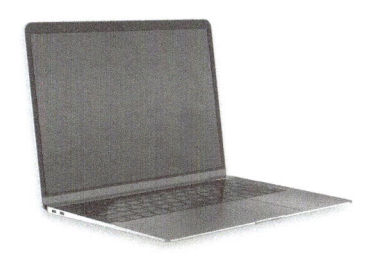

Open Discussion Boards

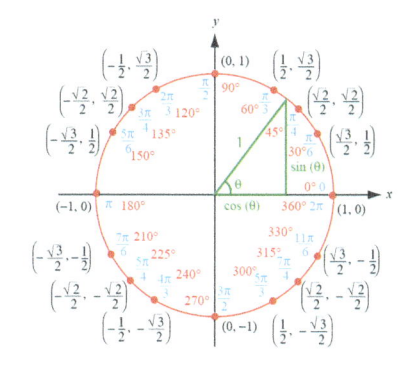

Special Guest

GAMSAT MATHS GM-153

5.1 Basic Trigonometric Functions

The trigonometric functions describe the relationship between the angles and sides of right triangles. The angle in question is generally denoted by θ, the Greek letter theta, but you will never see the right angle used as θ.

We call the leg connecting to the corner of θ: the *adjacent side* ("b" in the diagram); and the leg that does not touch: the *opposite side* ("a" in the diagram). The edge across from the right angle is called the *hypotenuse* ("c" in the diagram).

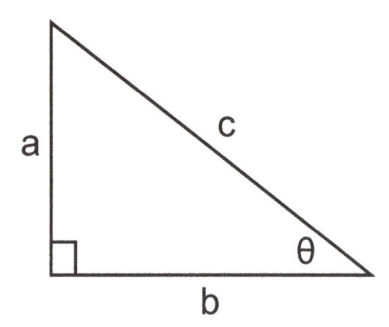

5.1.1 Sine

A lot of people like to use the mnemonic device "SOH-CAH-TOA" to remember how to evaluate the three basic trigonometric functions: Sine, cosine, and tangent. The first three letters, "SOH," refer to the first letter of each word in the following equation.

$$\text{Sine} = \frac{\text{Opposite}}{\text{Hypotenuse}}$$

Sine of an angle θ is written sin(θ). So to calculate this value, simply divide the length of the opposite side by the length of the hypotenuse.

EXAMPLE

What is sin(θ) in the following triangle?

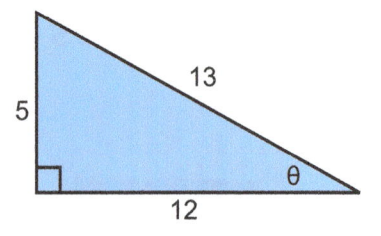

The opposite side has length 5, and the hypotenuse has length 13, so

$$\sin(\theta) = \frac{5}{13}$$

Low-level Importance

GM-154   CHAPTER 5: TRIGONOMETRY

5.1.2 Cosine

The second set of three letters in SOH-CAH-TOA refers to the equation for the cosine of an angle.

$$\text{Cosine} = \frac{\text{Adjacent}}{\text{Hypotenuse}}$$

The abbreviation for the cosine of an angle is $\cos(\theta)$.

EXAMPLE

In the 5–12–13 triangle in Section 5.1.1, what is $\cos(\theta)$?

Dividing the adjacent side by the hypotenuse, we obtain the following solution:

$$\cos(\theta) = \frac{12}{13}$$

5.1.3 Tangent

The final three letters in SOH-CAH-TOA refer to the equation for finding the tangent of an angle.

$$\text{Tangent} = \frac{\text{Opposite}}{\text{Adjacent}}$$

You can also find the tangent of an angle if you know the value for sine and cosine. Notice that the hypotenuse cancels out if you divide sine and cosine.

$$\text{Tangent} = \frac{\text{Sine}}{\text{Cosine}}$$

You can also manipulate this equation to express sine or cosine in terms of the tangent.

EXAMPLE

In the 5–12–13 triangle in Section 5.1.1, what is $\tan(\theta)$?

Dividing the opposite side by the adjacent side, we obtain:

$$\tan(\theta) = \frac{5}{12}$$

GAMSAT-Prep.com
GOLD STANDARD MATHS

5.1.4 Secant, Cosecant, and Cotangent

These three functions are far less commonly used than sine, cosine, and tangent, but you should still be familiar with them. They are not very hard to remember because they are just the reciprocals of the main three functions.

$$\text{Cosecant} = \frac{1}{\text{Sine}}$$

$$= \frac{\text{Hypotenuse}}{\text{Opposite}}$$

$$\text{Secant} = \frac{1}{\text{Cosine}}$$

$$= \frac{\text{Hypotenuse}}{\text{Adjacent}}$$

$$\text{Cotangent} = \frac{1}{\text{Tangent}}$$

$$= \frac{\text{Adjacent}}{\text{Opposite}}$$

The abbreviations for these functions are sec, csc, and cot, respectively. Unlike sine, cosine and tangent, you do not need to memorise these unusual functions.

5.2 The Unit Circle

5.2.1 Trig Functions on a Circle

As you can see from the equations in Section 5.1, the trigonometric functions are ratios of side lengths. This means that every angle has a value for each of the functions that *does not* depend on the scale of the triangle.

In Section 5.1 we looked at examples with a 5–12–13 triangle. Our solutions were as follows:

$$\sin(\theta) = \frac{5}{13}$$

$$\cos(\theta) = \frac{12}{13}$$

$$\tan(\theta) = \frac{5}{12}$$

Let's compare these results with the trigonometric functions for the similar triangle 10, 24, 26, which clearly has longer sides but the same angle θ:

Low-level Importance

GM-156 CHAPTER 5: TRIGONOMETRY

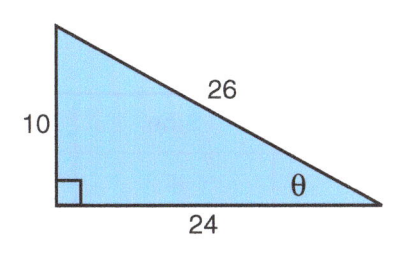

$$\sin(\theta) = \frac{10}{26} = \frac{5}{13}$$

$$\cos(\theta) = \frac{24}{26} = \frac{12}{13}$$

$$\tan(\theta) = \frac{10}{24} = \frac{5}{12}$$

obtain a circle of radius 1. This is known as the **unit circle**, as shown in the succeeding picture. The angle formed at the vertex of the x-axis is equal to θ.

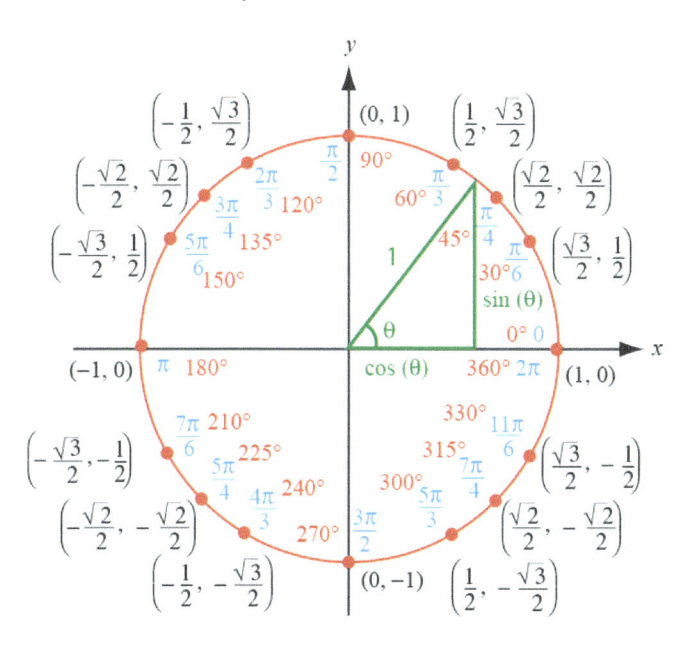

As you can see, the trigonometric values for the angle remain the same.

Also, the absolute value of sine and cosine is never greater than 1 for any angle. This makes perfect sense because the hypotenuse of a triangle is always its longest side, and for sine and cosine, the hypotenuse is in the denominator.

If we plot the graph of sine and cosine for θ from 0° to 360° in Cartesian Coordinates with $x = \cos(\theta)$ and $y = \sin(\theta)$, we

When simply dealing with right triangle figures, we never use negative numbers because negative length does not make sense. With the unit circle, though, legs of the triangle can be in negative space on the Cartesian plane. This can result in negative values for sine and cosine. You do not need to memorise the results of the unit circle.

5.2.2 Degrees and Radians

Up until this point, we have measured angles using degrees. When dealing with trigonometric functions, however, it is often more convenient to use the unit-less measurement of **radians**. There are 2π radians in 360°, so one trip around the unit circle is an increase in θ by 2π radians.

GAMSAT-Prep.com
GOLD STANDARD MATHS

2π radians = 360°

This translates to 1 radian = $\frac{360}{2\pi}$, but you will usually be working with radians in multiples of π, so it is not necessary to memorise this.

Here is a list of important angles (in degrees and radians) and their sine and cosine values that can be deduced from the unit circle:

Degrees	Radians	Sine	Cosine
0°	0	0	1
30°	$\frac{\pi}{6}$	$\frac{1}{2}$	$\frac{\sqrt{3}}{2}$
45°	$\frac{\pi}{4}$	$\frac{1}{\sqrt{2}}$	$\frac{1}{\sqrt{2}}$
60°	$\frac{\pi}{3}$	$\frac{\sqrt{3}}{2}$	$\frac{1}{2}$
90°	$\frac{\pi}{2}$	1	0

Note that $\frac{1}{\sqrt{2}}$ is the same as $\frac{\sqrt{2}}{2}$.

These major angles repeat for each quadrant of the unit circle, but the signs of the sine and cosine values change. Moving counterclockwise around the circle and beginning with the upper right, the quadrants are labelled I, II, III, and IV.

Quadrant	Sine	Cosine
I	+	+
II	+	−
III	−	−
IV	−	+

NOTE

How many degrees are there in $\frac{3(\pi)}{4}$ radians?

Because 2π radians = 360°, this makes 1(π) radian = 180°.

Solution:

1π radian = 180°

$\frac{3\pi}{4} = \frac{3\pi}{4} \times \frac{180°}{\pi}$

= 135°

How many radians are there in 270°?

Solution:

1π radian = 180°

$270° \times \frac{\pi}{180°} = \frac{3\pi}{2}$

GM-158 CHAPTER 5: TRIGONOMETRY

Low-level Importance

5.2.3 Graphing Trig Functions

Looking at the unit circle, it is very apparent that the trigonometric functions are **periodic**. This means that they continue to repeat the same cycle infinitely. After you go once around the circle, a full 360°, you end up right back at the beginning and begin to cycle through again. It is due to this *periodicity* that these functions are used to describe periodic motion (e.g. a pendulum or swing in motion, etc.) which we will explore in Physics Chapter 7.

A. Sine

As you can see from the table in 5.2.2, the sine function increases for the first 90°. For the next 90° it decreases while staying positive, then it continues to decrease into the negatives, and finally for the last 90°, it increases from −1 back to 0. From this information, we can picture the general shape of the graph, and we know that the period of the function is a full 360° or 2π radians.

The graph itself looks like this:

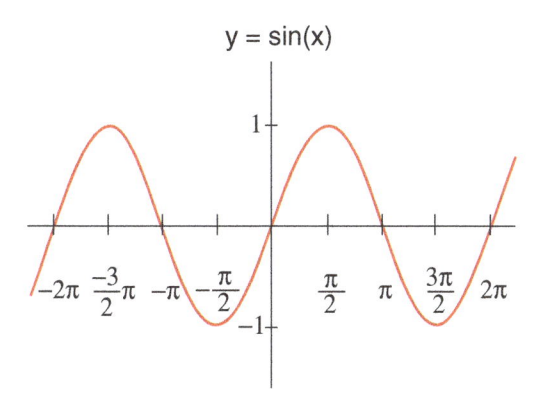

$y = \sin(x)$

As you can see in the graph, the sine function reaches a maximum at $\frac{\pi}{2} + 2\pi \times n$, has an x-intercept at $\pi \times n$, and a minimum at $\frac{3\pi}{2} + 2\pi \times n$ where n is any integer.

B. Cosine

The cosine function is identical to the sine function, except that it is shifted along the x-axis by half a period. So rather than starting at 0 and increasing, it starts at one and decreases. The period is still 2π radians.

The graph looks like this:

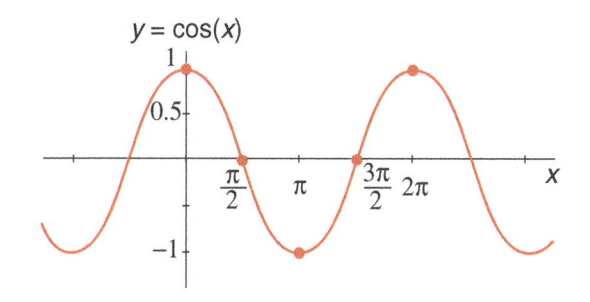

$y = \cos(x)$

Just like with the sine function, you can see where the maxima, minima, and intercepts of the cosine function are from the graph. It reaches a maximum at $2\pi \times n$, an x-intercept at $\frac{\pi}{2} + \pi \times n$, and a minimum at $2\pi \times n + \pi$ where n is any integer.

C. Tangent

The graph of the tangent function differs from sine and cosine graphs in a few important ways. First of all, the tangent function repeats itself every π radian instead of every 2π. So it is π-periodic rather than 2π-periodic. Also, it has vertical **asymptotes**, vertical lines that the function approaches but never crosses, at $(n)\left(\frac{\pi}{2}\right)$ for every odd integer n. The value of the tangent goes infinity as it approaches an asymptote from left to right; and negative infinity as it approaches from right to left.

> **NOTE**
> We will see the application of sine curves when we discuss Wave Characteristics and Periodic Motion in Physics Chapter 7.

Remember, the tangent function is the ratio of the sine function to the cosine function, so the asymptotes occur when the cosine of an angle is equal to zero, where $\cos(x) = 0$, because division by zero is undefined. 0/0 is never possible for the tangent function, so it is irrelevant.

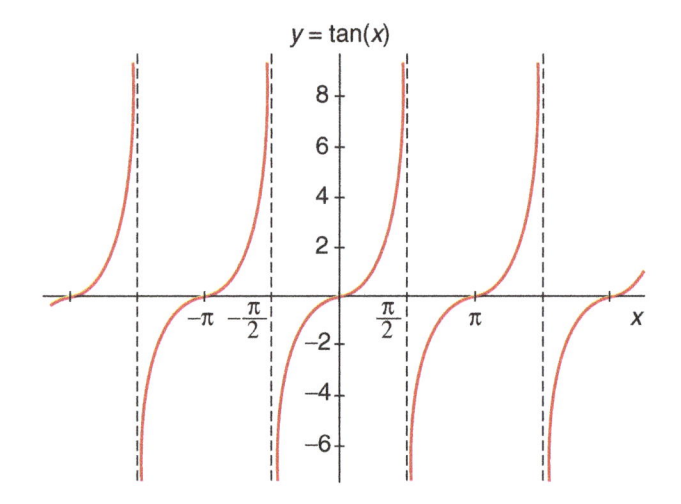

5.3 Trigonometric Problems

5.3.1 Inverse Trig Functions

We have discussed the formulas for finding the value of trigonometric functions for different angles, but how can you find the value of an angle if all you know is the value of one of the functions? This is where the inverse trigonometric functions come into play.

The **inverse** of a trigonometric function takes an input value x and outputs an angle. The value of the inverse trigonometric function of x is equal to the angle. To represent an inverse function, we write -1 in superscript like we would an exponent. But remember, this is not actually an exponent.

Inverse sine is represented as $\sin^{-1}$ and it is defined as such:

$$\sin(\sin^{-1}(x)) = x$$

So, $\sin(\theta) = x$ and $\sin^{-1}(x) = \theta$.

Now that we have inverse functions in our toolbox, we can begin to solve algebraic problems that contain trigonometric functions.

Solve the following equation for x.

$$\pi - \tan 2x = \left(\frac{4}{3}\right)\pi$$

$$\Rightarrow -\tan 2x = \left(\frac{1}{3}\right)\pi$$

$$\Rightarrow \tan 2x = \frac{-\pi}{3}$$

$$\Rightarrow 2x = \tan^{-1}\left(\frac{-\pi}{3}\right)$$

$$\Rightarrow x = \left(\frac{1}{2}\right)\tan^{-1}\left(\frac{-\pi}{3}\right)$$

GOLD STANDARD WARM-UP EXERCISES
CHAPTER 5: Trigonometry

NOTE

All these questions are "open book" practice questions. Please feel free to find information in this chapter to help you solve these problems. This type of practice helps to improve your deductive reasoning. Of course, please do not use a calculator.

1. What percentage of the unit circle is represented by the angle $8\pi/5$?
   A. 1.6%
   B. 80%
   C. 0.25%
   D. 160%

2. Which of the following is the value of $-\cos(\pi/2)$?
   A. 0
   B. -1
   C. 1
   D. $1/\sqrt{2}$

GAMSAT-Prep.com
GOLD STANDARD MATHS

3. The tangent of one of the acute angles in a right triangle is 3/2. If the leg opposite this angle has a length of 12, what is the length of the hypotenuse?
   A. 8
   B. $6\sqrt{13}$
   C. $4\sqrt{13}$
   D. 18

4. Given that the sine of an acute angle is equal to the cosine of its complement, and vice versa, the value of $\cos(\pi/6)$ equals the value of which of the following? (note: for complementary angles, see GM 4.1.3)
   A. $\sin(\pi/2)$
   B. $\sin(\pi/4)$
   C. $\sin(\pi/6)$
   D. $\sin(\pi/3)$

CHAPTER 5 WORKED SOLUTIONS

Question 1   B
See: GM 5.2, 5.2.1
A circle covers a total of 2π radians, and

$$\frac{\frac{8\pi}{5}}{2\pi} = \frac{4}{5}$$

which is equivalent to 80%.

Question 2   A
See: GM 5.1.2, 5.2

$$-\cos\left(\frac{\pi}{2}\right) = \cos\left(\frac{\pi}{2}\right) = 0$$

Question 3   C
See: GM 5.1, 5.1.3, 5.3, 5.3.3
In a right triangle, the tangent of an angle represents the ratio of sides $\frac{opposite}{adjacent}$, so the given values form the proportion $\frac{3}{2} = \frac{12}{x}$, where x is the side adjacent the angle in question. Cross-multiplication gives us 3x = 24, or x = 8, and we can find the length of the hypotenuse using the Pythagorean Theorem:

$$12^2 + 8^2 = c^2$$
$$144 + 64 = c^2$$
$$\sqrt{208} = c$$
$$\sqrt{4 \times 4 \times 13} = c$$
$$4\sqrt{13} = c$$

Question 4   D
See: GM 4.1.3, 5.2, 5.2.3
The cosine of an angle is equal to the sine of its complement. $\frac{\pi}{6}$, or $\left(\frac{\pi}{6}\right)\left(\frac{180°}{\pi}\right) = 30°$, is the complement of $\frac{\pi}{3} = 60°$.

CHAPTER 5: TRIGONOMETRY

GAMSAT MASTERS SERIES

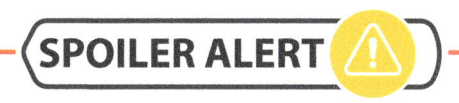

> **SPOILER ALERT** ⚠️
>
> Gold Standard has cross-referenced the content in this chapter to examples from ACER's official GAMSAT practice materials. It is for you to decide when you want to explore these questions since you may want to preserve some of ACER's materials for timed mock-exam practice.
>
> **Examples** – Pythagorean theorem and a little sine/cosine: Q44–47 of 2; note that even though the trigonometric functions are introduced in this unit by ACER, the passage guides you as to what information to use so rote learning would be irrelevant. Note that "Q" is followed by the question number, and, for example, "of 1" refers to booklet number 1 which is referenced in the Spoiler Alert table at the end of Chapter 1. The 10 full-length HEAPS GAMSAT practice tests (by Gold Standard and MediRed), exams 1 through 10, contain specific cross-references to this chapter within the worked solutions.

Chapter Checklist

- ☐ Reassess your 'learning objectives' for this chapter: Go back to the first page of this chapter and re-evaluate the top 3 boxes and the Introduction.

- ☐ Complete a maximum of 1 page of notes using symbols/abbreviations to represent the entire chapter based on your learning objectives. These are your Gold Notes.

- ☐ Consider your multimedia options based on your optimal way of learning:

    - ☐ Download the free Gold Standard GAMSAT app for your Android device or iPhone.
    - ☐ Create your own, tangible study cards or try the free app: Anki.
    - ☐ Record your voice reading your Gold Notes onto your smartphone (MP3s) and listen during exercise, transportation, etc.
    - ☐ Try out the Gold Standard GAMSAT Physics online videos at gamsat-prep.com which have heaps of calculations, or you can try other maths options on YouTube like Khan Academy or Leah4sciMCAT playlist for Maths Without a Calculator (the latter was produced for MCAT preparation but it remains helpful for GAMSAT).

- ☐ Reassess your schedule for your full-length GAMSAT practice tests: ACER and/or HEAPS exams. Ensure that you have scheduled one full day to complete a practice test and 1-2 days for a thorough assessment of worked solutions while adding to your abbreviated Gold Notes.

- ☐ Reassess your progress in scheduling and/or evaluating stress reduction techniques such as regular exercise (sports), yoga, meditation and/or mindfulness exercises (*see* YouTube for suggestions).

Low-level Importance

GOLD NOTES

PROBABILITY AND STATISTICS
Chapter 6

Memorise
* Formula for Average
* Formula for Probability

Understand
* Determining Probabilities
* Combining Probabilities of Multiple Events
* Mode, Median, Variance, Standard Deviation and its Corresponding Graph
* Correlation Coefficient
* Regression lines ("lines of best fit")

Importance
Low level: 1% of GAMSAT Section 3 maths-based questions released by ACER are related to content in this chapter (in our estimation).
* Note that approximately 90% of such questions are related to just 3 chapters: 1, 2, and 3.

GAMSAT-Prep.com

Introduction

The content in this chapter essentially provides you with some background information regarding graphs and research articles which you will likely be exposed to during the real exam. However, it is very unlikely that this content will be specifically tested.

Often research passages are presented as stimulus material for GAMSAT questions so a basic understanding of probability and statistics is useful. From the standpoint of performing calculations, probability and statistics are exceedingly minor subjects for the GAMSAT. This section will help you keep things straight such as when to multiply and when to add probabilities – simple questions that can often be the most confusing probabilities.

Additional Resources

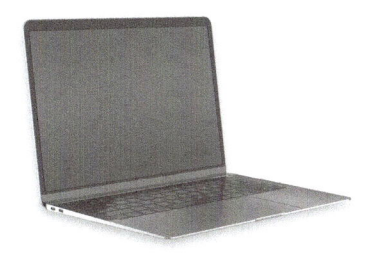

Open Discussion Boards

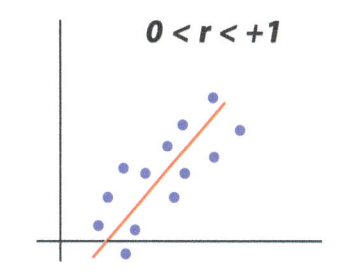

Special Guest

GAMSAT-Prep.com
GOLD STANDARD MATHS

6.1 Probability

6.1.1 What is Probability?

Probability is a measure of the likelihood that something will happen.

In mathematics, probability is represented as a ratio of two numbers. The second number - the denominator - corresponds to the total number of possible outcomes the situation can have. The first number - the numerator - corresponds to the number of ways the particular outcome in question can occur.

$$\text{Probability} = \frac{\text{(number of ways the outcome can occur)}}{\text{(number of possible outcomes)}}$$

Let's look at a simple example.

Let's consider the flipping of a coin. Of course, we know that there are only two possible outcomes of a coin flip, heads or tails. So the total number of outcomes is 2, which will be our denominator.

Say we want to find the probability that a flipped coin will be heads. There is only one way this outcome can come about, so the numerator will be 1. Therefore, the probability of flipping heads is 1 in 2:

$$\text{Probability of Heads} = \frac{1}{2}$$

It is important to note that the quantity in the numerator of a probability ratio is a subset of the quantity in the denominator. The number of ways an outcome can occur is always less than or equal to the total number of outcomes. This means that a probability will never be more than 1, since 1 would mean the outcome is the *only* possibility. Also, the sum of the probabilities of all possible outcomes will always be 1.

Let's look at a slightly more complicated example.

Say you have a typical six-sided die with the sides labelled 1 through 6. If you roll the die once, what is the probability that the number will not be divisible by 3?

Let's begin by finding the total number of outcomes. Be careful here. The only outcomes we wish to determine the probability of are rolls of numbers divisible by 3, but the total number of possible outcomes is not affected by this restriction. There are still 6 in total, one for each number it is possible to roll.

Now we want to know how many ways out of these 6 we can roll a number that is not divisible by 3. Well, the only two numbers that are divisible by 3 that are possibilities are 3 and 6. So 1, 2, 4, and 5 are not. This means that there are 4 ways for the outcome to occur.

GM-166   CHAPTER 6: PROBABILITY AND STATISTICS

$$\text{Probability} = \frac{4}{6}$$

Reducing fractions is usually fine when working with probability; just know that if you do, the numerator and denominator will not necessarily correspond to the number of possibilities anymore.

$$\text{Probability} = \frac{2}{3}$$

The simplest way to complicate a probability problem is to allow for multiple correct outcomes. To find the total probability, simply add the individual probabilities for each correct outcome. For the above example, the total probability is actually the sum of the probabilities of rolling 1, 2, 4, and 5.

6.1.2 Combining Probabilities

What if you are asked to find the probability that multiple events will occur?

The solution to such a problem will still be a ratio in which the numbers represent the same quantities as before. The new difficulty is figuring out how many different outcome possibilities there are. Luckily, there is an easy way to calculate this. All you have to do is find the probability of each individual event and then multiply them together.

Why does this work? Think about it this way: For each possible outcome of the first event, there is still every possible outcome for the second. So the total number of possibilities will be the number of outcomes in the first times the number of outcomes in the second.

EXAMPLE

Let's go back to the flipping coin! If you flip it twice, what is the probability that the first flip will turn up heads and the second tails?

When dealing with multiple events, always focus on one event at a time before combining. So start with the first flip. We know that the probability it will be heads is ½. Now for the second flip, the probability it will be tails is also ½.

Now to find the probability that both of the events will occur, we multiply the individual probabilities:

$$\text{Probability} = \frac{1}{2} \times \frac{1}{2}$$
$$= \frac{1}{4}$$

GAMSAT-Prep.com
GOLD STANDARD MATHS

Let's look at another coin flip example.

EXAMPLE

If you flip a coin twice, what is the probability that it will come up heads exactly one time?

This question seems almost identical to the previous example, but be careful! The difference is that the phrasing of this question does not specify particular outcomes for the individual events.

Let's solve this in two ways:

(i) Let's combine both events into one. To find the total number of possible outcomes, multiply the totals of each event, so there are 2 × 2 = 4 possibilities. Now count the number of ways we can flip heads once. Well, we could have heads on the first flip and tails on the second, so that is 1, or we could have tails then heads, so that is 2. Therefore, the probability of flipping heads exactly once is 2 to 4.

$$\text{Probability} = \frac{2}{4}$$

(ii) Now let's treat the events separately. Ask yourself: What are the odds that an outcome of the first event will be compatible with flipping heads once? The answer is $\frac{2}{2}$ since we can still achieve the overall desired outcome with the second flip no matter what the first flip is.

Now what are the odds that an outcome of the second event will be compatible with flipping heads once? Since you already have a first flip determined, there is only one outcome for the second flip that will give the desired result. If the first flip was heads we need a tails flip, and if the first flip was tails we need a heads flip. So the odds for the second flip are ½.

$$\text{Probability} = \frac{2}{2} \times \frac{1}{2}$$
$$= \frac{2}{4}$$

There are all kinds of confusing ways probability problems can be written. You have to be extra careful to break them down and determine exactly what is being asked because the test writers love to try and trick you. Double and triple-check that you have the setup right for probability problems because it is so easy to accidentally overlook something.

> **NOTE**
>
> When you want to know the probability of event A or B, the probabilities must be added. If you want to know the probability of events A and B, the probabilities must be multiplied.

6.2 Statistics

6.2.1 Averages

When given a collection of numbers, the **average** is the sum of the numbers divided by the total number of numbers.

$$\text{Average} = \frac{(\text{sum of numbers})}{(\text{number of numbers})}$$

EXAMPLE

What is the average of the set {4, 7, 6, 7}?

Add up the numbers and, since there are 4 of them, divide by 4.

$$\text{Average} = \frac{(4+7+6+7)}{4}$$
$$= \frac{24}{4}$$
$$= 6$$

The average may or may not actually appear in the set of numbers, but it is a common way to think of the typical value for the set.

6.2.2 Mode, Median, Mean

Here are a few other statistics terms you should know:

The **mode** of a set of values is the number that appears the most times. Mode can be bimodal or multimodal. Simply stated, bimodal means that two numbers are repeated the most while multimodal indicates two or more numbers are repeated the most.

The **median** of a set of values is the number that appears exactly in the center of the distribution. This means there are an equal number of values greater than and less than the median.

Arithmetic mean is just another name for the average of a set of numbers. The terms are interchangeable.

EXAMPLE

Find the mode, median, and mean of the following set: {3, 5, 11, 3, 8}.

Let's begin with the mode. All we need to do is see which value or values repeat the most times. In this case, the only one that repeats is 3.

Mode = 3

To find the median we always need to first arrange the set in numerical order.

{3, 3, 5, 8, 11}

Now the median is whichever number lies in the exact center.

Median = 5

Since the mean is the same as the average, we add the values and divide by 5.

$$\text{Mean} = \frac{(3+3+5+8+11)}{5}$$
$$= \frac{30}{5}$$
$$= 6$$

> **NOTE**
>
> If a set has an even number of values, there will be no value exactly in the center. In this case, the median is the average of the two values that straddle the center.
>
> **Example**
>
> Given: 3, 4, 5, 6, 6, 8, 9, 10, 10, 12
>
> The median is the average of the two middle data: $\frac{(6+8)}{2} = 7$

6.3 More Tools for Probability and Statistics

6.3.1 The Correlation Coefficient

The correlation coefficient r indicates whether two sets of data are associated or *correlated*. The value of r ranges from -1.0 to 1.0. The larger the absolute value of r, the stronger the association. Given two sets of data X and Y, a positive value for r indicates that as X increases, Y increases. A negative value for r indicates that as X increases, Y decreases.

GAMSAT MASTERS SERIES

Imagine that the weight (X) and height (Y) of everyone in the entire country was determined. There would be a strong positive correlation between a person's weight and their height. In general, as weight increases, height increases (*in a population*). However, the correlation would not be perfect (i.e. r < 1.0). After all, there would be some people who are very tall but very thin, and others who would be very short but overweight. We might find that r = 0.7. This would suggest there is a strong positive association between weight and height, but it is not a perfect association.

If two sets of data are correlated, does that mean that one *causes* the other? Not necessarily; simply because weight and height are correlated does not mean that if you gained weight you will necessarily gain height! Thus association does not imply causality.

Note that a correlation greater than 0.8 is generally described as strong, whereas a correlation that is less than 0.5 is generally described as weak. However, the interpretation and use of these values can vary based upon the "type" of data being examined. For example, a study based on chemical or biological data may require a stronger correlation than a study using social science data. You will regularly see regression lines with well-correlated data in ACER's practice materials and during the real GAMSAT.

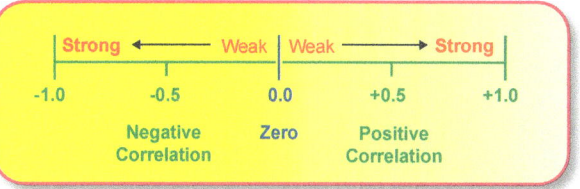

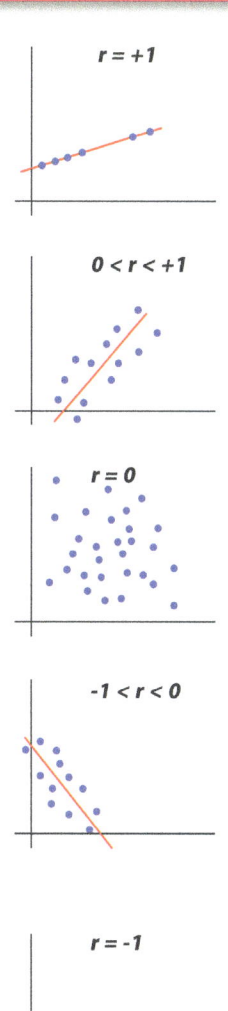

Varying values of the correlation coefficient (r) based on data plotted for two variables (= scatter diagrams). In red is the line of "best fit" (= *regression line*). One purpose of the regression line is to predict what would likely occur outside of the experimental data (meaning, you can extrapolate beyond what is shown).

Low-level Importance

GAMSAT MATHS GM-171

6.3.2 The Standard Deviation

When given a set of data, it is often useful to know the average value, *the mean*, and the *range* of values. As previously discussed, the mean is simply the sum of the data values divided by the number of data values. The range is the numerical difference between the largest value and the smallest value.

Another useful measurement is the *standard deviation*. The standard deviation indicates the dispersion of values around the mean. Given a bell-shaped distribution of data (e.g., the height and weight of a population, the GPA of undergraduate students, etc.), each standard deviation (SD) includes a given percentage of data. For example, the mean +/− 1 SD includes approximately 68% of the data values, the mean +/− 2 SD includes 95% of the data values, and the mean +/− 3 SD includes 99.7% of the data values.

> **NOTE**
>
> To see a Normal Curve displaying GAMSAT score results, go to www.GAMSAT-prep.com/GAMSAT-scores.

For example, imagine that you read that the mean GPA required for admission to Belcurve University's Dental School is 3.5 with a standard deviation of 0.2 (SD = 0.2). Thus approximately 68% of the students admitted have a GPA of 3.5 +/− 0.2, which means between 3.3 and 3.7. We can also conclude that approximately 95% of the students admitted have a GPA of 3.5 +/− 2(0.2), which means between 3.1 and 3.9. Therefore the standard deviation becomes a useful measure of the dispersion of values around the mean 3.5.

- Green Area = 68% or 1 Standard Deviation
- Green + Blue = 95% or 2 Standard Deviations
- Green + Blue + Red = 99% or 3 Standard Deviations

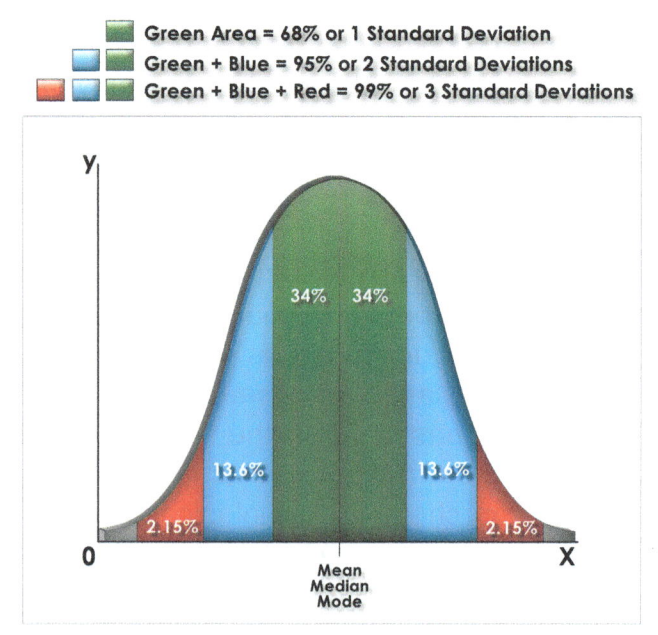

Figure 6.1: The Normal Curve (also referred to as: the Normal Distribution Curve).

6.3.3 Variance

Variance is another measure of how far a set of numbers is spread out or, in other words, how far numbers are from the mean. Thus variance is calculated as the average of the squared differences from the mean.

There are three steps to calculate the variance:

1. Determine the mean (the simple average of all the numbers)
2. For each number: subtract the mean and square the result (the squared difference)
3. Determine the average of those squared differences

The variance is also defined as the square of the standard deviation. Thus unlike standard deviation, the variance has units that are the square of the units of the variable itself.

For example, a variable measured in metres will have a variance measured in metres squared.

You are unlikely to need to calculate the standard deviation nor the variance. But having a basic understanding of these statistical measures can help when reading passages or analysing graphs (e.g., with error bars; GM 3.5.5) during the GAMSAT.

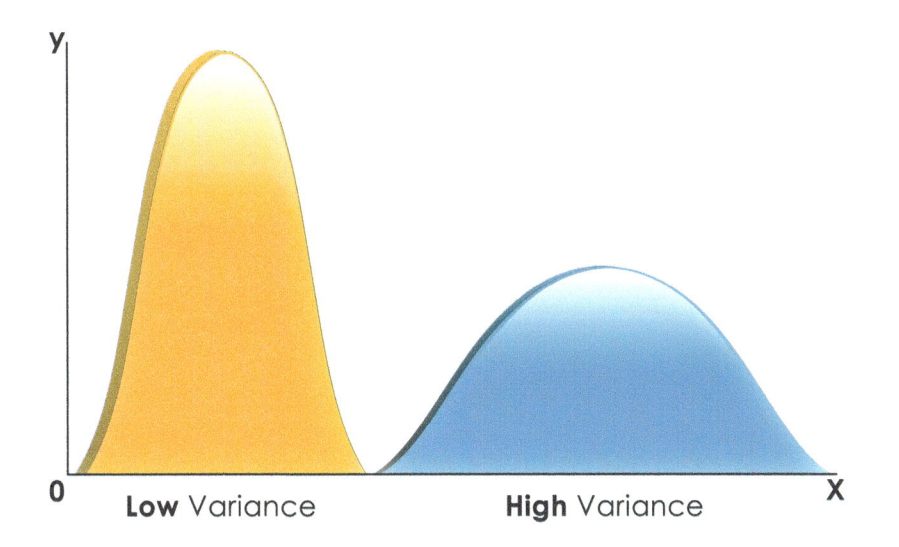

Figure 6.2: Variance.

6.3.4 Simple Probability Revisited

Let's apply a formula to simple probability. If a phenomenon or experiment has *n* equally likely outcomes, *s* of which are called successes, then the probability *P* of success is given by $P = \frac{s}{n}$.

EXAMPLE

- if "heads" in a coin toss is considered a success, then
$P(\text{success}) = \frac{1}{2}$;

- if a card is drawn from a deck and diamonds are considered successes, then
$P(\text{success}) = \frac{13}{52}$. It follows that $P(\text{success}) = 1 - P(\text{failure})$.

NOTE

Any of the 4 GAMSAT sciences may require the use of simple probability but it most often presents itself in Genetics (Biology Chapter 15).

GOLD STANDARD WARM-UP EXERCISES

CHAPTER 6: Probability and Statistics

1. A jar contains 4 red marbles and 6 blue marbles. What is the probability that a marble chosen at random will be red?
   A. 4/6
   B. 4/10
   C. 2/6
   D. 6/10

2. A box contains 6 yellow balls and 4 green balls. Two balls are chosen at random without replacement. What is the probability that the first ball is yellow and the second ball is green?
   A. 5/12
   B. 1/10
   C. 6/25
   D. 4/15

3. An English teacher wants to prepare a class reading list that includes 1 philosophy book, 1 work of historical fiction, and 1 biography. She has 3 philosophy books, 2 works of historical fiction, and 4 biographies to choose from. How many different combinations of books can she put together for her list?
   A. 32
   B. 288
   C. 9
   D. 24

4. A medical training survey shows that the distribution of the residents' annual income is a bell curve. 2,516 residents are within one standard deviation of the average annual income. How many residents were in the survey's sample?
   A. 3,700
   B. 2,648
   C. 2,524
   D. 2,523

5. The average time it takes 3 students to complete a test is 35 minutes. If 1 student takes 41 minutes to complete the test and another takes 37 minutes, how many minutes does the third student take to complete the test?
   A. 4
   B. 38
   C. 27
   D. 39

6. A small library receives a shipment of grey books, blue books, black books, and brown books. If the librarian decides to shelve all the books of one colour on Monday, all of the books of another colour on Tuesday, and the rest of the books on Wednesday, in how many different ways can the book shelving be completed?
   A. 3
   B. 4
   C. 8
   D. 12

7. When you roll a die, what is the probability to first get a 3 and then a 1 or a 2?
   A. 1/6
   B. 1/8
   C. 1/32
   D. 1/18

GAMSAT-Prep.com
GOLD STANDARD MATHS

CHAPTER 6 WORKED SOLUTIONS

Question 1   B
See: GM 6.1.1
There are four red marbles, and a total of 4 red + 6 blue = 10 marbles, so the probability is $\frac{4}{10}$.

Question 2   D
See: GM 6.1, 6.1.2
With a total of 10 balls and 6 yellow balls, the probability that the first ball is yellow is $\frac{6}{10} = \frac{3}{5}$. After the first ball is chosen, there are 9 left, of which 4 are green. The probability of choosing a green ball at this point is therefore $\frac{4}{9}$. The total probability is $\left(\frac{3}{5}\right)\left(\frac{4}{9}\right) = \frac{4}{15}$

Question 3   D
See: GM 6.3, 6.3.4
Multiply all possible choices: $3 \times 2 \times 4 = 24$

Question 4   A
See: GM 6.3.2
The 2516 residents represent 68% of the total number of residents x:

$$2516 = 0.68x = (2/3)x \text{ (approx.)}$$
$$x = 2516/(2/3) = (2516 \times 3)/2 = 7548/2 = 3774$$

Question 5   C
See: GM 6.2, 6.2.1
If the third student takes x minutes to complete the test:

$$\frac{41 + 37 + x}{3} = 35$$
$$78 + x = 105$$
$$x = 27$$

Question 6   D
See: GM 6.3.4
There are 4 different book colours, so there are 4 different choices for books to shelve on Monday. There are only 3 choices on Tuesday. On Wednesday, the rest of the books will be shelved, so there is only 1 choice. This gives a total of $4 \times 3 \times 1 = 12$ different ways to shelve the books.

Question 7   D
See: GM 6.1, 6.1.2
A die has a total of 6 possible sides. There is only one side that displays a 3, so the probability of rolling a 3 is $\frac{1}{6}$. Similarly, the probability of rolling any other number is also $\frac{1}{6}$. The probability of rolling a 1 or a 2 is the sum of their individual probabilities: $\frac{1}{6} + \frac{1}{6} = \frac{1}{3}$. Because this probability is independent of the probability of first rolling a 3, we multiply the results to get the total probability: $\left(\frac{1}{6}\right)\left(\frac{1}{3}\right) = \frac{1}{18}$.

GAMSAT MASTERS SERIES

⚠ SPOILER ALERT

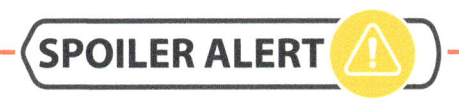

Gold Standard has cross-referenced the content in this chapter to examples from ACER's official GAMSAT practice materials. It is for you to decide when you want to explore these questions since you may want to preserve some of ACER's materials for timed mock-exam practice.

Examples – There are a few genetics units that would benefit from a very elementary understanding of probability/statistics such Q54-56 of 5. Note that "Q" is followed by the question number, and, for example, "of 1" refers to booklet number 1 which is referenced in the Spoiler Alert table at the end of Chapter 1. The 10 full-length HEAPS GAMSAT practice tests (by Gold Standard and MediRed), exams 1 through 10, contain specific cross-references to this chapter within the worked solutions. Note that we will cover probability/statistics from a genetics perspective in Biology Chapter 15 of the Masters Series.

Chapter Checklist

- [ ] Reassess your 'learning objectives' for this chapter: Go back to the first page of this chapter and re-evaluate the top 3 boxes and the Introduction.

- [ ] Complete a maximum of 1 page of notes using symbols/abbreviations to represent the entire chapter based on your learning objectives. These are your Gold Notes.

- [ ] Consider your multimedia options based on your optimal way of learning:
    - [ ] Download the free Gold Standard GAMSAT app for your Android device or iPhone.
    - [ ] Create your own, tangible study cards or try the free app: Anki.
    - [ ] Record your voice reading your Gold Notes onto your smartphone (MP3s) and listen during exercise, transportation, etc.
    - [ ] Try out the Gold Standard GAMSAT Physics online videos at gamsat-prep.com which have heaps of calculations, or you can try other maths options on YouTube like Khan Academy or Leah4sciMCAT playlist for Maths Without a Calculator (the latter was produced for MCAT preparation but it remains helpful for GAMSAT).

- [ ] Reassess your schedule for your full-length GAMSAT practice tests: ACER and/or HEAPS exams. Ensure that you have scheduled one full day to complete a practice test and 1-2 days for a thorough assessment of worked solutions while adding to your abbreviated Gold Notes.

- [ ] Reassess your progress in scheduling and/or evaluating stress reduction techniques such as regular exercise (sports), yoga, meditation and/or mindfulness exercises (*see* YouTube for suggestions).

Low-level Importance

GOLD NOTES

GAMSAT PHYSICS
5 Sections • 12 Chapters

01 FORCES AND ENERGY
Chapter 1: Translational Motion
Chapter 2: Force, Motion and Gravitation
Chapter 3: Particle Dynamics
Chapter 4: Equilibrium
Chapter 5: Work and Energy

02 FLUIDS AND SOLIDS
Chapter 6: Fluids and Solids

03 WAVES AND SOUND
Chapter 7: Wave Characteristics and Periodic Motion
Chapter 8: Sound

04 ELECTRICITY
Chapter 9: Electrostatics and Electromagnetism
Chapter 10: Electric Circuits

05 LIGHT, OPTICS AND THE ATOM
Chapter 11: Light and Geometric Optics
Chapter 12: Atomic and Nuclear Structure

GAMSAT-prep.com

TRANSLATIONAL MOTION
Chapter 1

Memorise
* Trigonometric functions: definitions
* Pythagorean theorem
* Define: displacement, velocity, acceleration
* Equations: kinematics (optional)

Understand
* Scalar vs. vector
* Add, subtract, resolve vectors
* Determine common values of functions
* Displacement, velocity, acceleration (avg. and instant.) including graphs

Importance
High level: 10% of GAMSAT Physics questions released by ACER are related to content in this chapter (in our estimation).
* Note that approximately 75% of the questions in GAMSAT Physics are related to just 6 chapters: 1, 4, 6, 9, 11 and 12.

GAMSAT-Prep.com

Introduction

Translational motion is the movement of an object (or particle) through space without turning (rotation). Displacement, velocity and acceleration are key vectors — specified by magnitude and direction — often used to describe translational motion. Being able to manipulate and resolve vectors is helpful for problem-solving in GAMSAT Physics.

Whether science or non-science background: (1) please complete the GAMSAT Maths chapters prior to starting Physics; (2) closely consider information underlined, in italics, in red boxes or highlighted in yellow; (3) the *Need for Speed* exercises, the chapter-ending questions, Spoiler Alert and your Chapter Checklist are all designed to help you focus on your keys for success: learn, revise and practice. Let's begin!

Multimedia Resources at GAMSAT-Prep.com

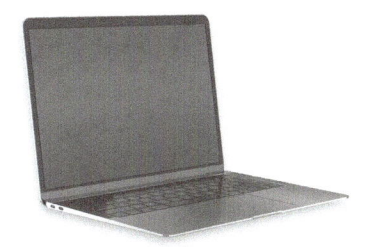

Open Discussion Boards 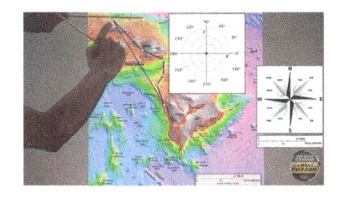   Foundational Videos   Flashcards 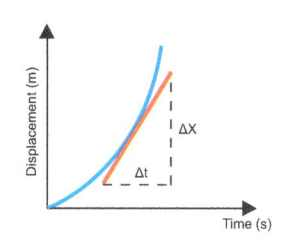   Special Guest

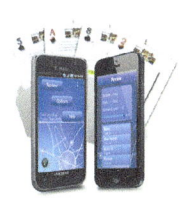

THE PHYSICAL SCIENCES   PHY-03

* The real GAMSAT may have advanced-level information presented (i.e. in a passage) but previous knowledge of said information is not required to answer the questions that would follow. Practice questions at the end of this chapter, as well as ACER and GS (HEAPS) practice GAMSATs can help you clarify this point.

GAMSAT-Prep.com
GOLD STANDARD PHYSICS

1.0 GAMSAT has a *Need for Speed*!

Before you begin your time in the GAMSAT Physics gym, we want to remind you that you have been here already! As long as you have completed the exercises in GAMSAT Maths, you have already completed the most important part of your GAMSAT Physics, General Chemistry and Biology preparation (Organic Chemistry is a different story!). You have completed many equation manipulations using numbers and/or variables. You have completed an examination of the most important SI units. You have completed dimensional analysis including for the Law of Gravitation. You have been exposed to GAMSAT-level graph analysis including the quite famous velocity-time graph (GM 3.8). Logs, sound, trigonometric functions and so much more!

As you have done for the first 3 chapters of GAMSAT Maths, please attempt the *Need for Speed* exercises either before or after reading through the content of this chapter. And, as before, you can be guided by the section numbers and the pink highlighter throughout the chapter so that you can quickly identify the practice questions from the table in order to check your answers and to find the worked solutions.

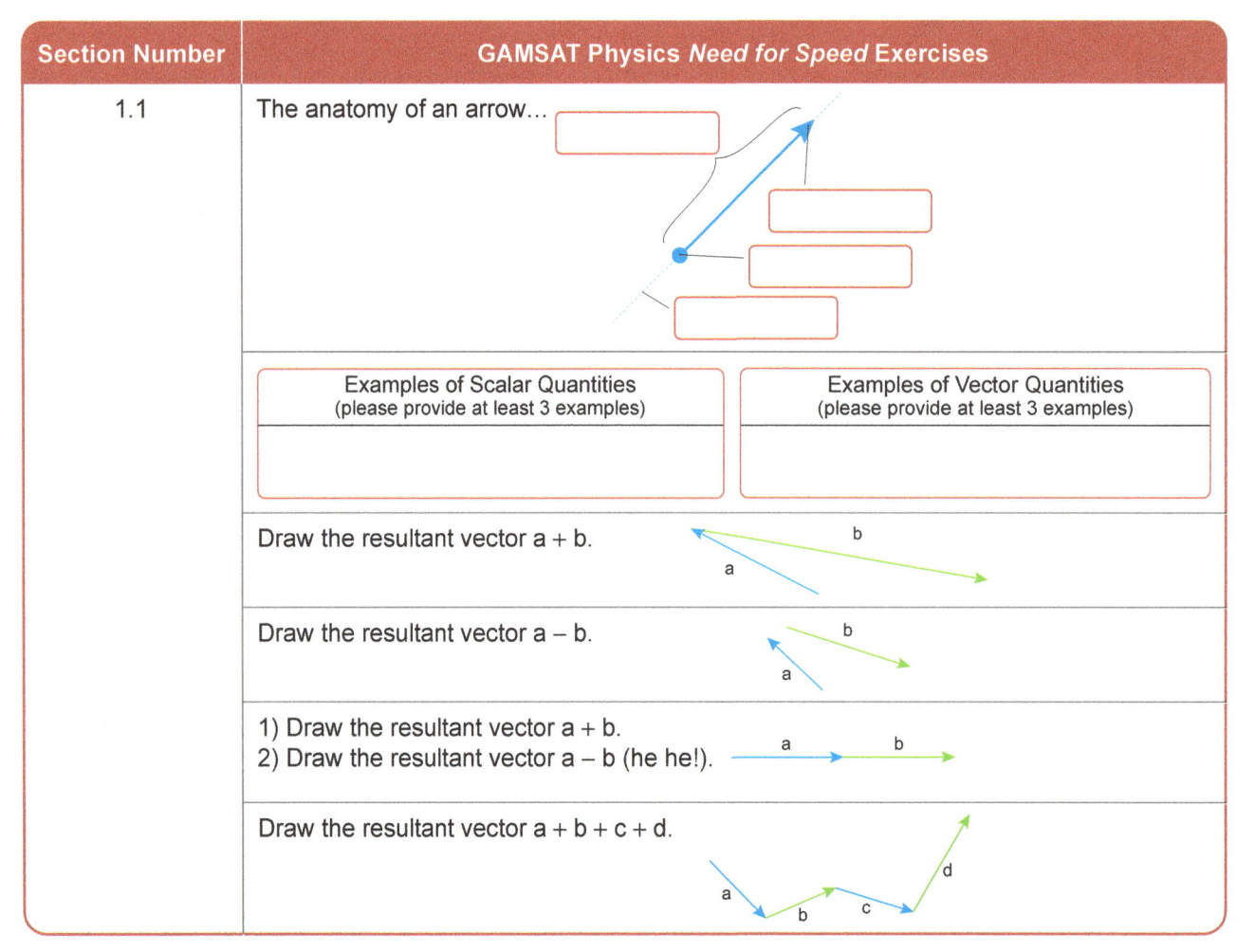

Section Number	GAMSAT Physics *Need for Speed* Exercises
1.1	The anatomy of an arrow…
	Examples of Scalar Quantities (please provide at least 3 examples) / Examples of Vector Quantities (please provide at least 3 examples)
	Draw the resultant vector a + b.
	Draw the resultant vector a − b.
	1) Draw the resultant vector a + b. 2) Draw the resultant vector a − b (he he!).
	Draw the resultant vector a + b + c + d.

PHY-04   CHAPTER 1: TRANSLATIONAL MOTION

GAMSAT MASTERS SERIES

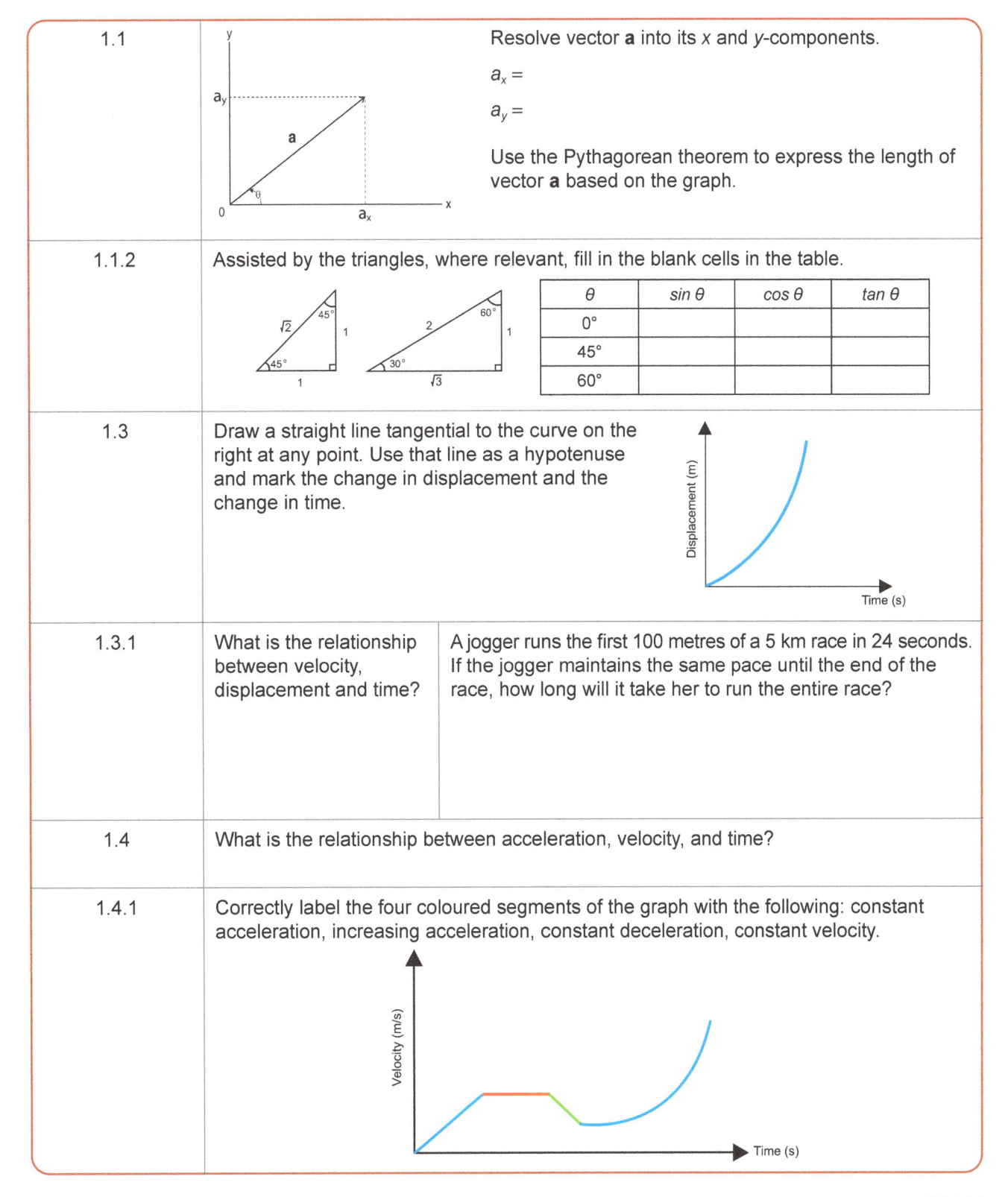

1.1		Resolve vector **a** into its *x* and *y*-components.
	*(diagram of vector **a** with components a_x, a_y and angle θ)*	$a_x =$ $a_y =$ Use the Pythagorean theorem to express the length of vector **a** based on the graph.

1.1.2	Assisted by the triangles, where relevant, fill in the blank cells in the table.

(Triangle 1: 45°-45°-90° with sides 1, 1, √2)
(Triangle 2: 30°-60°-90° with sides 1, √3, 2)

θ	sin θ	cos θ	tan θ
0°			
45°			
60°			

1.3	Draw a straight line tangential to the curve on the right at any point. Use that line as a hypotenuse and mark the change in displacement and the change in time.	*(Displacement (m) vs Time (s) graph showing an upward curving line)*

1.3.1	What is the relationship between velocity, displacement and time?	A jogger runs the first 100 metres of a 5 km race in 24 seconds. If the jogger maintains the same pace until the end of the race, how long will it take her to run the entire race?

1.4	What is the relationship between acceleration, velocity, and time?

1.4.1	Correctly label the four coloured segments of the graph with the following: constant acceleration, increasing acceleration, constant deceleration, constant velocity.

(Velocity (m/s) vs Time (s) graph with four coloured segments)

High-level Importance

THE PHYSICAL SCIENCES — PHY-05

1.1 Scalars and Vectors

High-level Importance

Observation: People generally move! The first five chapters in GAMSAT Physics are concerned with the movement of objects (and people!), as well as the associated forces and energy. Motion that results in a change of location is *translational*. That may sound silly but we will later explore movement where objects continually return to their original position (periodic motion, simple harmonic motion).

Let us take a snapshot of your translational motion from yesterday. Let's say that you woke up from bed, and left your humble abode to do some shopping, and then returned home to prepare some food in the kitchen. How far did you travel? Physics has 2 answers. The first answer is intuitive: The total distance that you travelled including bed to shop and shop to kitchen. Your GPS and/or step tracker could give you a rather accurate assessment of the total distance: It is a *scalar* quantity because it only has a number with some unit, like metres (SI unit) or kilometres.

Physics' second answer: The sum total of your movement yesterday only depends on your initial position (your bed!) and your final position (your kitchen). Those few metres (or less, if you happen to sleep in your kitchen) would be defined as your *displacement*. Similar to distance, we can assess your displacement with a number and some unit, like metres or kilometres (tiny fraction thereof). However, in Physics, displacement has something that distance does not have: Direction. We can represent your displacement with a number, a unit, and a direction which basically specifies the direct way to go from bed to kitchen (no twists, no turns, a straight line as if there is no barrier). Thus displacement is a *vector*.

And so, we have our first, simple vector. It is an arrow pointing from your bed to your kitchen, and the length of that arrow represents the direct distance (the amount or *magnitude*) in, for example, metres. Of course, we could indicate your direction by other means: We could use a modern implement like a compass! We could determine that your kitchen is in a north-east direction from your room. However, if we want to summarise the magnitude and direction of your displacement vector, we need to learn the anatomy of an arrow…

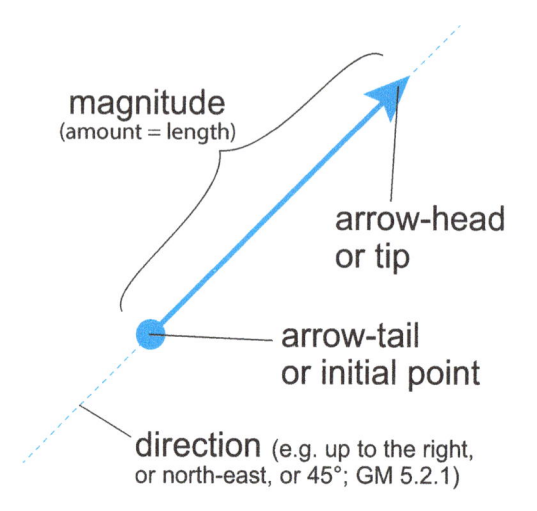

magnitude (amount = length)
arrow-head or tip
arrow-tail or initial point
direction (e.g. up to the right, or north-east, or 45°; GM 5.2.1)

We will now foreshadow the scalar and vector quantities that we will be exploring over the 12 Physics chapters. You may already have a sense as to the logic of the classification but, if not, after you have completed Physics, please return to this section to confirm.

PHY-06 CHAPTER 1: TRANSLATIONAL MOTION

Examples of Scalar Quantities
distance, speed, time, temperature, mass, area, volume, energy, entropy, electric charge

Examples of Vector Quantities
displacement, velocity, acceleration, force, momentum, gravitational field, electrical field

The Big Picture: *Scalars*, such as speed, have magnitude only and are specified by a number with a unit (55 miles/hour). Scalars obey the rules of ordinary algebra (i.e. GM Chap. 2 and 3). *Vectors*, like velocity, have both magnitude **and** direction (100 km/hour, west). Vectors are represented by arrows where: **i)** the length of the arrow indicates the magnitude of the vector, and **ii)** the arrow-head indicates the direction of the vector. Vectors obey the special rules of vector algebra. Vectors can be moved in space but their orientation must be kept the same.

Addition of Vectors: Two vectors **a** and **b** can be added geometrically by drawing them to a common scale and placing them head to tail. The vector connecting the tail of **a** to the head of **b** is the sum or *resultant* vector **r**.

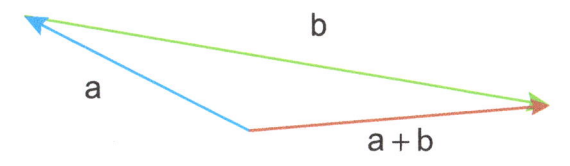

Figure III.B.1.1: The vector sum a + b = r. Notice that the bigger, green vector has the bigger effect on the direction of the resultant vector.

Subtraction of Vectors: To subtract the vector **b** from **a**, reverse the direction of **b** then add to **a**.

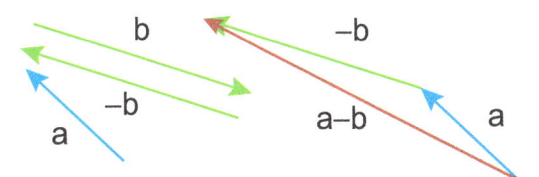

Figure III.B.1.2: The vector difference a − b = a + (−b) = r.

What happens if the vectors are in the same direction? Just sum their magnitudes and the direction remains the same.

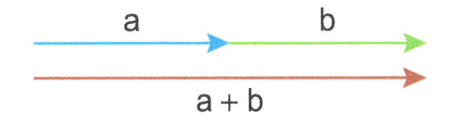

Why didn't we draw the red arrow from the tail of the blue arrow to the head of the green arrow? We wanted to avoid an overlapping rainbow and to remind you of the rule: "vectors can be moved in space but their orientation must be kept the same." For the vectors above, what would **a** − **b** look like? Nothing! Being the same length but opposite directions, they would exactly cancel.

What if there are many vectors? Again, draw to a common scale, place the arrows head to tail, and the vector connecting the tail of the first to the head of the last is the resultant vector (notice that the resultant depends on the initial position and the final position as opposed to every twist and turn on the way to the shop!):

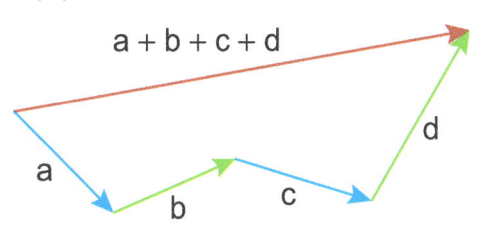

GAMSAT-Prep.com
GOLD STANDARD PHYSICS

High-level Importance

Imagine playing billiards or pool and every shot you intend to take is perfectly and directly lined up with a pocket. Wake up! Real life is usually a bit more chaotic than that. Normally you have to consider vectors: What angle should I hit that ball so that it moves at yet a different angle to head in the direction of the pocket? Once you have the direction lined up, you must contemplate the magnitude: Should I strike the ball with great strength or softly?

Air traffic controllers sometimes use the phrase "expect vectors for the visual approach..." when the plane nears the airport. When you dive into a pool, direction and magnitude can have a splash effect. Football, basketball, tennis – all sports are dependent on the direction and magnitude of velocity, acceleration, force, etc. Vectors at angles permeate life. How can we simplify the complexity? Sometimes the solution is to change the vector into its *x*-part and its *y*-part (*x* and *y*-components) so that we can compare everything happening in the *x*-direction in isolation, and then everything happening in the *y*-direction in isolation.

<u>Resolution of Vectors</u>: Perpendicular projections of a vector can be made on a coordinate axis. Thus the vector **a** can be *resolved* into its *x*-component (a_x) and its *y*-component (a_y).

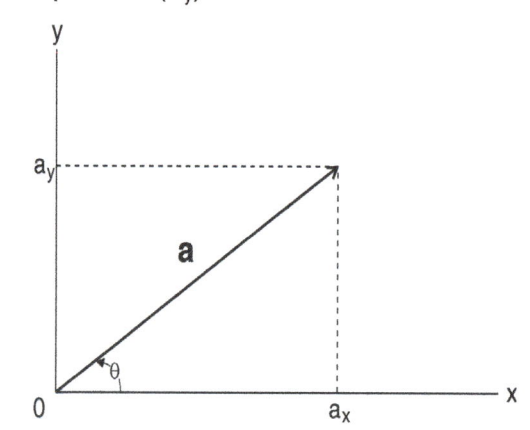

Figure III.B.1.3: The resolution of a vector into its scalar components in a coordinate system.

As an example, the cosine (*see* reminder PHY 1.1.1) of the angle θ gives the adjacent side (a_x) divided by the hypotenuse (**a**): $cos\ θ = a_x/a$. Multiply through by **a**, then follow the rules for sine, and you get:

$$a_x = a\ cos\ θ \quad \text{and} \quad a_y = a\ sin\ θ$$

Conversely, given the components, we can reconstruct vector **a** (thanks Pythagoras!):

$$a = \sqrt{a_x^2 + a_y^2} \quad \text{and} \quad tan\ θ = a_y/a_x$$

If you have not used vectors before, please consider trying the vector-related exercises in *Need for Speed* now, and then you can try the first 5 Foundational GAMSAT practice questions at the end of this chapter.

1.1.1 Trigonometric Functions: A Quick Reminder

The power in trigonometric functions lies in their ability to relate an angle to the ratio of scalar components or *sides* of a triangle. These functions may be defined as follows:

$$sin\ θ = opp/hyp = y/r$$
$$cos\ θ = adj/hyp = x/r$$

PHY-08   CHAPTER 1: TRANSLATIONAL MOTION

[*opp* = the length of the side opposite to angle θ, *adj* = the length of the side *adjacent* to angle θ, *hyp* = the length of the hypotenuse]

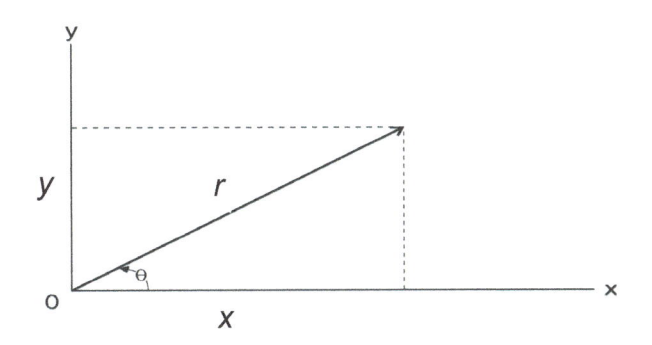

Thus sine (*r*sin θ) gives the *y*-component and cosine (*r*cos θ) gives the *x*-component of vector r. The tangent function (*tan* θ) relates sine and cosine:

$$\tan \theta = \sin \theta / \cos \theta = opp/adj = y/x$$

The Pythagorean theorem relates the sides of a right angle triangle according to the following:

$$r^2 = x^2 + y^2.$$

1.1.2 Common Values of Trigonometric Functions

There are special angles which produce standard values of the trigonometric functions. Several of the values are derived from the unit circle (GM 5.2) and can be resolved using the following triangles (you do not need to commit any of these values to memory; however, given the triangles, you should be able to confirm the values in the table):

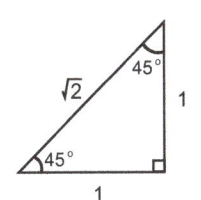

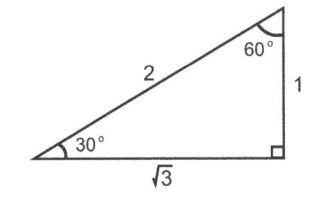

θ	sin θ	cos θ	tan θ
0°	0	1	0
30°	1/2	$\sqrt{3}/2$	$1/\sqrt{3}$
45°	$1/\sqrt{2}$	$1/\sqrt{2}$	1
60°	$\sqrt{3}/2$	1/2	$\sqrt{3}$
90°	1	0	-
180°	0	-1	0

Each trigonometric function (i.e. sine) contains an inverse function (i.e. $\sin^{-1}$), where if sin θ = x, θ = $\sin^{-1}$ x. Thus cos 60° = 1/2, and 60° = $\cos^{-1}$ (1/2). Some texts denote the inverse function with "arc" as a prefix. Thus arcsec (2) = $\sec^{-1}$ (2). {GM 5.3.1}

Table III.B.1.1:
Common values of trigonometric functions. The angle θ may be given in radians (R) where $2\pi^R$ = 360°= 1 revolution. Recall $\sqrt{3} \approx 1.7, \sqrt{2} \approx 1.4$ (GM 1.1.2, 1.5.6).

Note that 1° = 60 arcminutes, 1 arcminute = 60 arcseconds. These conversions do not need to be memorised because they would be given on the exam, if needed.

1.2 Distance and Displacement

Distance is the amount of separation between two points in space. As we have discussed, distance has a magnitude but no direction. It is a scalar quantity and is always positive.

Displacement of an object between two points is the difference between the final position and the initial position of the object in a given referential system (AKA, *frame of reference*; e.g. a coordinate system with an *x*-axis and a *y*-axis; or use a compass!). Thus, a displacement has an origin, a direction and a magnitude. It is a vector.

The sign of the coordinates of the vector displacement depends on the system under study and the chosen referential system. The sign will be positive (+) if the system is moving towards the positive axis of the referential system and negative (–) if not.

The units of distance and displacement are expressed in length units such as *feet (ft), metres (m), miles* and *kilometres (km)*. The International System of Units (SI), the standard for the GAMSAT and science in general, uses the metre for length (*see* GM 2.1.3).

1.3 Speed and Velocity

Speed is the rate of change of distance with respect to time. It is a scalar quantity, it has a magnitude but no direction, like distance, and it is always positive.

Velocity is the rate of change of displacement with respect to time. It is a vector, and like the displacement, it has a direction and a magnitude. Its value depends on the position of the object. The sign of the coordinates of the vector velocity is the same as that of the displacement.

The instantaneous velocity of a system at a given time is the slope of the graph of the displacement of that system vs. time at that time. The magnitude of the velocity decreases if the vector velocity and the vector acceleration have opposite directions.

The units of speed and velocity are expressed in length divided by time such as *feet/sec., metres/sec. (m/s)* and *miles/hour*.

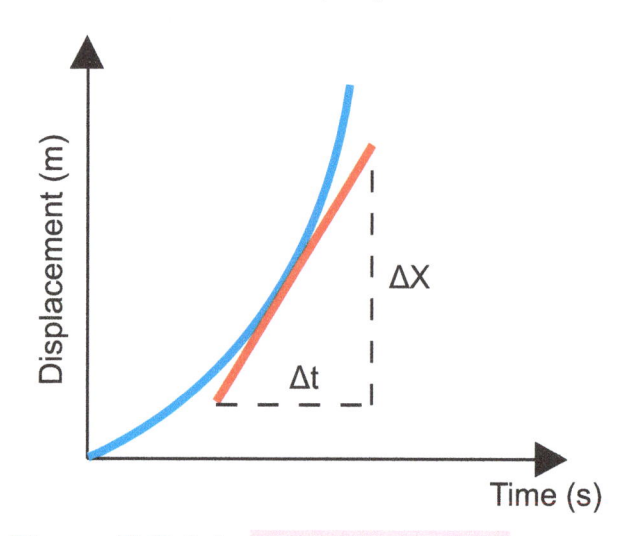

Figure III.B.1.4: Displacement vs. time. The capital letter X denotes displacement as opposed to referring to the *x*-axis (small letter *x*) which is time.

Dimensional Analysis: remember from GAMSAT Maths (GM 3.5.1) that a slope is "rise over run" meaning it is the change in the y-axis divided by the change in the x-axis. So, when we consider the units in Fig. III.B.1.4, we get m/s for the slope which is velocity in SI units (compare with the graph analysis of the velocity vs. time graph in GM 3.5.4).

1.3.1 Displacement, Time and Velocity

We will now transfer the words from PHY 1.3 into what is, or should become, an intuitive equation for you. Why? Because the following equation is literally saying, in SI units, m/s = m/s!

$$\text{Velocity} = \frac{\text{Displacement}}{\text{Time}}$$

You can use this equation to solve for any one of the three values if you know the other two.

EXAMPLE

A jogger runs the first 100 metres of a 5 km race in 24 seconds. If the jogger maintains the same pace until the end of the race, how long will it take her to run the entire race? *{Please work it out on your scratch paper before looking at the worked solution. If you have a strong science background, do not worry, kinematics and GAMSAT-level practice questions are coming in just a few more pages!}*

We are given a distance and a time, so we can easily find the velocity of the jogger.

$$v = \frac{100 \text{ m}}{24 \text{ s}}$$

The distance in question is in kilometres, so we could convert this velocity.

$$v = \frac{.1 \text{ km}}{24 \text{ s}}$$

Now we need to apply our velocity formula once more. We have a velocity and a distance, but we ultimately want to find the time.

$$\frac{.1 \text{ km}}{24 \text{ s}} = \frac{5 \text{ km}}{t}$$

$$\Rightarrow 5 \text{ km} \times 24 \text{ s} = .1 \text{ km} \times t$$

$$\Rightarrow \frac{(5 \times 24 \text{ s})}{.1} = \frac{120 \text{ s}}{\left(\frac{1}{10}\right)} = 120(10) \text{ s} = 1200 \text{ s} = t$$

By dimensional analysis (GM 2.2):

1200 s × (1 min./60 s) = 1200/60 = 120/6 = 20 min.

There are a half-dozen other ways to solve this problem, so as long as you have the correct answer, you can forge ahead because a lot more practice awaits you at the end of this chapter.

1.4 Acceleration, Deceleration: Speeding Up, Slowing Down

Acceleration (a) is the rate of change of the velocity (v) with respect to time (t):

$$a = \Delta v / \Delta t$$

Like the velocity, it is a vector and it has a direction and a magnitude. {Note that the Greek letter Δ is the symbol for 'change in'.}

The sign of the vector acceleration depends on the net force applied to the system and the chosen referential system. The units of acceleration are expressed as velocity divided by time such as metres/sec² (m/s²; SI units). The term for negative acceleration is deceleration.

Sports commentators will sometimes say that an athlete is accelerating if the person is moving fast. However, acceleration has nothing to do with going fast. A person can be moving very fast and still not be accelerating. Acceleration is related to the change in how fast a person or an object is moving. If there is no change in velocity, then the object is not accelerating.

1.4.1 Average and Instantaneous Acceleration

Anyone who has been in a car, bus, train or plane is acutely aware that constant acceleration is a rare, real-world experience. Speed up, slow down, turn, stop and repeat (to a different extent) ad nauseum. Measures that are somewhat more realistic than constant acceleration include the *average acceleration* and the *instantaneous acceleration* (we calculated the latter in GM 3.5.4).

The average acceleration a_v of any object is related to the change in velocity (v) over a given interval of time (t):

$$a_v = \frac{\Delta v}{\Delta t}$$

The instantaneous acceleration can be determined either by calculating the **slope** (*see* GM 3.5.4) of a velocity vs. time graph at any time, or by taking the limit when Δt approaches zero of the preceding expression.

$$a_v = \lim_{\Delta t \to 0} \frac{\Delta v}{\Delta t}$$

Maths involving "limits" does not exist on the GAMSAT. So let's discuss what this definition is describing in informal terms. The limit is the value of the change in velocity over the change in time as the time approaches 0. It's like saying that the change in velocity is happening in an instant. This allows us to talk about the acceleration in that incredibly fast moment: the instantaneous acceleration which can be determined graphically.

Consider the following events illustrated in the graph (Fig. III.B.1.5): your car starts at rest (0 velocity and time = 0); you steadily accelerate out of the parking lot (the change in velocity increases over time = acceleration); you are driving down the street at constant velocity (change in velocity = 0 and thus acceleration is 0 divided by the change in time which means: $a = 0$); you see a cat dart across the street which made you slow down temporarily (change in velocity is negative thus negative acceleration which, by definition, is deceleration; note to self: the cat is fine); you now enter the on-ramp for the highway so your velocity is now increasing at a faster and faster rate (increasing acceleration). You can examine the instantaneous acceleration at any one point (or instant) during the period that your acceleration is increasing.

To determine the displacement (*not* distance), take the area under the graph or curve. After all, if you multiply the units from the *y*-axis by those of the *x*-axis, we get m/s × s = m, which is the SI unit for displacement.

To calculate area: a rectangle is base (b) times height (h); a triangle is ½b × h; and for a curve, they can use graph paper and expect you would count the boxes under the curve to estimate the area (GM 3.5.4, Question 2), or, the curve may have a shape that can be approximated by a triangle, a rectangle, or some combination thereof (practice is coming!).

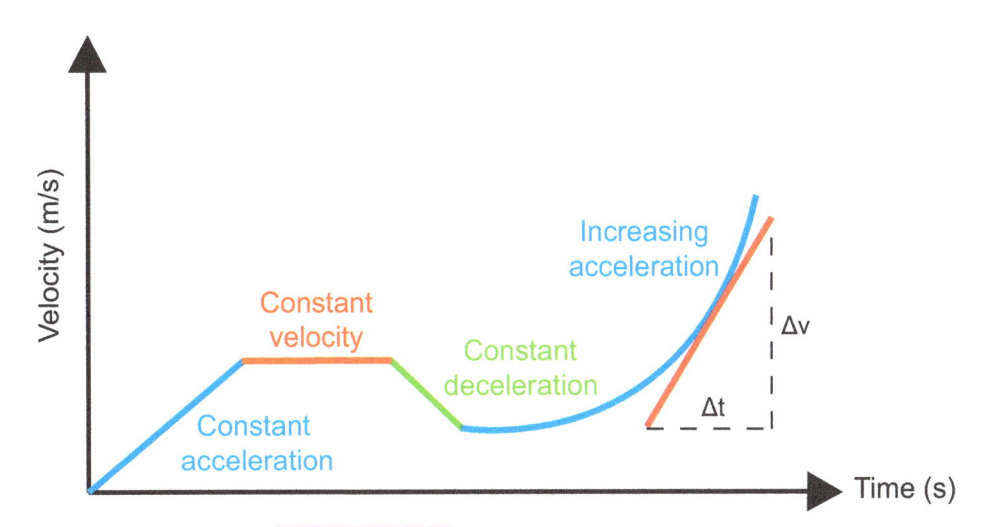

Figure III.B.1.5: Velocity vs. time. Note that at constant velocity, the slope and thus the acceleration are both equal to zero. Also note that during the period of increasing acceleration, to determine the instantaneous acceleration, one must be given the time and mark that point on the curve to generate a line tangential to the curve. The next step is to determine the slope of that line which comes from the change in *y*, velocity, over the change in *x*, time (GM 3.4.4, 3.5.4).

1.5 Uniformly Accelerated Motion

The magnitude and direction of the acceleration of a system are solely determined by the exterior forces acting upon the system. If the magnitude of these forces is constant, the magnitude of the acceleration will be constant and the resulting motion is a *uniformly accelerated motion*. The initial displacement, the velocity and the acceleration at any given time contribute to the over-all displacement of the system:

$x = x_0$ – displacement due to the initial displacement x_0.

$x = v_0 t$ – displacement due to the initial velocity v_0 at time t.

$x = \frac{1}{2}at^2$ – displacement due to the acceleration at time t.

The total displacement of the uniformly-accelerated motion is given by the following formula:

$$x = x_0 + v_0 t + \frac{1}{2}at^2$$

The translational motion is the motion of the centre of gravity (PHY 2.1) of a system through space, illustrated by the above equation.

1.6 Equations of Kinematics

Kinematics is the study of objects in motion with respect to space and time. There are three related equations and it is your choice as to whether or not to commit these 3 equations to memory. You will see in the Spoiler Alert references at the end of this chapter that ACER will normally provide these equations when needed. The first equation is in the preceding section (PHY 1.5), the others are:

$$v = v_0 + at \quad \text{and}$$
$$v^2 = v_0^2 + 2ax$$

where v is the final velocity; we will put these equations to use in PHY 2.6, and again in the GAMSAT-level practice questions at the end of Physics Chapter 2 (Questions 12, 13 and 14).

What's next? Perhaps a little break for exercise or coffee followed by 10 Foundational GAMSAT practice questions, followed by 10 GAMSAT-level practice questions. Do not worry about making mistakes. This is a process and you are building the foundations for something bigger.

CHAPTER 1: Translational Motion

GOLD STANDARD FOUNDATIONAL GAMSAT PRACTICE QUESTIONS

1) What is the SI unit for distance?

   A. kilometres
   C. centimetres
   B. metres
   D. m/s

2) All of the following are true EXCEPT one. Which one is the EXCEPTION?

   A. Vectors can be represented by an arrow on a scaled diagram; the length of the arrow represents the vector's magnitude and the direction it points represents the vector's direction.
   B. Scalar quantities have no direction and are never negative.
   C. Vectors can be added to vectors; scalars can be added to scalars.
   D. Vector and scalar quantities always have an associated direction.

3) Three little girls each pull on the same object with a 10 N force as shown below. The resultant force will be:

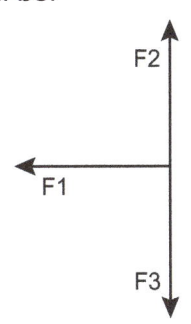

   A. zero
   C. 10 N to the right
   B. 10 N up or down
   D. 10 N to the left

4) An object experiences 3 forces: (i) 8 N south; (ii) 11 N north; (iii) 4 N east. What is the magnitude of the resultant force?

   A. 3 N
   C. 7 N
   B. 5 N
   D. 23 N

5) Consider the vectors **P** and **Q**.

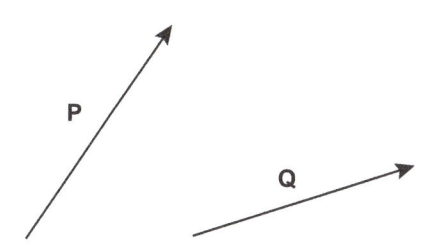

   Which of the following vectors is consistent with the resultant vector of **P** − **Q** ?

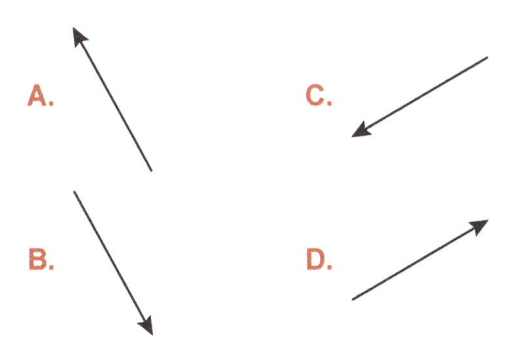

   A.
   B.
   C.
   D.

6) Which of the following represents a displacement (X) vs time (t) graph for a car driving at uniform speed?

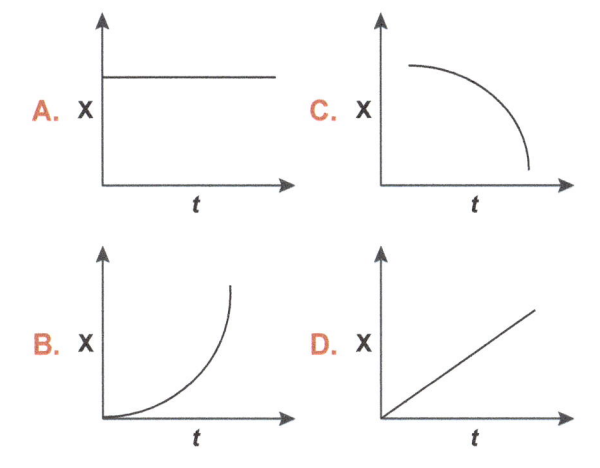

   A. X
   B. X
   C. X
   D. X

Questions 7-9

An Olympic athlete is performing running exercises that are timed and graphed by her trainers. Consider the results in Figure 1 for the next 3 questions.

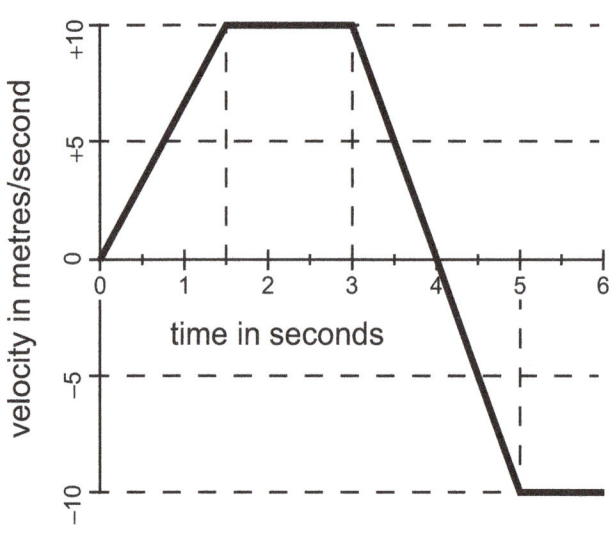

Figure 1

7) For *only* the time period 0 < t < 1.5 seconds, which of the following graphs represents the acceleration (*a*) versus time (*t*)?

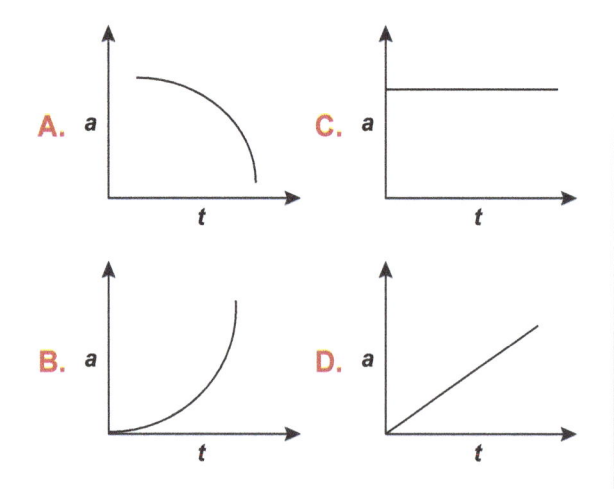

A. *a*
B. *a*
C. *a*
D. *a*

8) Based on Figure 1, for *only* the time period 0 < t < 1.5 seconds, which of the graphs below represents the displacement (X) travelled versus time (*t*)?

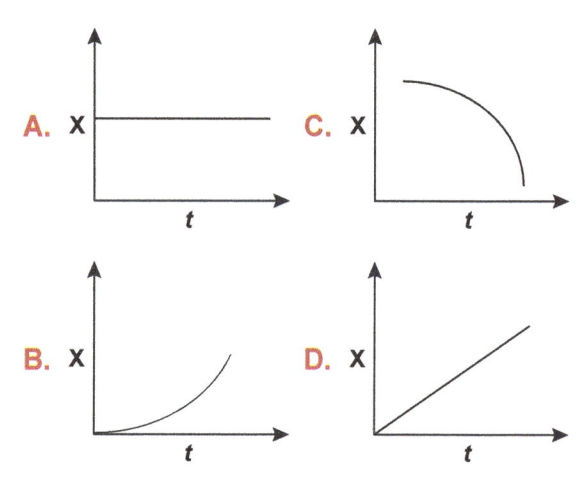

A. X
B. X
C. X
D. X

9) The runner starts at position X = 0. What is the final position (as measured from X = 0) after she runs through the motion described by Figure 1, from t = 0 seconds to t = 5 seconds?

A. 22.5 m
B. 25 m
C. 27.5 m
D. 32.5 m

10) Where in the figure shown below is the velocity positive?

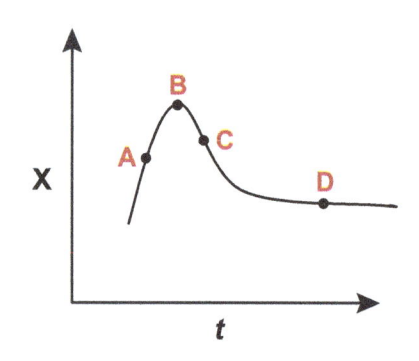

PHY-16   CHAPTER 1: TRANSLATIONAL MOTION

GAMSAT MASTERS SERIES

GOLD STANDARD GAMSAT-LEVEL PRACTICE QUESTIONS

Questions 11–15

Motor vehicle crashes account for nearly 1.3 million deaths worldwide every year and is the 9th leading cause of death. While the first mass-produced car was sold in 1903, it wasn't until the mid-1960s when vehicle safety standards started to become implemented, including the use of crash-test dummies.

Crash-test dummies, which are anthropomorphic devices used in simulated car crashes, allow companies to measure the forces a driver experiences during and after impact. These tests help car manufacturers design cars to keep passengers safe by minimising the amount of force they feel during a collision. In a research study sponsored by the National Highway Traffic Safety Administration (NHTSA), a test dummy in a Dodge Grand Caravan SE was crashed into a barrier with an impact velocity of 56.3 km/h (kph). The test dummy was prepared with a head accelerometer which recorded the "driver's" head velocity as a function of time as shown in Figure 1.

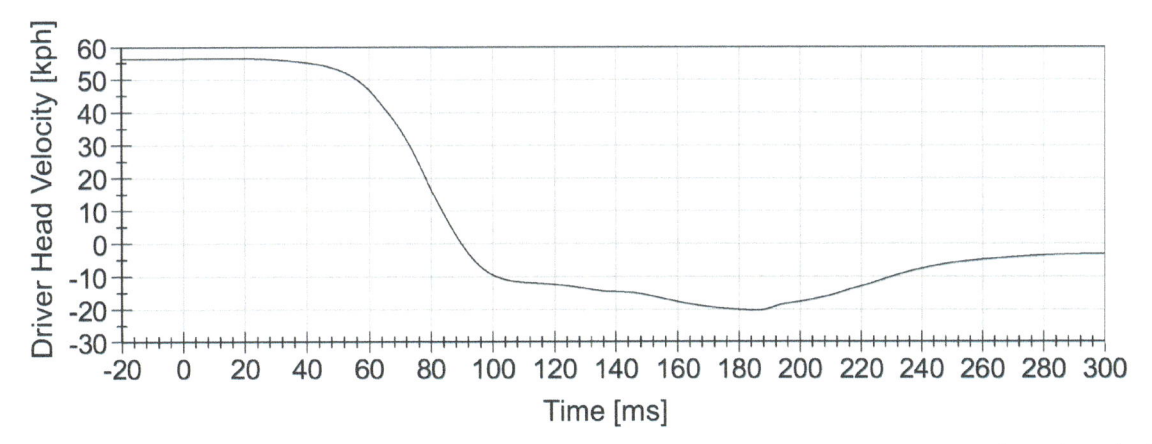

Figure 1: Velocity [kph] vs. time [ms] of the translational motion [along one axis] of the head of the test dummy. The car crash occurs at time = 0 ms.

Car manufacturers use measures such as the Head Injury Criterion (HIC) to determine the likelihood of a head injury in a collision. The HIC is proportional to the force the driver feels and the time duration of the acceleration. Crash-test dummies provide a means for measuring the HIC of various cars and are used to determine the NHTSA star rating for automobile safety. Cars with larger HIC values are ranked less safe.

11) During which time interval did the driver experience the highest risk of a head injury?

   A. 10-20 ms
   B. 70-80 ms
   C. 100-110 ms
   D. 180-190 ms

12) According to Figure 1, which of the following is the closest estimate of the maximum deceleration felt by the driver?

   A. 0.5 km/s^2
   B. 1 km/s^2
   C. 10 km/s^2
   D. 100 km/s^2

GAMSAT-Prep.com
GOLD STANDARD PHYSICS

High-level Importance

13) Given that the collision starts at t = 0 ms, what is the total distance the driver's head travels while decelerating?

A. 0.04 m
B. 0.4 m
C. 4 m
D. 40 m

14) Which of the following graphs best illustrates the driver's head deceleration after the impact?

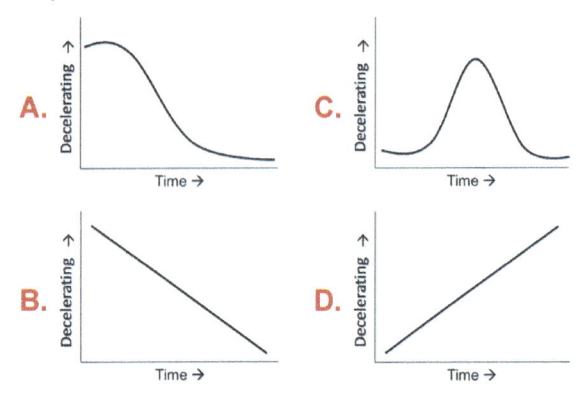

A. [graph: decelerating vs time, curve starting high, plateau then decreasing]
B. [graph: decelerating vs time, linear decreasing]
C. [graph: decelerating vs time, bell-shaped peak]
D. [graph: decelerating vs time, linear increasing]

15) Impulse is the change of momentum (Δp) of an object when the object is acted upon by a force (F) for an interval of time (Δt). So, with impulse, you can calculate the change in momentum, or you can use impulse to calculate the average impact force of a collision.

$$p = m\,\Delta v = F\,\Delta t$$

where the momentum (m Δv) is the product of mass (m) and the change in velocity (Δv).

Airbags are designed to inflate during a collision when the car slows down and deflate when the driver hits the airbag. Airbag deflation helps protect the driver by accomplishing which of the following?

A. Decreasing the contact time between the driver and the airbag
B. Decreasing the driver's change in momentum
C. Increasing the pressure on the driver
D. Increasing the collision time between the driver and the airbag

16) Fluoroscopy is an imaging technique that uses X-rays to obtain real-time moving images of the interior of the body. A patient was asked to perform cycles of deep inspiration and deep expiration. Fluoroscopy was used to measure the linear velocity of the movement of the diaphragm and the data was plotted against time. The origin in Figure 1 is the reference time 0 when the diaphragm was essentially in its equilibrium position.

Based on Figure 1, at what time after t = 0 is the total displacement of the diaphragm at a minimum?

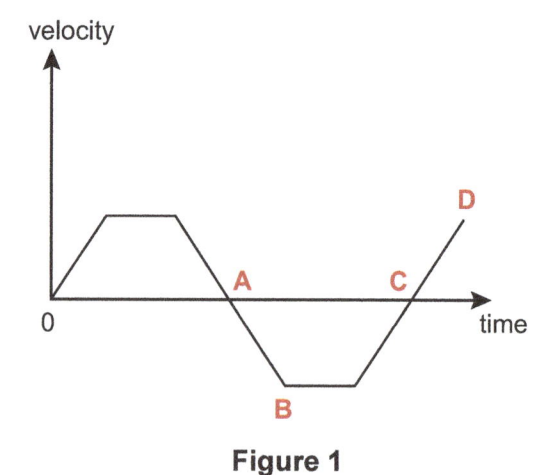

[Figure 1: velocity vs time graph showing points A (positive peak region returning to axis), B (negative trough), C (crossing axis), D (positive peak)]

Figure 1

17) A Doppler study of a patient's aorta was used to determine the speed of blood flow at 0.40 m/s in the thoracic aorta and then at a point 0.4 m away, 0.20 m/s in the abdominal aorta. Assuming that the blood flow slowed at a constant rate, what is the rate that the blood slowed between the 2 points measured along the aorta?

A. 0.15 m/s²
B. 0.30 m/s²
C. 1.50 m/s²
D. 3.00 m/s²

PHY-18 CHAPTER 1: TRANSLATIONAL MOTION

Questions 18–20

Hubble's law is the observation in cosmology that galaxies are moving away from the Earth at speeds proportional to their distance. Hubble's law is often expressed by the following equation:

$$v = H \times D$$

with H being the constant of proportionality—Hubble's constant—between the distance D to a galaxy, and its speed of separation v.

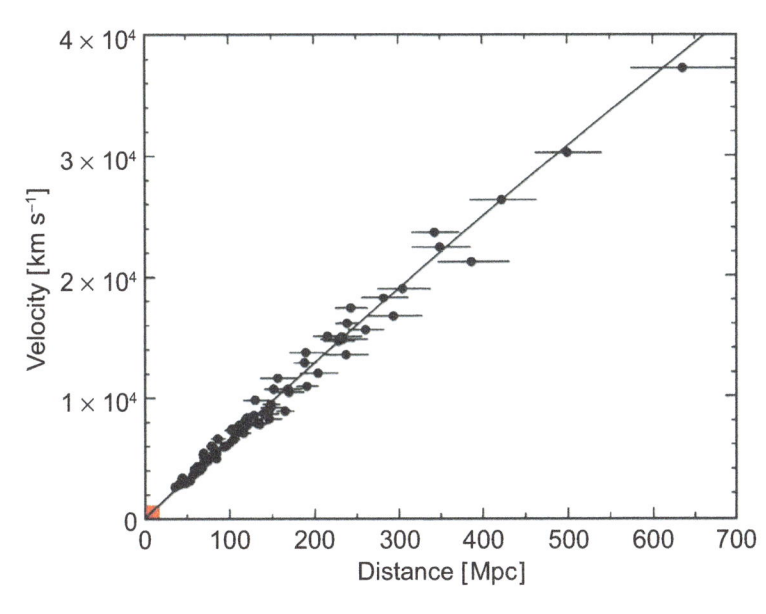

Figure 1: Hubble Diagram for Type Ia Supernovae. The very small red area represents the original data from Edwin Hubble used to make predictions about the universe. (redrawn after Kirshner 2004, National Academy of Sciences)

Note that:
- A megaparsec (Mpc) is one million parsecs, or about 3 260 000 light years.
- A light year is the distance that light travels in one year, approximately 1×10^{13} km.

18) Based on Figure 1, what are the units of Hubble's constant?

A. km s⁻¹ Mpc⁻¹
B. km s Mpc
C. (km/s) Mpc⁻¹
D. (km/s) Mpc⁻²

19) Using the units of Figure 1, the value of Hubble's constant can be approximated by which of the following?

A. 0.6
B. 6
C. 60
D. 120

20) Figure 1 presents data most consistent with which of the following?

A. There is a constant velocity at which galaxies are moving away irrespective of distance.
B. A velocity of 6000 km/s corresponds to a distance of approximately 3.3×10^{21} m.
C. A higher than expected Hubble's constant would suggest that at a given velocity, the distance is greater than anticipated.
D. The farther the galaxies, the faster they are moving away from Earth.

GAMSAT-Prep.com
GOLD STANDARD PHYSICS

SPOILER ALERT ⚠️

Gold Standard has cross-referenced the content in this chapter to examples from ACER's official GAMSAT practice materials (note that only ACER sells their eBooks brand new). It is for you to decide when you want to explore these questions since you may want to preserve some of ACER's materials for timed mock-exam practice.

Number	1	2	3	4	5
Title	GAMSAT Practice Questions	GAMSAT Sample Questions	GAMSAT Practice Test	GAMSAT Practice Test 2	GAMSAT Practice Test 3
Colour	Orange/Red	Blue	Green	Purple	Pink

Examples – Deceleration in a blood vessel: Q12 of 1; vectors, sin/cos but torque (PHY 4): Q44-47 of 2; equations of kinematics, graphs and dimensional analysis: Q36-41 of 4; light year calculation Q87 of 5. Note that "Q" is followed by the question number, and, for example, "of 1" refers to booklet number 1 in the table above. Also note that your gamsat-prep.com Masters Series online account has direct links to the step-by-step worked solutions for all of ACER's Section 3 practice questions (the solutions can also be found in the Gold Standard GAMSAT YouTube Channel). The 10 full-length HEAPS GAMSAT practice tests (by Gold Standard and MediRed), exams 1 through 10, contain specific cross-references to this chapter within the worked solutions. Note that the motor vehicle crash unit is from HEAPS-3. We will be exploring the use of kinematics equations in the GAMSAT-level practice questions in Physics Chapter 2.

Chapter Checklist

☐ Access your free online account at www.gamsat-prep.com/gamsat-maths-physics to view answers, worked solutions and discussion boards for chapter-ending practice questions.

☐ Reassess your 'learning objectives' for this chapter: Go back to the first page of this chapter and re-evaluate the top 3 boxes and the Introduction.

  ☐ Please be sure that you have completed the *Need for Speed* exercises at the beginning of this chapter.

☐ Complete a maximum of 1 page of notes using symbols/abbreviations to represent the entire chapter based on your learning objectives. These are your Gold Notes.

☐ Consider your multimedia options based on your optimal way of learning:

  ☐ Download the free Gold Standard GAMSAT app for your Android device or iPhone.
  ☐ Create your own, tangible study cards or try the free app: Anki.
  ☐ Record your voice reading your Gold Notes onto your smartphone (MP3s) and listen during exercise, transportation, etc.
  ☐ Try out the Gold Standard GAMSAT online videos at gamsat-prep.com, or you can try other options on YouTube like Khan Academy or Crash Course Physics.

☐ Schedule your full-length GAMSAT practice tests: ACER and/or HEAPS exams. Schedule one full day to complete a practice test and 1-2 days for a thorough assessment of worked solutions while adding to your abbreviated Gold Notes.

☐ Schedule and/or evaluate stress reduction techniques such as regular exercise (sports), yoga, meditation and/or mindfulness exercises (*see* YouTube for suggestions).

FORCE, MOTION, AND GRAVITATION
Chapter 2

Memorise
* Define with units: weight, mass
* Newton's laws, Law of Gravitation

Understand
* Mass, weight, centre of gravity
* Newton's laws
* Law of Gravitation, free-fall motion
* Projectile motion equations and calculations

Importance
Medium level: 6% of GAMSAT Physics questions released by ACER are related to content in this chapter (in our estimation).
* Note that approximately **75%** of the questions in GAMSAT Physics are related to just 6 chapters: 1, 4, 6, 9, 11 and 12.

GAMSAT-Prep.com

Introduction

Force is a vector (often a push or pull) that can cause a mass to change velocity, thus motion. Forces can be due to gravity, magnetism, or anything that causes a mass to accelerate including you! You can push or pull (which demands an examination of Newton's laws!), or you can drop something (*free-fall motion*), or perhaps you might want to throw this book through the air (*projectile motion*, which is often simplified by resolving vectors into *x* and *y*-components). We will examine all of these possibilities before experiencing some GAMSAT-level practice!

Multimedia Resources at GAMSAT-Prep.com

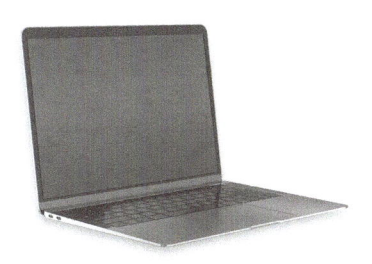

Open Discussion Boards   Foundational Videos   Flashcards   Special Guest

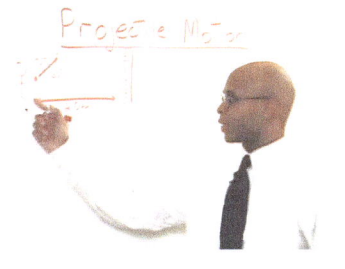

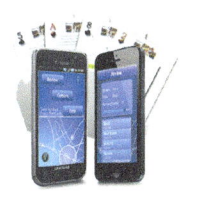

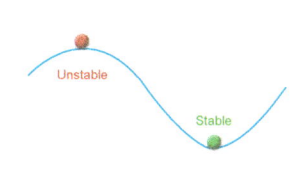

* The real GAMSAT may have advanced-level information presented (i.e. in a passage) but previous knowledge of said information is not required to answer the questions that would follow. Practice questions at the end of this chapter, as well as ACER and GS (HEAPS) practice GAMSATs can help you clarify this point.

GAMSAT-Prep.com
GOLD STANDARD PHYSICS

2.0 GAMSAT has a *Need for Speed*!

Section Number	GAMSAT Physics *Need for Speed* Exercises
2.1	The motion of an object can be described as depending on what point? (*two answers are possible*)
	How is weight related to mass?
2.2	How is force related to acceleration (Newton's 2nd law)?
2.3	Newton's 3rd law, complete the expression: For every action, there is…
2.4	The Law of Gravitation is an inverse square law, where F =
2.5	When an object drops (free fall), in the absence of air resistance, does its acceleration change?
	Approximate the acceleration due to gravity in SI units:
2.6 (*projectile motion*) Note: Only the 'initial speed' and 'magnitude' equations are essential.	initial speed in the *y*-direction as it relates to the initial speed V_o and the angle α with the horizontal: V_{oy} =
	displacement at time t as it relates to V_{oy} and g: y =
	speed at any time t as it relates to V_{oy} and g: V_y =
	magnitude of the initial velocity as it relates to the initial velocities in the *x* and *y*-directions (hint: Pythagoras; PHY 1.1.1): $|V_o|$ =
	When an object is thrown in the air, what is its vertical velocity (V_y) at its highest point (Y_{max})?
	Neglecting air resistance, how is the final velocity in the *x*-direction (V_x) related to the original velocity in the *x*-direction (V_{ox})?
	If you throw an object in the air, at what angle to the ground should you throw it so that it goes as far as possible (i.e. the greatest horizontal distance, or *range*)?

Medium-level Importance

PHY-22 CHAPTER 2: FORCE, MOTION, AND GRAVITATION

2.1 Mass, Centre of Mass, Weight

The mass (*m*) of an object is its measure of inertia. It is the measure of the capacity of that object to remain motionless or to move with a constant velocity if the sum of the forces acting upon it is zero. This definition is derived from Newton's first law.

The *centre of mass* of an object is a point whose motion can be described as the motion of a particle through space. The centre of mass of an object: 1) always has the simplest motion of all the points of that object; 2) is always in the middle of an object with an even distribution of mass (*uniform*).

The *centre of gravity* (COG) is the centre of mass seen as the centre of application of all the gravitational forces acting on the object. For example, for a uniform plank hanging horizontally, the COG is at half the length of the plank. {Note: For GAMSAT, the centre of mass and COG are the same.}

The COG can be determined experimentally by suspending an object by a string at different points and noting that the direction of the string passes through the COG.

The intersection of the projected lines in the different suspensions is the COG.

An object is in *stable equilibrium* if the COG is as low as possible and any change in orientation will lead to an elevation of the COG. An object is in *unstable equilibrium* if the COG is high relative to the support point or surface and any change in orientation will lead to a lowering of the COG.

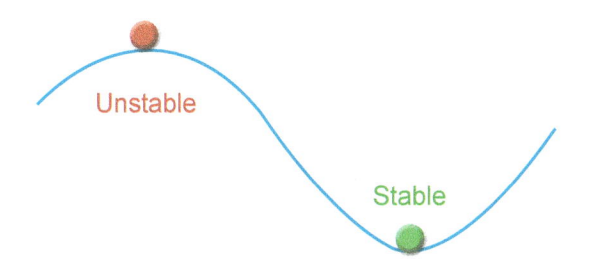

Unstable

Stable

The *weight* is a force (i.e. newtons, pounds). It is a vector unlike the *mass* which is a scalar (i.e. kilograms, slugs). The weight is proportional to the mass. It is the product of the mass by the vector gravitational acceleration *g*.

$$W = m \times g$$

2.2 Newton's Second Law

Newton's second law states that the sum (Σ) of all the exterior forces (*F*) acting upon the centre of mass of a system is equal to the product of the mass (*m*) of the system by the acceleration (*a*) of its centre of mass.

Therefore, if there is a net force, the object must accelerate. It is a vectorial equality which asserts that a net force against an object *must* result in acceleration:

$$\Sigma F = m \times a$$

GAMSAT-Prep.com
GOLD STANDARD PHYSICS

It is important to note that for a system in complex motion, Newton's second law can only determine the acceleration of the centre of mass. It does not give any indication about the motion of the other parts of the system.

Whereas, for a system in translational motion, Newton's second law gives the acceleration of the system.

In your daily life, you would already have the sense that objects with a greater mass (m) require a greater force (F) to get it to move with increasing speed (a). If you maintain a net force on an object, it will not only move, it must accelerate. We will be exploring more consequences of Newton's second law both in this and later chapters.

2.3 Newton's Third Law

Newton's third law states that for every action there is an equal and opposite reaction. If one object exerts a force, F, on a second object, the second object exerts a force, F', on the first object. F and F' have opposite direction but the same magnitude.

One conclusion would be that forces are found in pairs. Consider the time you sit in a chair. Your body exerts a force downward (mg, your weight) and that chair needs to exert an equal force upward (the normal force N) or the chair will collapse. There is symmetry. Acting forces encounter other forces in the opposite direction. Consider shooting a cannonball. When the explosion fires the cannonball through the air, the cannon is pushed backward. The force pushing the ball out is equal to the force pushing the cannon back, but the effect on the cannon is less noticeable because it has a much larger mass and it may be restrained. Similarly, a gun experiences a "kick" backwards when a bullet is fired forward.

2.4 The Law of Gravitation

The Law of Gravitation states that there is a force of attraction existing between any two bodies of masses m_1 and m_2. The force is proportional to the product of the masses and inversely proportional to the square of the distance between them (reminder: we explored a GAMSAT-level practice question based on the Law of Gravitation in GM 2.2.1).

$$F = K_G(m_1 m_2 / r^2)$$

r is the distance between the bodies (NOT the radius of either mass); K_G is the universal constant of gravitation, and its value depends on the units being used.

2.5 Free-fall Motion

The free-fall motion of an object is the upward or downward vertical motion of that object with reference to the earth.

The motion is always uniformly accelerated with the acceleration g: vertical, directed towards the centre of the earth and the magnitude is considered constant during the free-fall motion.

Also, during free-fall motion, the air resistance is considered negligible. The equation of the motion can easily be derived from Newton's second law.

$$\Sigma F = ma$$

Where ΣF represents the sum of all the forces acting on the object, m is the mass of the object and a is the acceleration of the centre of mass of the object. Hence, a can be replaced by g since $a = g$, by definition. In free-fall motion, the only force acting on the object is the gravitational force, which gives the following equality:

$$K_G m_{object} \frac{M_{earth}}{r^2_{earth}} = m_{object}\, g$$

dividing both sides by m_{object} we get:

$$g = K_G \frac{M_{earth}}{r^2_{earth}}$$

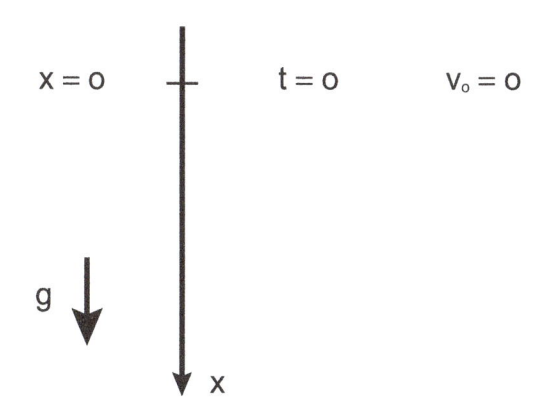

Figure III.B.2.1: Free-fall motion.

(x = 0, t = 0, v_0 = 0, g directed downward along x)

The value of g in SI units is 9.8 m/s², though usually ACER will let you use the estimate of 10 m/s². The equation for uniformly accelerated motion (PHY 1.5) is applicable by replacing a by g:

$$x = x_0 + v_0 t + 1/2 g t^2$$

$$v = gt$$

$$a = g$$

Before doing any calculation, the reference point and a positive direction must be chosen. In the free fall of an actual object, the value of g is modified by the buoyancy (PHY 6.1.2) of air and resistance of air. This results in a *drag force* which depends on the location on earth, shape and size of the object, and the velocity of the object (as free-fall velocity increases, the drag force increases). When the drag force reaches the force of gravity, the object reaches a final velocity called the terminal velocity and continues to fall at that velocity.

2.6 Projectile Motion

The *projectile motion* is the motion of any object fired or launched at some angle α from the horizontal (Figure III.B.2.2). The motion defines a parabola (*see* GM 3.5.2) in the plane O-x-y that contains the initial (*original*) vector velocity v_o.

The motion can be decomposed into two distinct motions: a vertical (up and down, y) component, affected by g, and a horizontal (i.e. a viewer might see the motion as side to side; x), independent of g. Algebra and trigonometry help to resolve vectors into their x and y-components, which (believe it or not!) simplifies the problem (PHY 2.6.1).

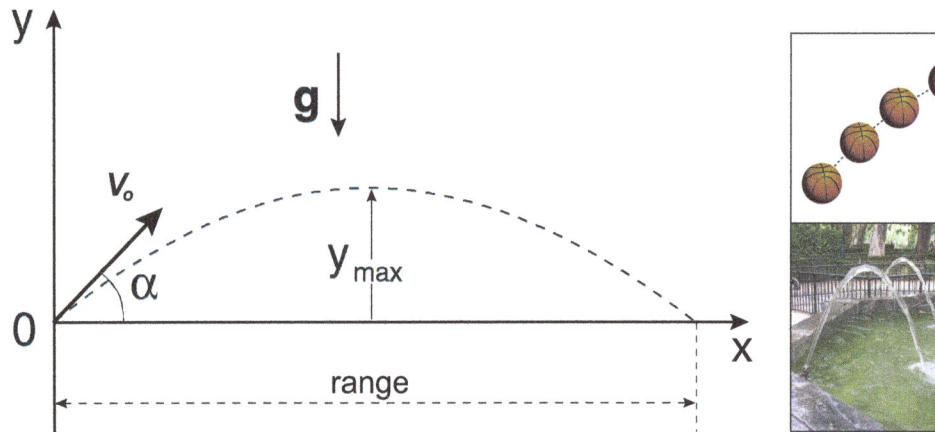

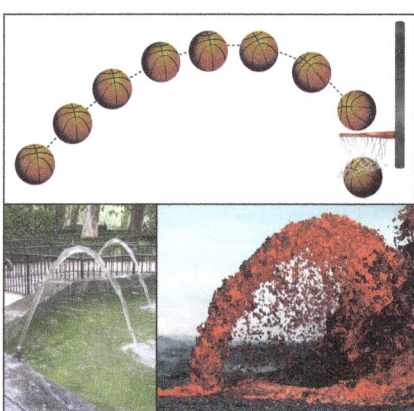

Figure III.B.2.2: Projectile motion: Graph deconstructing the main features with analysis below. Inset images demonstrating parabolic motion (GM 3.5.2): a basketball (all net!); a fountain's water in Madrid (GuidoB, Wikimedia Commons); and a volcano's lava in Hawaii (Griggs, usgs.gov).

Vertical component (free fall)
- initial speed : $V_{oy} = V_o \sin α$
- displacement at time t: $y = V_{oy}t + 1/2gt^2$
- speed at any time t: $V_y = V_{oy} + gt$

Initial velocity (*see* PHY 1.1.1)
- magnitude: $|V_o| = \sqrt{V_{ox}^2 + V_{oy}^2}$
- direction: *alpha*: $\tan α = V_{oy} / V_{ox}$
- important points to consider:

1) Neglecting air resistance, there is no acceleration in the horizontal direction: V_x is constant.
2) V_y is zero at Y_{max}, then $V_y = 0 = V_{oy} + gt_{up}$ or $-V_{oy} = gt_{up}$ can be solved for t.

Horizontal component (linear with constant speed)
- initial speed : $V_{ox} = V_o \cos α$
- displacement at any time t: $x = V_{ox}t$
- speed at any time t: $V_x = V_{ox}$ (speed is constant)

3) Also, by eliminating the variables y and t in the equations, we can get the following equality:

$$x = \frac{V_o^2 \sin 2α}{g}$$

The horizontal distance from the origin to where the object strikes the ground (= *the range*) is maximum for a given V_o when $\sin 2α = 1$, hence for $2α = (π/2)^R$ => $α = (π/4)^R$ or $α = 45$ degrees.

2.6.1 Projectile Motion Problem (Imperial units)

In the Rugby World Cup, a player kicks the ball at an angle of 30° from the horizontal with an initial speed of 75 ft/s. Assume that the ball moves in a vertical plane and that air resistance is negligible.

Note that:
- acceleration due to gravity: 32 ft/s²
- there are 3 feet in 1 yard
- feel free to return to PHY 1.1.2 to find the solution to any trigonometric function you believe would help solve this problem.

(a) *Find the time at which the ball reaches the highest point of its trajectory.*

{key: height refers to the y-component, and we can define gravity as a negative vector since it is directed downwards; note that when the projectile reaches the maximum height, it stops moving up and starts falling. In other words, its vertical velocity component changes from positive to negative, which means it must be equal to 0 for a very brief moment in time.}

V_y is zero at Y_{max} (= the highest point), thus:

$V_y = 0$, $V_o = 75$ ft/s, $\alpha = 30°$, $g = -32$ ft/s²

$V_y = V_o \sin \alpha + gt_{up}$, $\sin 30° = 1/2$ (PHY 1.1.2)

Isolate t_{up}:

$$t_{up} = \frac{V_y - V_o \sin \alpha}{g} = \frac{-75(\sin 30°)}{-32}$$

$= 75(\frac{1}{2})/32 = 75/64 = 1\frac{11}{64} = 1.2$ s

(b) *How high does the ball go?*

$Y_{max} = V_o (\sin \alpha) t_{up} + 1/2 g t_{up}^2$

$Y_{max} = 75(\sin 30°)1.2 + 1/2(-32)(1.2)^2$

$= 75(0.6) - 32(0.72) = 45 - 23 = 22$ feet

(c) *How long is the ball in the air and what is its range?*

{key: time is the same for x- and y-components, range = x-component}

Once the ball strikes the ground its vertical displacement y = 0, thus:

$y = 0 = V_o (\sin \alpha) t + 1/2 g t^2$

Divide through by t then isolate:

$t = 2V_o(\sin \alpha)/g = 2.4$ seconds.

Since $t = 2t_{up}$, we can conclude that the time required for the ball to go up to Y_{max} is the same as the time required to come back down: 1.2 seconds in either direction.

The range $x = V_o(\cos \alpha)t$

$x = 75(\cos 30°)2.4 \approx 150$ feet, or:

$x \approx 150$ ft (1 yd/ 3 ft) = 50 yards

{Had the player kicked the ball at 45° from the horizontal he would have maximised his range (see the last paragraph in PHY 2.6). He should be benched for not having done his physics!}

GAMSAT-Prep.com
GOLD STANDARD PHYSICS

(d) *What is the velocity of the ball as it strikes the ground?*

{*key:* **velocity** is the resultant vector of V_x and V_y - the final velocities in the x and y directions}

$V_x = V_o \cos α = 75(\cos 30°) = 65$ ft/s

$V_y = V_o \sin α + gt$

$\quad = 75(\sin 30°) + (-32)(2.4) = -39$ ft/s

$V = \sqrt{V_x^2 + V_y^2} = \sqrt{(65)^2 + (-39)^2}$

$\quad = \sqrt{(13 \times 5)^2 + (13 \times -3)^2}$

$V = 13\sqrt{(5)^2 + (-3)^2} = 13\sqrt{34}$

To estimate $\sqrt{34}$ we must first recognise that the answer must be at least 5 ($5^2 = 25$) but closer to 6 ($6^2 = 36$). Try squaring 5.7, 5.8, 5.9. Squaring 5.8 is the closest estimate (= *33.6*), thus

$V = 13(5.8) = 75$ ft/s.

Please note:
- With no air resistance and a symmetric problem (the ball is launched and returns to the same vertical point), the initial and final speeds are the same (75 ft/s).
- Usually ACER will use SI units in GAMSAT problems, but many problems on the real GAMSAT are solved using dimensional analysis, with or without SI units.
- Please be sure you can do all the preceding calculations efficiently. To learn more about SI units, *see* GM 2.1.3.

Medium-level Importance

It's time for a fireside chat!

Usually, variables used in equations are English or Greek letters, such as x or θ. One of the frustrations that some students have when learning or revising Physics, is that they begin to notice that the variables used in equations, for the same parameters, are not consistent. Distance is d, but sometimes D, or x, or X (some textbooks use S), and then there's r (but it is not necessarily the radius), and coming later in the book, distances: i, f, o, λ, and so on.

F is not ma. They are just symbols, models, abbreviations for the big idea: the acceleration of an object is directly related to the net force and inversely related to its mass. That makes sense. Or, considered another way: A net force results in a mass undergoing acceleration. F = ma is like saying Bugs Bunny is an accurate representation of a rabbit. There are key similarities, but nothing trumps the true concept. Do not get attached to variables, they are cartoons. Try, when possible, to get a sense of the meaning. It is usually relatable, well, until we get to the last chapter and talk about atoms!

This discussion is only relevant because some examiners (and yes, occasionally ACER does this) set traps for students trying to commit to memory an idea that they do not understand. Forewarned is forearmed!

PHY-28   CHAPTER 2: FORCE, MOTION, AND GRAVITATION

GAMSAT MASTERS SERIES

CHAPTER 2: Force, Motion, and Gravitation

GOLD STANDARD FOUNDATIONAL GAMSAT PRACTICE QUESTIONS

1) Consider a situation where you accidentally bump into a vase which then tilts briefly, but then returns to the upright position. When you initially bumped the vase, its centre of gravity moved (note: gravitational potential energy is given by weight, mg, times height):

   A. upward and its gravitational potential energy increased.
   B. downward and its gravitational potential energy decreased.
   C. downward and its gravitational potential energy increased.
   D. upward and its gravitational potential energy decreased.

2) A torus of revolution is ring-shaped and can be generated by revolving a circle in three-dimensional space about an axis. A torus of revolution was constructed from a uniform aluminum frame and laid on the ground on its side as shown in the diagram.

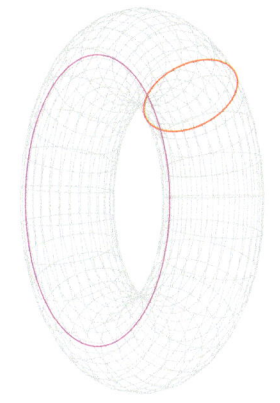

   The diameter of the red circle used to generate the torus is 2 m. The distance from the centre of the tube to the centre of the torus is 6 m. Which of the following best approximates the centre of gravity of the torus as measured from the ground?

   A. 1 m
   B. 2 m
   C. 6 m
   D. 7 m

3) Which unit is equivalent to N/kg (newton per kilogram)?

   A. J • s
   B. m/s^2
   C. kg • m/s
   D. m/s

4) Newton's second law states that the net force is equal to the product of mass and acceleration (F = ma). Consider a net force of 10 N that accelerates an object to 5.0 m/s^2. What net force would be required to accelerate the same object to 1.0 m/s^2?

   A. 2.0 N
   B. 3.0 N
   C. 4.0 N
   D. 5.0 N

5) A 1.0 kg cart and a 2.0 kg cart are pushed apart by an expanding spring. If the average force on the 1.0 kg cart is 1.0 N, what is the average force on the 2.0 kg cart?

   A. 0.0 N
   B. 0.5 N
   C. 1.0 N
   D. 2.0 N

THE PHYSICAL SCIENCES PHY-29

6) A woman travels to a planet that has twice the radius of Earth and twice the mass. Her weight on that planet compared to her weight on Earth is:

   A. doubled.
   B. quartered.
   C. halved.
   D. cannot be determined with the information given.

7) If an object is moved from the surface of the Earth to a location two Earth-radii above the surface of the Earth, then the force of gravitational attraction between the object and the Earth will be what fraction of the magnitude as if it were on Earth's surface?

   A. One-half
   B. One-fourth
   C. One-ninth
   D. One-sixteenth

8) Four balls leave a cliff at the same time, launched from the same height. Their initial horizontal (v_{ox}) and vertical (v_{oy}) velocities in m/s are shown. Air resistance is negligible.

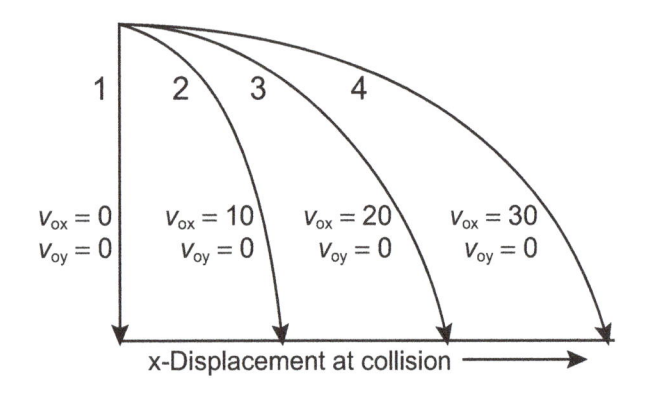

   Ball 1: $v_{ox} = 0$, $v_{oy} = 0$
   Ball 2: $v_{ox} = 10$, $v_{oy} = 0$
   Ball 3: $v_{ox} = 20$, $v_{oy} = 0$
   Ball 4: $v_{ox} = 30$, $v_{oy} = 0$

   x-Displacement at collision →

   Which ball hits the ground first?

   A. Ball 1
   B. Ball 2 or 3
   C. Ball 4
   D. All four projectiles will hit the ground at the same time.

9) An object is launched at 45 degrees from the horizontal. Neglecting air resistance, the final horizontal velocity would be equal to:

   A. (displacement)(sine 45°).
   B. (displacement)(cosine 45°).
   C. (1/2) the initial horizontal velocity.
   D. the initial horizontal velocity.

10) In the absence of air resistance, a cricket ball is thrown from point **A** and follows a parabolic path, as shown in the diagram, in which the highest point reached is point **B**.

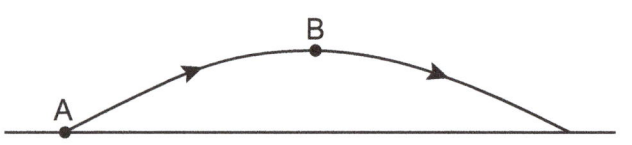

   The vertical component of acceleration of the cricket ball, as it follows this path, is:

   A. zero at **B**.
   B. greatest at **A**.
   C. greatest at **B**.
   D. the same at **A** as at **B**.

GAMSAT MASTERS SERIES

GOLD STANDARD GAMSAT-LEVEL PRACTICE QUESTIONS

Note that irrespective of the Percent Importance for a chapter, GAMSAT-level practice questions are always ranked as High-level Importance.

11) Two tennis-ball launchers project balls at the same time, initial speed and angle from different floors of a sports hall. The two tennis balls land in a field below. Air resistance is negligible.

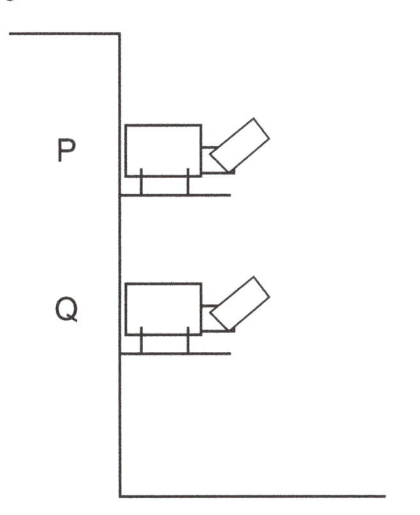

Which of the following is true regarding the flight of the 2 tennis balls?

A. Tennis ball Q will hit the ground farther from the base of the building as compared to tennis ball P.
B. Tennis ball P will experience a greater acceleration at some point during the flight.
C. At their maximum heights, the 2 tennis balls would have a significant difference in their speeds.
D. Just before striking the ground, the 2 tennis balls will be experiencing the maximum difference in their speeds.

Questions 12–14

You may consider the following equations for the questions in this unit.

$$v = v_o + at$$
$$v^2 = v_o^2 + 2ax$$
$$x = x_o + v_o t + \tfrac{1}{2}at^2$$

where v is the final velocity, v_o is the original velocity, a is the acceleration, t is the time, and x is the displacement.

12) A ball is shot from a canon vertically with an initial velocity of 45 m/s. If gravity pulls the ball at a constant rate of -10 m/s^2, how long will it take for the ball to come back to its initial position?

A. 7 seconds
B. 8 seconds
C. 9 seconds
D. 10 seconds

13) Suppose that an object is held at rest over a surface and dropped. The velocity on impact with the surface is 10 m/s. Neglecting air resistance, from approximately what height above the surface was the object dropped? (Gravitational acceleration = 9.8 m/s^2)

A. 5 m
B. 9.8 m
C. 19.8 m
D. Cannot be determined without being provided the mass of the object.

14) A stone is dropped into a well. Ten seconds later a splash is heard. How deep is the water level below the well opening (ignoring the time taken for sound to travel)?

A. 1000 m
B. 500 m
C. 50 m
D. 200 m

GAMSAT-Prep.com
GOLD STANDARD PHYSICS

High-level Importance

Questions 15–18

Escape velocity is the minimum speed needed for an object to escape from the gravitational influence of a massive body and, essentially, achieve an infinite distance from it. Escape velocity v_e is a function of the mass of the celestial body M and the radius of the mass of the body r:

$$v_e = \sqrt{\frac{2GM}{r}}$$

G is the universal gravitational constant.

Consider Figure 1 and Table 1.

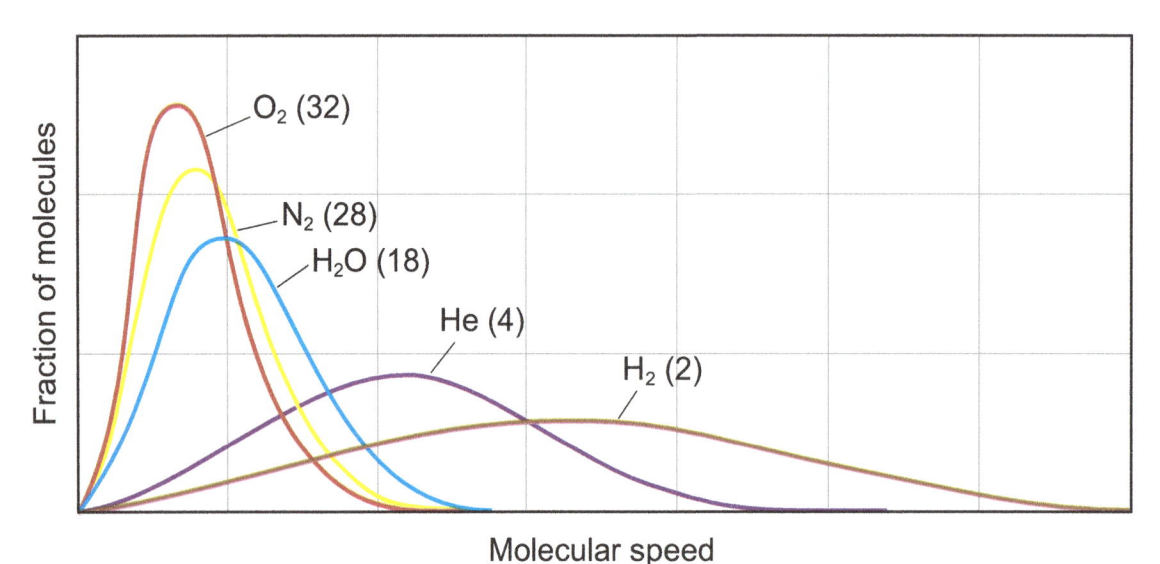

Figure 1: Maxwell Plot revealing the speed probability of common gases at standard temperature. Note the numbers in brackets represent the relative molecular weights.

	Mercury	Venus	Earth	Mars	Jupiter	Saturn	Uranus	Neptune	Pluto
Mass (× 10^{24} kg)	0.330	4.87	5.97	0.642	1898	568	86.8	102	0.0146
Escape Velocity (km/s)	4.3	10.4	11.2	5.0	59.5	35.5	21.3	23.5	1.3

Table 1: The mass and escape velocity of planets in Earth's solar system.

PHY-32 CHAPTER 2: FORCE, MOTION, AND GRAVITATION

15) Which of the following molecules would have the greatest difficulty to escape from Earth's atmosphere?

   A. O_2
   B. N_2
   C. H_2O
   D. H_2

16) Based on the information provided, which of the following pairs of planets would be expected to have the most similar radii?

   A. Jupiter and Neptune
   B. Uranus and Saturn
   C. Jupiter and Saturn
   D. Earth and Saturn

17) According to the information provided, the atmosphere of which of the following planets would be expected to contain the greatest concentration of gases?

   A. Earth
   B. Mars
   C. Saturn
   D. Jupiter

18) Stars may appear as simple dots in the night sky but they are actually huge celestial bodies shining due to thermonuclear fusion of hydrogen (H_2) into helium (He) in their core. Based on the information provided, as compared to the planets in Earth's solar system, what would be expected in terms of the relative mass and relative radii of average-sized stars, respectively?

   A. Large, large
   B. Large, small
   C. Small, large
   D. Small, small

19) A student throws a rock at a 60° angle over a lake. The rock leaves his hand at a velocity of 20 m/s. How far away from the student will the rock shadow appear on the ground after 1 second, assuming the shadow projects straight down from the rock? (Note that the sine of 60° is 0.87; cosine 60° is 0.5).

   A. 5 m
   B. 7 m
   C. 10 m
   D. 12 m

20) A planet is in orbit with its moon. A sudden event results in the planet's radius increasing 3-fold with no change in mass and the distance to its moon remains unchanged. Which of the following best describes the new force of gravity on the surface of the planet and the force of gravity between the planet and the moon, respectively, as compared to prior to the increase in radius?

   A. Decreased, decreased
   B. Increased, decreased
   C. Decreased, unchanged
   D. Unchanged, decreased

GAMSAT-Prep.com
GOLD STANDARD PHYSICS

High-level Importance

> ## ⚠ SPOILER ALERT
>
> Gold Standard has cross-referenced the content in this chapter to examples from ACER's official GAMSAT practice materials. It is for you to decide when you want to explore these questions since you may want to preserve some of ACER's materials for timed mock-exam practice.
>
> **Examples** – Conservation of energy (Physics Chapter 5) unit but the answer depends on choosing the correct centre of gravity: Q8 of 2; torque (Physics Chapter 4) unit but the answer depends on understanding weight: Q47 of 2; equations of kinematics with graphs: Q36-41 of 3; gravitation and the moon but mostly maths: Q57-60 of 5. Note that "Q" is followed by the question number, and, for example, "of 1" refers to booklet number 1 which is referenced in the Spoiler Alert table at the end of Chapter 1. The 10 full-length HEAPS GAMSAT practice tests (by Gold Standard and MediRed), exams 1 through 10, contain specific cross-references to this chapter within the worked solutions. Note that HEAPS-2 and HEAPS-4 have multiple units with gravitation, kinematics equations and related graphs.

Chapter Checklist

- ☐ Access your online account to view answers, worked solutions and discussion boards.
- ☐ Reassess your 'learning objectives' for this chapter: Go back to the first page of this chapter and re-evaluate the top 3 boxes and the Introduction.
  - ☐ Please be sure that you have completed the *Need for Speed* exercises at the beginning of this chapter.
- ☐ Complete a maximum of 1 page of notes using symbols/abbreviations to represent the entire chapter based on your learning objectives. These are your Gold Notes.
- ☐ Consider your multimedia options based on your optimal way of learning:
  - ☐ Download the free Gold Standard GAMSAT app for your Android device or iPhone.
  - ☐ Create your own, tangible study cards or try the free app: Anki.
  - ☐ Record your voice reading your Gold Notes onto your smartphone (MP3s) and listen during exercise, transportation, etc.
  - ☐ Try out the Gold Standard GAMSAT online videos at gamsat-prep.com, or you can try other options on YouTube like Khan Academy or Crash Course Physics.
- ☐ Reassess your schedule for your full-length GAMSAT practice tests: ACER and/or HEAPS exams. Ensure that you have scheduled one full day to complete a practice test and 1-2 days for a thorough assessment of worked solutions while adding to your abbreviated Gold Notes.
- ☐ Reassess your progress in scheduling and/or evaluating stress reduction techniques such as regular exercise (sports), yoga, meditation and/or mindfulness exercises (*see* YouTube for suggestions).

PARTICLE DYNAMICS
Chapter 3

Memorise
* Centripetal force and acceleration
* Circumference and area of a circle

Understand
* Equations: f_{max}, μ
* Static vs. kinetic friction
* Resolving vectors
* Uniform circular motion
* Solve pulley system, free-body diagram

Importance
Low level: 2% of GAMSAT Physics questions released by ACER are related to content in this chapter (in our estimation).
* Note that approximately 75% of the questions in GAMSAT Physics are related to just 6 chapters: 1, 4, 6, 9, 11 and 12.

GAMSAT-Prep.com

Introduction

Particle dynamics is concerned with the physics of motion. Among other topics, particle dynamics includes Newton's laws, frictional forces, and problems dealing with incline planes, uniform circular motion and pulley systems.

Reminder: The 'Importance level' refers to assumed knowledge and is NOT related to the practice questions. The questions at the end of this chapter use reasoning, equation manipulation and graph analysis which are all skills that will benefit you even when the questions are not based on the content of this chapter.

Multimedia Resources at GAMSAT-Prep.com

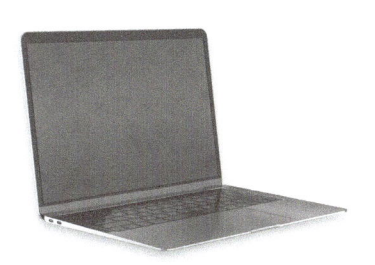

Open Discussion Boards   Foundational Videos   Flashcards   Special Guest

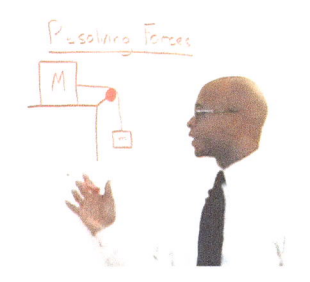

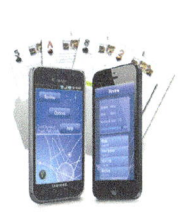

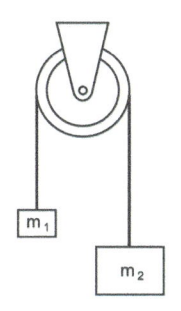

THE PHYSICAL SCIENCES   PHY-35

* The real GAMSAT may have advanced-level information presented (i.e. in a passage) but previous knowledge of said information is not required to answer the questions that would follow. Practice questions at the end of this chapter, as well as ACER and GS (HEAPS) practice GAMSATs can help you clarify this point.

GAMSAT-Prep.com
GOLD STANDARD PHYSICS

3.1 GAMSAT has a *Need for Speed*!

Section Number	GAMSAT Physics *Need for Speed* Exercises
3.2	The maximal frictional force f_{max} =
	Describe the direction of the normal force vector N.
3.3	During uniform circular motion, the magnitude of the centripetal acceleration is given by:
	The circumference of a circle:
	The area of a circle:

3.2 Frictional Forces

Friction is a force between two surfaces that are sliding, or trying to slide, past each other. In the language of Physics, frictional forces are nonconservative (mechanical energy is not conserved; PHY 5.6) and are caused by molecular adhesion between tangential surfaces but are independent of the area of contact of the surfaces. Frictional forces always oppose the motion. The maximal frictional force has the following expression: $f_{max} = \mu N$, where μ is the coefficient of friction and N is the normal force to the surface on which the object rests, it is the reaction of that surface against the weight of the object. Thus N always acts perpendicular to the surface.

Static friction is when the object is not moving, and it must be overcome for motion to begin. The coefficient of static friction μ_s is given as:

$$\mu_s = \tan \alpha$$

where α is the angle at which the object first begins to move on an inclined *plane* (= flat surface) as the angle is increased from 0 degrees to α degrees (*see Figure III.B.3.2*). There is also a coefficient of kinetic friction, μ_k, which exists when surfaces are in motion; $\mu_k < \mu_s$ always.

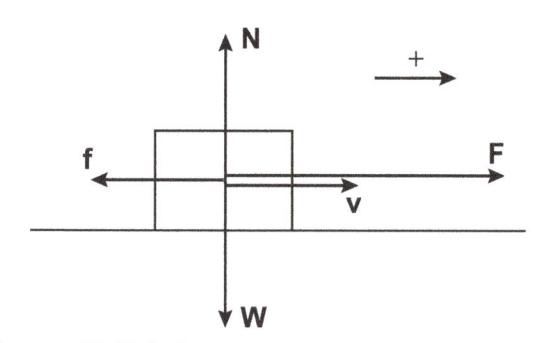

Figure III.B.3.1: Frictional force f, pulling force F, velocity v, weight W, and force normal N.

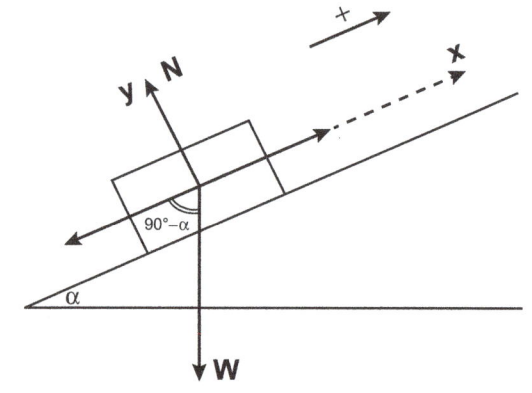

Figure III.B.3.2: Analysis of motion on an incline. To understand the relationship of the angles in the diagram, *see* Geometry GM 4.1.3.

Low-level Importance

PHY-36   CHAPTER 3: PARTICLE DYNAMICS

The weight (W) due to gravity (g) may be sufficient to cause motion if friction is overcome. The reference axes are usually chosen as shown such that one (the *x*) is along the surface of the incline.

Note that W is directed downward and N is directed upward but *perpendicular* to the surface of the incline (i.e. in the positive *y* direction).

3.2.1 Incline Plane Problem with Friction (SI units)

A 50 kilogram block is on an incline of 45°. The coefficient of sliding (= *kinetic*) friction between the block and the plane is 0.10. Take *g* as 9.8 m/s².

Determine the acceleration of the block. {*key: motion* is along the plane, so only the x-components of the force is relevant to the acceleration}

Begin with Newton's second law (PHY 2.2):

$$F = m \times a$$

thus

$$F_x = f_k - W\sin\alpha = \mu_k N - W\sin\alpha = m \times a$$

The force normal (N) can be determined by summing the forces in the *y*-direction where the acceleration is zero:

$$F_y = N - W\cos\alpha = m \times a = 0$$

Therefore,

$$N = W\cos\alpha$$

Solving for *a* and combining our first and last equations we get (recall: $W = mg$):

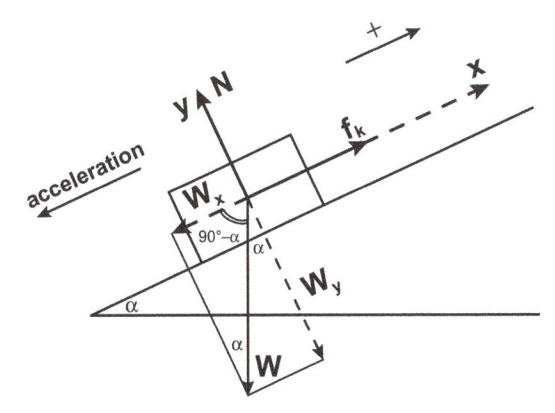

Figure III.B.3.3: Resolving the weight W into its x-component ($W\sin\alpha$) and its y-component ($W\cos\alpha$).

$$a = (\mu_k W\cos\alpha - W\sin\alpha)/m$$
$$= mg(\mu_k\cos\alpha - \sin\alpha)/m = g(\mu_k\cos\alpha - \sin\alpha)$$

Substituting the values:

$$a = 9.8 \text{ m/s}^2(0.10\cos 45° - \sin 45°) = -6.2 \text{ m/s}^2$$

- Thus the block accelerates at 6.2 m/s² down the plane. Also note that the *mass* of the block is irrelevant. {Resolving vectors is a 'GAMSAT 100' topic. In other words, it is a rare enough GAMSAT topic that it should only be pursued by students aiming for a perfect Section 3 score. If you wish to see the steps to resolve the forces, go to the very last page of this chapter.}

GAMSAT-Prep.com
GOLD STANDARD PHYSICS

3.3 Uniform Circular Motion

In Chapter 1, we saw that acceleration is due to a change in velocity (PHY 1.4). For a particle moving in a circle at constant speed (= *uniform circular motion*), the velocity vector changes continuously in direction but the magnitude remains the same.

The velocity is always tangent to the circle and since it is always changing (i.e. *direction*) it creates an acceleration directed radially inward called the *centripetal* acceleration (a_c). The magnitude of the acceleration a_c is given by v^2/r where r is the radius of the circle.

Every accelerated particle must have a force acting on it according to Newton's second law (PHY 2.2). Thus we can calculate the *centripetal* force,

$$F_c = ma_c = mv^2/r.$$

The centripetal force can be produced in many ways: a taut string which is holding a ball at the end that is spinning in a circle (Fig. III.B.3.4a); a radially directed frictional force like when a car drives around a curve on an unbanked road; a contact force exerted by another body like driving around a curve on a banked road (Fig. III.B.3.4b, c), or like the wall of an amusement park rotor.

Any particle moving in a circle with *non-uniform* speed will experience both centripetal *and* tangential forces and accelerations. {Reminder: the circumference of a circle is $2\pi r$ and the area is πr^2, GM 4.2.3}

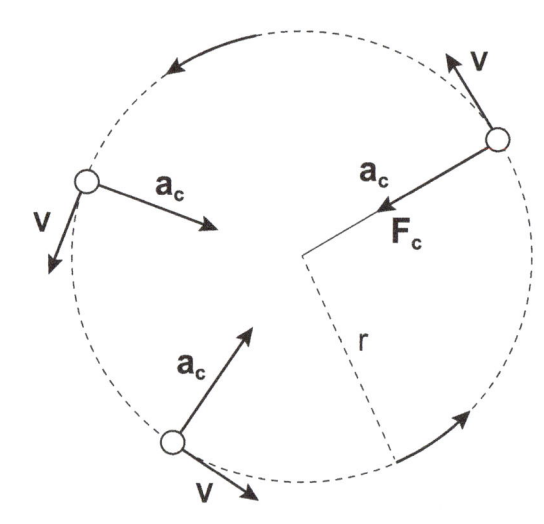

Figure III.B.3.4a: Uniform Circular Motion.

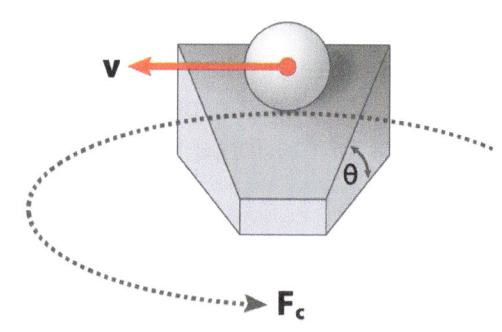

Figure III.B.3.4b: A ball in uniform circular motion on a banked curve at angle θ from the horizontal, analogous to driving on a banked, slippery road. The ball will slide to the centre unless it travels fast enough (e.g. roulette, the casino game).

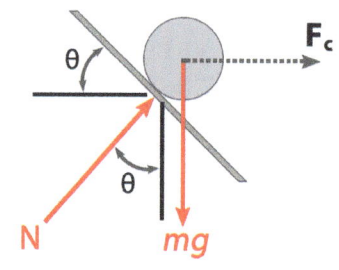

Figure III.B.3.4c: The net force on the ball due to vector addition of the normal force N exerted by the road and vertical force mg due to gravity must equal the centripetal force F_c to continue to travel the circular path.

3.4 Pulley Systems

Consider two unequal masses connected by a string which passes over a frictionless, massless pulley (see Figure III.B.3.5). Let us determine the following parameters: **i)** the tension T in the string which is a force and **ii)** the acceleration of the masses given that m_2 is greater than m_1.

Always begin by drawing vector or *free-body* diagrams of a problem (although, often ACER will draw one for you). The position of each mass will lie at the origin O of their respective axes. Now we assign positivity or negativity to the directions of motion. We can arbitrarily define the upward direction as positive. Thus if the acceleration of m_1 is a then the acceleration of m_2 must be $-a$.

Using Newton's second law we can derive the equation of motion for m_1:

$$F = T - m_1 g = m_1 a$$

and for m_2:

$$F = T - m_2 g = - m_2 a$$

Subtracting one equation from the other eliminates T then we can solve for a:

$$a = \frac{m_2 - m_1}{m_2 + m_1} g$$

Solve for a using the equations of motion, equate the formulas, then we can solve for T:

$$T = \frac{2 m_1 m_2}{m_1 + m_2} g$$

{Only if you are unable to complete the manipulations above, go to the very last page of this chapter.}

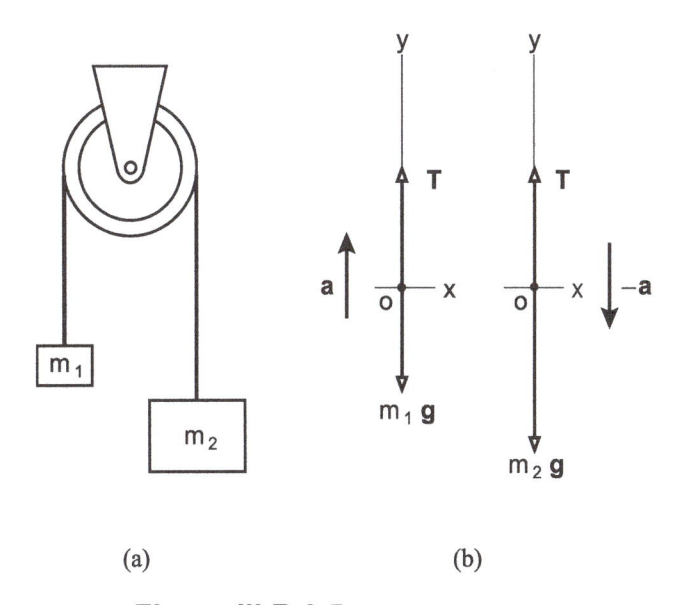

Figure III.B.3.5: A Pulley System. (a) Two unequal masses suspended by a string from a pulley. (b) Free-body diagrams for m_1 and m_2.

Consider solving the problem yourself given $g = 10$ m/s² and where m_2 is 3.0 kg ($W_2 = m_2 g$ = 30 N) and m_1 is 1.0 kg ($W_1 = m_1 g = 10$ N):

$$a = \frac{3.0 - 1.0}{3.0 + 1.0} g = g/2 = 5 \text{ m/s}^2$$

and

$$T = \frac{2(1.0)(3.0)}{1.0 + 3.0}(10) = 15 \text{ N}$$

- Note that T is always between the weight of mass m_1 and that of m_2. The reason is that T must exceed $m_1 g$ to give m_1 an upward acceleration, and $m_2 g$ must exceed T to give m_2 a downward acceleration. {If you wish to see a step-by-step analysis, go to gamsat-prep.com/forum, Masters Series GAMSAT Section 3 Physics, and then Chapter 3: Particle Dynamics.}

CHAPTER 3: Particle Dynamics

GOLD STANDARD FOUNDATIONAL GAMSAT PRACTICE QUESTIONS

1) Which of the following is consistent with the SI unit for frictional force and weight?

   A. J•s
   B. kg•m/s^2
   C. kg•m/s
   D. The pound

2) A 75 N force is used to push a refrigerator weighing 400 N. The refrigerator does not move. What is the frictional force exerted by the floor on the refrigerator?

   A. Less than 75 N
   B. Exactly 75 N
   C. Between 75 N and 400 N
   D. Exactly 400 N

3) Compared to the force needed to start sliding an object across a rough flat (i.e. not inclined) floor, the force required to keep the object sliding once it is moving is:

   A. more.
   B. less.
   C. the same.
   D. more or less, depending on how rough the floor is.

4) A 5 kg box is at rest on an inclined plane at 45 degrees to the horizontal. Friction is present, gravity can be estimated at 10 m/s^2. The net force in newtons acting on the object is which of the following?

   A. 0 N
   B. 25 N
   C. 50 N
   D. 75 N

5) A 1500 kg race car is driving around a horizontal circular track and has a constant speed of 14 m/s. The direction of the centripetal force is:

   A. tangent to the track in the direction of motion.
   B. tangent to the track opposite to the direction of motion.
   C. away from the centre of the track.
   D. toward the centre of the track.

6) A mass is attached to a string in an orbiting space station and placed in uniform circular motion at constant speed. Which diagram is most consistent with the direction of the velocity and the centripetal force of the mass at a given instant?

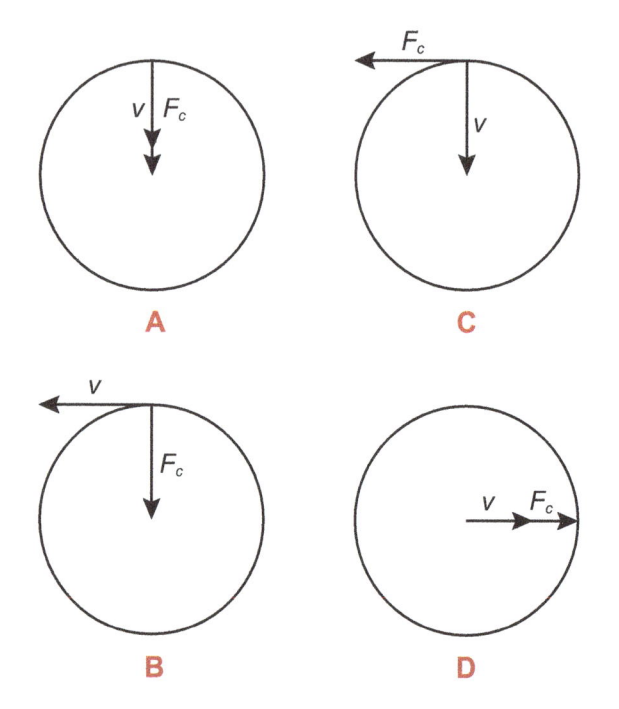

7) The figure below shows a rough semicircular track whose ends are at a vertical height *h*. A block placed at point *R* at one end of the track is released from rest and slides past the bottom of the track. Which of the following is true of the height to which the block rises on the other side of the track?

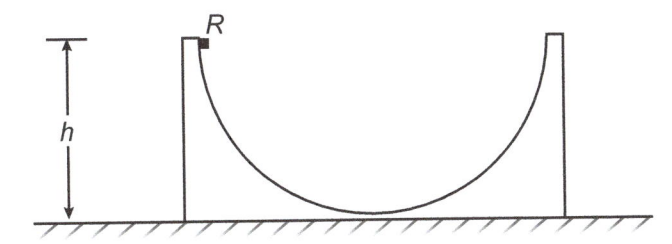

A. It is equal to *h*/2.
B. It is equal to *h*.
C. It is equal to *h*/2π.
D. It is equal to a number between zero and *h*, the exact magnitude depends on how much energy was lost to friction.

8) Two identical masses m are connected to a massless string which is hung over two frictionless pulleys as shown in the diagram. If everything is at rest, what is the tension in the cord?

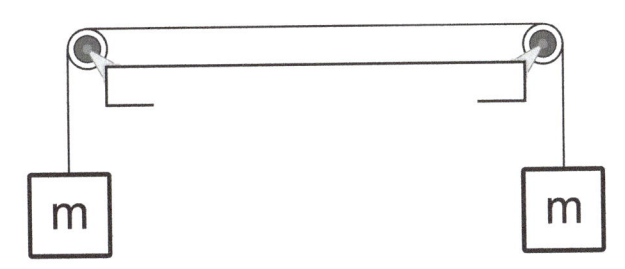

A. Exactly 2 mg
B. Less than mg
C. More than mg but less than 2 mg
D. Exactly mg

9) The driver of a 1000 kg car tries to turn through a circle of radius 100 m on an unbanked curve at a speed of 10 m/s. The maximum frictional force between the tires and the slippery road is 900 N. The car will:

A. Slide off to the outside of the curve.
B. Make the turn.
C. Make the turn only if it speeds up.
D. Slow down due to the centrifugal force.

10) The hammer throw is an Olympic sport where participants throw a metal ball attached by a steel wire to a grip.

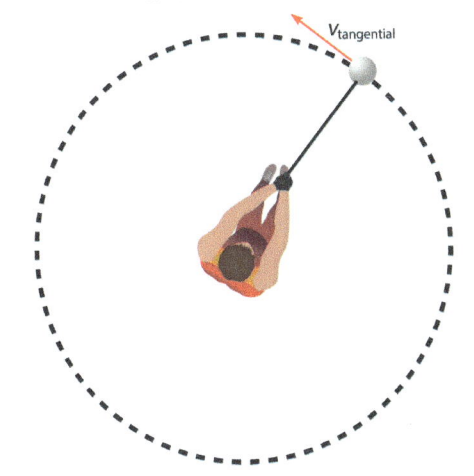

Note that:
- centripetal acceleration is given by v^2/r.
- the circumference of a circle is $2\pi r$ and the area is πr^2.
- T is the period, which is the time needed to complete one revolution.

Which of the following is consistent with the centripetal acceleration of the hammer moving in the circle in relation to the time needed to complete a revolution?

A. $a_c = 4\pi^2 r T^{-2}$
B. $a_c = 4\pi^2 r^{-1} T^{-2}$
C. $a_c = 4\pi^2 r^2 T^{-2}$
D. $a_c = 4\pi^2 T^2$

GOLD STANDARD GAMSAT-LEVEL PRACTICE QUESTIONS

Questions 11–12

A glider is a fixed-wing aircraft that is supported in flight by the reaction of the air against its lifting surfaces, and whose free flight does not depend on an engine. It is common for gliders to engage in a circular motion in order to gain altitude (i.e. *soar*). Typically, the glider's wings will tilt which creates an angle of bank with the horizon. Figure 1 demonstrates the interplay of certain variables as the glider is soaring in circular motion.

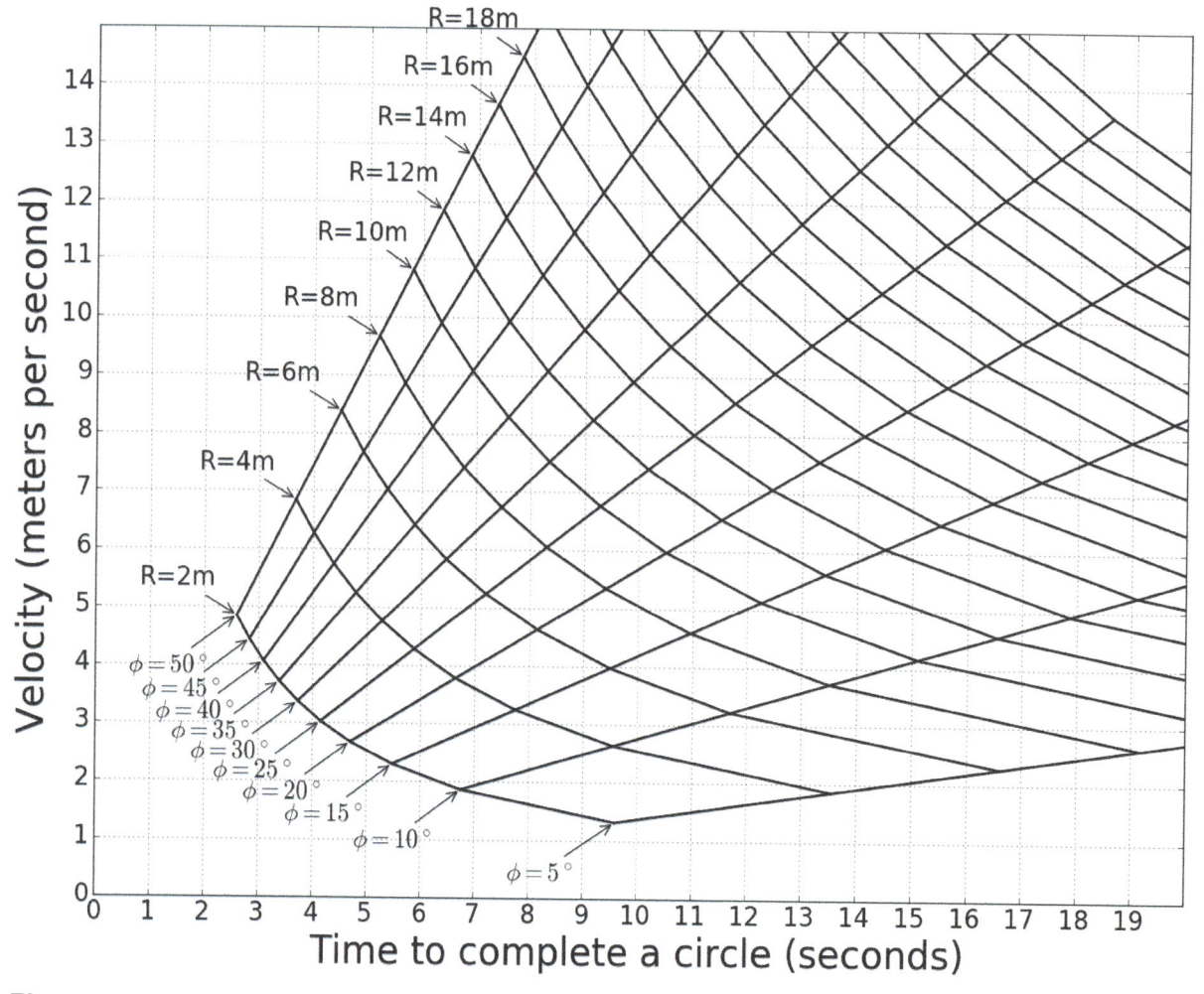

Figure 1: Computer generated graph illustrating the interplay between time, velocity, radius R of the circle, and angle of banking. As an example, to complete a circle in 7 seconds with a velocity of 9 m/s, the radius would be 10 m and the angle of banking would be 40°.

11) According to Figure 1, given the glider's velocity of 9 m/s and 9 seconds to complete a circle, which of the following would be the most accurate estimate of the glider's banking angle?

A. 30°
B. 32.5°
C. 35°
D. 37.5°

12) According to Figure 1, given the glider's velocity of 9 m/s and 9 seconds to complete a circle, which of the following would be the most accurate estimate of the glider's circle radius?

A. 11 m
B. 12 m
C. 13 m
D. 14 m

13) The following system includes a frictionless pulley and a cord of negligible mass. Since the system is at rest, what can be said about the force of friction between the platform and the large weight?

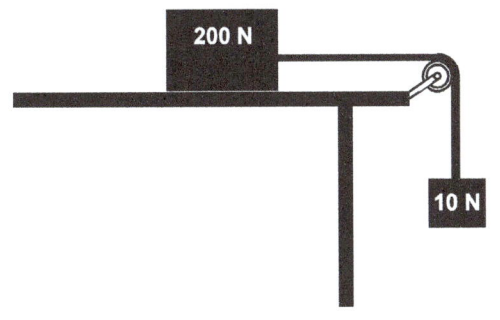

A. It is 200 N.
B. It is 10 N.
C. It is 190 N.
D. In this case, the force of friction is not necessarily present.

Questions 14–16

14) A centrifuge is a device with a motor in it, which is used to spin an object with high speed. This spinning at high speed forces objects with greater density outwards as the centripetal force F_c is directed inwards towards the centre of the circle. This force is used in medical laboratories so that serum can be separated from blood cells.

The following equations may be of value:

- $F_c = mv^2/r$, where m is the mass, v is the velocity, and r is the radius (note that this equation derives from Newton's 2nd law where force is mass times acceleration)
- $\omega = 2\pi/T$, where ω is the angular velocity (rotational speed), T is the period (the time for one rotation)
- $v = r\omega$

Which of the following expressions is consistent with the time period T?

A. $[2\pi \cdot mr/F_c]^{1/2}$
B. $[4\pi \cdot mr/F_c]^{1/2}$
C. $[4\pi^2 mr/F_c]^{1/2}$
D. $[4\pi^2 m/F_c]^{1/2}$

15) Donor blood is placed in a centrifuge and is spun at 12 000 revolutions per minute (rpm). Given this information, what would be the time period T?

A. 0.005 s
B. 0.5 s
C. 20 s
D. 200

16) If the identical centrifuge from the previous question has its rotational speed changed to 6000 rpm, how would that affect its centripetal acceleration?

   A. The new centripetal acceleration would be 1/4 of the original.
   B. The new centripetal acceleration would be 1/2 of the original.
   C. The new centripetal acceleration would be twice the original.
   D. The new centripetal acceleration would be 4 times the original.

17) Mary stands on a scale in the lift (GAMSAT is so realistic!). She notices that the scale reading is lower than her usual weight. Which of the following is the best description of the possible motion of the lift?

   A. It is moving up with constant speed.
   B. It is moving down and slowing down.
   C. It is moving down at constant speed.
   D. It is moving up and slowing down.

Questions 18–20

The Froude number (Fr) has been widely used in anthropology to adjust for size differences when comparing gait parameters or other locomotor variables (such as optimal walking speed or speed at gait transitions) among humans, nonhuman primates, and fossil hominins.

$$\mathrm{Fr} = \frac{u}{\sqrt{gL}}$$

where u is the organism's velocity, g is the acceleration due to gravity, and L is the characteristic length from hip to ground (all normally reported in SI units).

18) What are the dimensions of the Froude number?

   A. s
   B. m^2/s^2
   C. m^3/s^2
   D. It is dimensionless.

19) Two hominins were found to have approximately the same Froude number. Species A has a hip length of 0.5 m and an optimal-walking speed of 1.0 m/s, and Species B has a hip length of 0.7 m. What is the approximate optimal-walking speed of Species B?

   A. 0.8 m/s
   B. 1.0 m/s
   C. 1.2 m/s
   D. 1.6 m/s

20) One study concluded that the walk-run transition speeds for humans, nonhuman primates, and hominins occurs at a Froude number of approximately 1.0. What would be the predicted walk-run transition speed for Species A?

   A. 1.8 m/s
   B. 2.2 m/s
   C. 2.6 m/s
   D. 3.0 m/s

GAMSAT MASTERS SERIES

⚠ SPOILER ALERT

Gold Standard has cross-referenced the content in this chapter to examples from ACER's official GAMSAT practice materials. It is for you to decide when you want to explore these questions since you may want to preserve some of ACER's materials for timed mock-exam practice.

Examples – Froude number with a pretty graph Q34-35 of 1; angle of bank nomogram with centripetal force/acceleration: Q67-68 of 5. Note that "Q" is followed by the question number, and, for example, "of 1" refers to booklet number 1 which is referenced in the Spoiler Alert table at the end of Chapter 1. The 10 full-length HEAPS GAMSAT practice tests (by Gold Standard and MediRed), exams 1 through 10, contain specific cross-references to this chapter within the worked solutions. Note that the angle of bank nomogram makes an appearance in HEAPS-1 but with a different topic and different questions; the pulley system at rest is in HEAPS-6. HEAPS-2 has a pulley system with a broken leg (ouch!); and HEAPS-4 has friction with the equations of kinematics.

High-level Importance

Chapter Checklist

- ☐ Access your online account to view answers, worked solutions and discussion boards.
- ☐ Reassess your 'learning objectives' for this chapter: Go back to the first page of this chapter and re-evaluate the top 3 boxes and the Introduction.
    - ☐ Please be sure that you have completed the *Need for Speed* exercises at the beginning of this chapter.
- ☐ Complete a maximum of 1 page of notes using symbols/abbreviations to represent the entire chapter based on your learning objectives. These are your Gold Notes.
- ☐ Consider your multimedia options based on your optimal way of learning:
    - ☐ Download the free Gold Standard GAMSAT app for your Android device or iPhone.
    - ☐ Create your own, tangible study cards or try the free app: Anki.
    - ☐ Record your voice reading your Gold Notes onto your smartphone (MP3s) and listen during exercise, transportation, etc.
    - ☐ Try out the Gold Standard GAMSAT online videos at gamsat-prep.com, or you can try other options on YouTube like Khan Academy or Crash Course Physics.
- ☐ Reassess your schedule for your full-length GAMSAT practice tests: ACER and/or HEAPS exams. Ensure that you have scheduled one full day to complete a practice test and 1-2 days for a thorough assessment of worked solutions while adding to your abbreviated Gold Notes.
- ☐ Reassess your progress in scheduling and/or evaluating stress reduction techniques such as regular exercise (sports), yoga, meditation and/or mindfulness exercises (*see* YouTube for suggestions).

Chapter 3 Additional Details: Manipulating Equations

RE: PHY 3.2.1

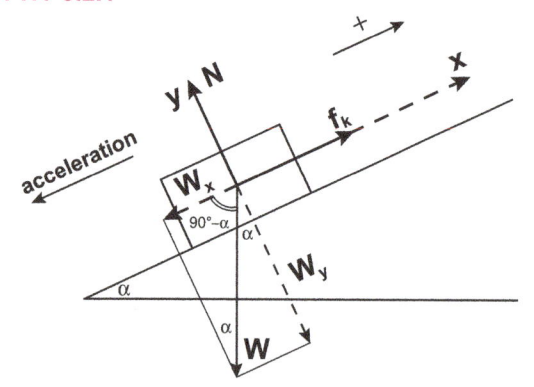

Figure III.B.3.3: Resolving the weight W into its *x*-component (W sinα) and its *y*-component (W cosα).

Look carefully at the diagram. Notice that there is an x-axis identified and it is represented as a positive arrow (vector) pointing parallel to the inclined plane (up and to the right in the diagram).

Once a direction is identified then everything else can fall into place.

Resolving the forces (capital letter F) in the x-direction (= F_x) gives us one force pointing in the positive x-direction (the kinetic friction, small letter f, f_k) and one force pointing in the negative x-direction (the x-component of the weight W, W_x). So we get:

Sum of forces in the x direction: $F_x = f_k - W_x$

Using "sine is opposite/hypotenuse":

$\sin α = W_x/W$

so

$W_x = W\sin α$

thus

$F_x = f_k - W\sin α$

and according to Newton's second law:

$ma = f_k - W\sin α$

Now examining all forces in the y-direction (which by definition is perpendicular to the x-axis already identified):

N points up, W_y points down. We can define 'up' as positive. I think you would agree that the object is incapable of moving, let alone accelerating, in the y-axis (because the inclined plane itself is in the way) so we get:

Sum of forces $F = ma = 0$

$N - W_y = 0$

$N = W_y$

Using "cosine is adjacent/hypotenuse":

$N = W\cos α$

If you wish to explore any more details, go to gamsat-prep.com/forum, Masters Series Physics, Chapter 3.

RE: PHY 3.4

Note that we discussed solving equations with multiple variables in GM 3.3.2.

$T - m_1g = m_1a$

and

$T - m_2g = -m_2a$

If we are looking for the acceleration then we can eliminate the tension T by subtracting the 2nd equation from the first:

$\quad T - m_1g = m_1a$
$-(T - m_2g = -m_2a)$

$0 - m_1g + m_2g = m_1a + m_2a$ (remember that a minus times a minus is positive; GM 1.2.1.1)

Now we resolve: $g(-m_1 + m_2) = a(m_1 + m_2)$

Isolate the acceleration: $g(m_2 - m_1)/(m_1 + m_2) = a$

Now to resolve for tension T, the first step is to isolate the acceleration a:

Since $T - m_1g = m_1a$, then: $(T - m_1g)/m_1 = a$

and

$T - m_2g = -m_2a$, then: $(T - m_2g)/-m_2 = a$

Since both equations are equal to 'a', we can equate them (*try the equation manipulation yourself prior to examining the worked solution below*):

$(T - m_1g)/m_1 = (T - m_2g)/-m_2$

To get rid of the denominators, multiply through by $(-m_2m_1)$, or cross multiply (GM 1.4.2):

$-m_2(T - m_1g) = m_1(T - m_2g)$

Extract and then isolate T:

$T(-m_2) + m_1m_2g = T(m_1) - m_1m_2g$

$2m_1m_2g = T(m_1) - T(-m_2) = T(m_1 + m_2)$

$2m_1m_2g / (m_1 + m_2) = T$

If you wish to explore any more details, go to gamsat-prep.com/forum, Masters Series Physics, Chapter 3. Note that anytime ACER has a question that would normally take more than 2 minutes, it is usually preceded by 1-2 very easy questions.

EQUILIBRIUM
Chapter 4

Memorise
* Definitions and equations to solve torque problems
* Newton's first law, inertia

Understand
* Solve torque, collision problems
* Choosing an appropriate pivot point
* Create vector diagrams
* Elastic vs. inelastic vs. conservation of energy
* Solve momentum problem

Importance
High level: 12% of GAMSAT Physics questions released by ACER are related to content in this chapter (in our estimation).
* Note that approximately 75% of the questions in GAMSAT Physics are related to just 6 chapters: 1, 4, 6, 9, 11 and 12.

GAMSAT-Prep.com

Introduction

Equilibrium exists when a mass is at rest or moves with constant velocity. Translational (straight line) and rotational (turning) equilibria can be resolved using linear forces, torque forces, Newton's first law and inertia. Momentum is a vector that can be used to solve problems involving elastic (bouncy) or inelastic (sticky) collisions.

Multimedia Resources at GAMSAT-Prep.com

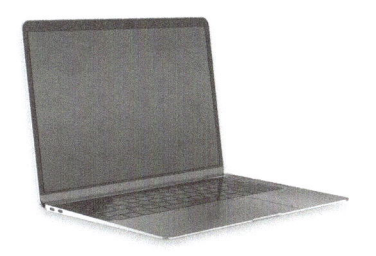

Open Discussion Boards

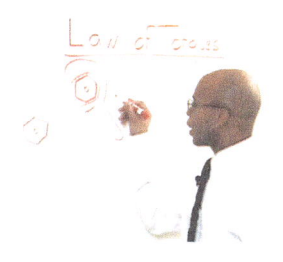

Foundational Videos

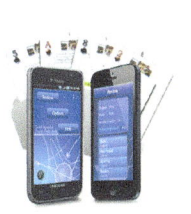

Flashcards

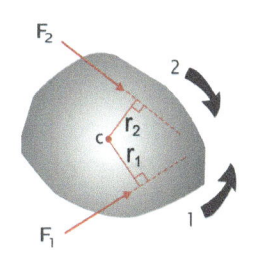

Special Guest

THE PHYSICAL SCIENCES   PHY-47

* The real GAMSAT may have advanced-level information presented (i.e. in a passage) but previous knowledge of said information is not required to answer the questions that would follow. Practice questions at the end of this chapter, as well as ACER and GS (HEAPS) practice GAMSATs can help you clarify this point.

GAMSAT-Prep.com
GOLD STANDARD PHYSICS

4.0 GAMSAT has a *Need for Speed*!

High-level Importance

Section Number	GAMSAT Physics *Need for Speed* Exercises
4.1	How would you describe a torque force?
	How can you calculate a torque force?
4.2	How would you describe inertia?
4.3	How would you describe impulse (this is Physics!)?
4.4	*(see sub-table below)*

Process • no external force • ideal	Objects stick together?	Momentum conserved?	Kinetic energy conserved?	Good example? • at least one example • perfection is unnecessary!
Elastic collision				
Inelastic collision				

4.1 Translational, Rotational and Complex Motion

When a force acts upon an object, the object will undergo translational (Chapter 1), rotational (*turning*) or complex (translational and rotational) motion.

Rotational motion of an object about an axis is the rotation of that object around that axis caused by perpendicular forces to that axis. The effective force causing rotation about an axis is the torque (*L*).

The torque is like a *turning force*. Consider a hinged door. If you were to apply a force *F* at the pivot point (*the hinge*), the door

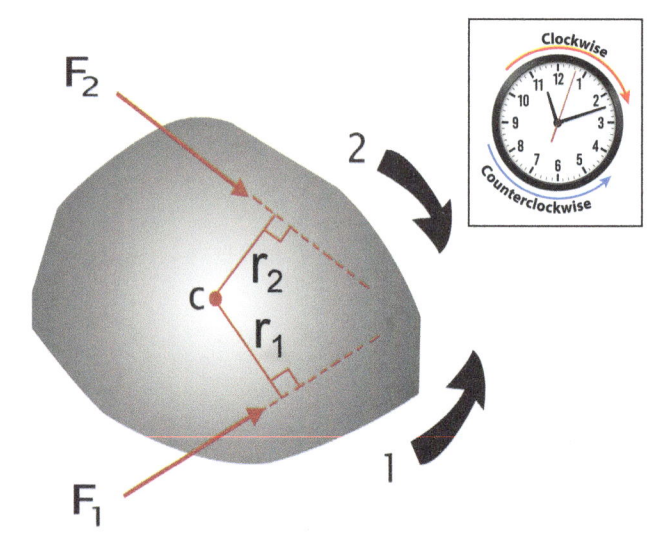

Figure III.B.4.1: Rotational Motion.

PHY-48 CHAPTER 4: EQUILIBRIUM

would not turn ($L=0$). If you apply the *same* force further and further from the pivot point, the turning force multiplies and the acceleration of the door increases. Thus the torque can be defined as the force applied multiplied by the perpendicular distance from the pivot point (= *lever or moment arm = r*).

$$L = (\text{force}) \times (\text{lever arm})$$

Thus according to Figure III.B.4.1:

$$L_1 = F_1 \times r_1 = \text{counterclockwise (or anticlockwise) torque (1) = positive}$$

and

$$L_2 = F_2 \times r_2 = \text{clockwise torque (2) = negative.}$$

Positivity and negativity are arbitrary designations of the two opposite directions of motion. To determine the direction of rotation caused by the torque, imagine the direction the object would rotate if the force is pushing its moment arm at right angles. The net torques acting upon an object is obtained by summing the counterclockwise (+) and the clockwise (−) torques. An object is at equilibrium when the net forces and the net torques acting upon the object is zero. Thus, the object is either motionless or moving at a constant velocity due to its internal inertia.

The conditions of equilibrium are:

For translational equilibrium:

$$\Sigma F_x = 0 \text{ and } \Sigma F_y = 0$$

For rotational equilibrium:

$$\Sigma L = 0$$

In terms of translational equilibrium, the meaning of the equations can be summarised as: all upward forces equal all downward forces (*y*-axis), all forces to the left equal all forces to the right (*x*-axis), all forces towards you equals all forces away from you (*z*-axis, $\Sigma F_z = 0$; the latter is possible, but not likely to be found as a GAMSAT question).

In terms of rotational equilibrium, if the torques sum to zero about one point in an object, they will sum to zero about any point in the object. If the point chosen as reference (= *pivot point or fulcrum*) includes the line of action of one of the forces, that force need not be included in calculating torques. {*The issue here is that torque is force times distance from the pivot point; so at the pivot point, the distance from itself is zero so the torque at the pivot point must be zero. This is akin to applying a force at the hinge of a door: It will not open.*}

4.1.1 Torque Problem (SI units)

A 70 kg person sits 50 cm from the edge of a non-uniform plank (a long, thin, flat piece of wood) which weighs 100 N and is 2.0 m long (*see Figure III.B.4.2*). The weight supported by point B is 250 N. Find the centre of gravity (COG) of the plank.

{key: draw a vector diagram then choose an unknown value as the pivot point i.e. point A; see PHY 2.1 for a definition of COG}

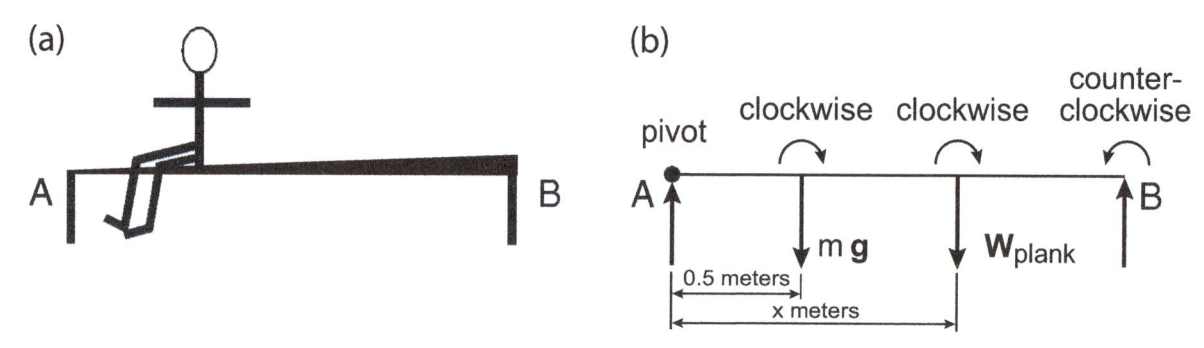

Figure III.B.4.2: Torque Problem.
(a) A person sitting on a non-uniform bench which is composed of a plank with two supports A and B. (b) Vector diagram with point A as the reference point. The torque force at point A is zero since its distance from itself is zero.

The counterclockwise torque (CCW) is given by the force at point B multiplied by its distance from the reference point A:

$$CCW = F_B r_B = 250(2.0) = 500 \text{ Nm}$$

The clockwise torques (CW) are given by the force exerted by the person (= the weight *mg*) multiplied by the distance from the pivot point (r = 50 cm = 0.5 m) *and* the force exerted by the plank (= the weight) multiplied by the distance from the pivot point where the weight of the plank acts (= COG):

$$CW = mgr + W(COG) = 70(10)0.5 + 100(COG)$$
$$= 350 + 100(COG)$$

Gravity was estimated as 10 m/s². Now we have:

$$\Sigma L = CCW - CW = 500 - 350 - 100(COG) = 0$$

Isolate COG

$$COG = 150/100 = 1.5 \text{ m from point } A.$$

• Note that had the plank been uniform its COG would be at its centre which is 1.0 m from either end.

• Had the problem requested the weight supported at point A, it would be easy to determine since $\Sigma F_y = 0$. If we define upward forces as positive, we get:

$$\Sigma F_y = F_A + F_B - mg - W_{plank} = 0$$

Isolate F_A

$$F_A = 70(10) + 100 - 250 = 550 \text{ N}.$$

4.2 Newton's First Law

Newton's first law states that objects in motion or at rest tend to remain as such unless acted upon by an outside force. That is, objects have inertia (i.e. the resistance to any change in the object's velocity, which of course includes a change from a velocity of 0). For translational motion, the mass (m) is a measure of inertia.

For rotational motion, a quantity derived from the mass called the moment of inertia (I) is the measure of inertia. In general $I = \Sigma mr^2$ where r is the distance from the axis of rotation. However, the exact formulation depends on the structure of the object (if needed, ACER would provide any relevant equation and would define the variables).

4.3 Momentum

The momentum (M, though sometimes symbolised as P) is a vector quantity. The momentum of an object is the product of its mass and its velocity.

$$M = m\,v$$

Linear momentum is a measure of the tendency of an object to maintain motion in a straight line. The greater the momentum (M), the greater the tendency of the object to remain moving along a straight line in the same direction. The momentum (M) is also a measure of the force needed to stop or change the direction of the object.

The impulse I is a measure of the change of the momentum of an object. It is the product of the force applied by the time during which the force was applied to change the momentum.

$$I = F\,\Delta t = \Delta M$$

where F is the acting force and Δt is the elapsed time during which the force was acting. Momentum is also conserved just like energy (PHY 4.3.1). The total linear momentum of a system is constant when the resultant external force acting on the system is zero.

4.3.1 Understanding Conservation

Conservation in Physics refers to something which does not change. This means that the variable in an equation which represents a *conserved* quantity is constant over time. It has the same value both before and after an event.

There are many conserved quantities in Physics that are very good approximations of reality. Complicated problems can be simplified by the understanding that the overall energy and momentum are conserved.

GAMSAT-Prep.com
GOLD STANDARD PHYSICS

High-level Importance

Overall energy, as we will examine more closely in the next chapter, refers to the total energy of a system. When objects move around over time, the energy associated with them—e.g., kinetic, gravitational potential, sound, heat—might change forms, but if energy is conserved, then the total energy will remain the same.

Although total energy is conserved, as we will see in the next section, it is possible that one of the specific forms of energy might change in a collision (i.e. it may transfer from one type of energy to another).

Note that non-conservative forces are dissipative forces (meaning they lose a form of energy, usually as heat) such as friction (PHY 3.2) or air resistance. These forces take energy away from the system as the system progresses, energy that you cannot get back.

4.4 Collisions

During motion, objects can collide. There are two kinds of collisions: *elastic* and *inelastic*. During an elastic collision (objects rebound off each other), there is a conservation of momentum and conservation of kinetic energy. Whereas, during an inelastic collision (objects stick together), there is conservation of momentum but not conservation of kinetic energy. Kinetic energy is lost as heat or sound, so total energy is conserved.

Process • no external force • ideal	Objects stick together?	Momentum conserved?	Kinetic energy conserved?
Elastic collision	No	Yes	Yes
Inelastic collision	Yes	Yes	No

{Note: the facts in this table represent a rare, direct-knowledge ACER GAMSAT question revealed in the Spoiler Alert section at the end of this chapter.}

Examples of elastic collisions include 2 rubber balls colliding, a ball at a billiard table hits another ball, particle collisions in ideal gases, and the sling-shot type gravitational interactions between satellites and planets popularised in science fiction movies. Examples of inelastic collisions include 2 cars colliding at high speed becoming stuck together, a dropped ball of clay does not rebound (note that its kinetic energy gets lost through deformation when it hits the ground and changes shape), and a ballistic pendulum which can be a huge chunk of wood used to measure the speed of a moving object (i.e. bullet) which becomes completely embedded in the wood. If, however, the bullet were to emerge from the wood block, then it would be an elastic collision since the objects did not stick together.

Imagine two spheres with masses m_1 and m_2 and the velocity components before the collision v_{1i} and v_{2i} and after the collision v_{1f} and v_{2f}. If the momentum and the velocity

PHY-52 CHAPTER 4: EQUILIBRIUM

are in the same directions, and we define that direction as positive, from the conservation of momentum we obtain:

$$m_1v_{1i} + m_2v_{2i} = m_1v_{1f} + m_2v_{2f}.$$

If the directions are not the same then each momentum must be resolved into x- and y-components as necessary.

4.4.1 Collision Problem (CGS units)

A bullet of mass 10 g and a speed of 5.0×10^4 cm/s strikes a 700 g wooden block at rest on a very smooth surface. The bullet emerges with its speed reduced to 3.5×10^4 cm/s.

Find the resulting speed of the block. {CGS uses <u>c</u>entimetres, <u>g</u>rams, and <u>s</u>econds as units; the CGS unit of force is a *dyne*. You do not need to commit any of the preceding to memory, the information will be provided by ACER, if needed}.

Let m_1 = the mass of the bullet (10 g), v_{1i} = the speed of the bullet before the collision (5.0×10^4 cm/s), m_2 = the mass of the wooden block (700 g), v_{2i} = the speed of the block before the collision (0 cm/s), v_{1f} = the speed of the bullet after the collision (3.5×10^4 cm/s), and v_{2f} = the speed of the block after the collision (*unknown*), now we have:

$$m_1v_{1i} + m_2v_{2i} = m_1v_{1f} + m_2v_{2f}$$

- In the explosion of an object at rest, the total momentum of all the fragments must sum to zero because of the conservation of momentum and because the original momentum was zero.
- If one object collides with a second identical object that is at rest, there is a total transfer of kinetic energy, that is the first object comes to rest and the second object moves off with the momentum of the first one.

Solving for v_{2f}

$$\begin{aligned}v_{2f} &= (m_1v_{1i} - m_1v_{1f})/m_2 \\ &= (5.0 \times 10^5 - 3.5 \times 10^5)/(700) \\ &= 2.1 \times 10^2 \text{ cm/s.}\end{aligned}$$

- Note: the least precise figures that we are given in the problem contain at least two digits or <u>significant figures</u>. Thus our answer can not be more precise than two significant figures. The exponent 10^x is not considered when counting significant figures unless you are *told* that the measurement was more precise than is evident {For more on significant figures *see* GM 1.4.3, 1.5.2 and PHY 8.5.1}.
- Note: Sometimes, during the exam, you will want to convert to SI units (i.e. metres, kilograms, etc.; GM 2.1, 2.2); however, depending on the answer choices and the nature of the equation or any constants, it may be faster to avoid any conversions. Experience with practice questions will enable you to decide efficiently.

CHAPTER 4: Equilibrium

GOLD STANDARD FOUNDATIONAL GAMSAT PRACTICE QUESTIONS

1) Consider the improvised diving board made of uniform material shown in Figure 1 where the distance d is measured from the centre of mass of the assembly. What is the maximum weight of a person who can slowly walk to the far-right end of the board without falling?

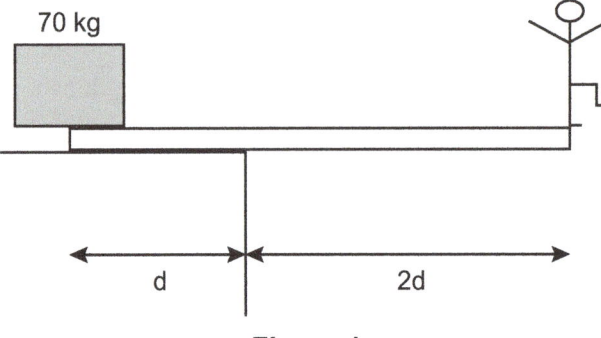

Figure 1

A. 20 kg
B. 25 kg
C. 30 kg
D. 35 kg

2) Momentum is mass times velocity, and impulse is the change in momentum. Which of the following is consistent with the SI units for impulse?

A. N•s
B. kg•m/s
C. Both **A** and **B**
D. None of the above

3) If a small particle is undergoing erratic motion with no external force acting on it, the direction of the particle's momentum at every point in its motion must always be:

A. the same as the direction of its acceleration.
B. the same as the direction of its net force.
C. the same as the direction of its velocity.
D. the same as the direction of its kinetic energy.

4) A mass 2m has a velocity v before it strikes a mass 3m at rest. The masses stick together and move off with what velocity?

A. 5v/2
B. 3v/5
C. v/5
D. 2v/5

5) A clown, standing motionless on a frictionless surface, throws a ball away from herself. If the ball weighs 5 kg, and she throws it at the speed of 3 m/s, how fast will the clown be moving afterward? The clown weighs 50 kg.

A. 0.1 m/s
B. 0.25 m/s
C. 0.3 m/s
D. 0.5 m/s

Questions 6–8

Undergraduate Physics labs routinely ask students to explore frictionless collisions with the use of air tables. In one such experiment, students float disks above an air table covered by plain newspaper-grade paper. As the disks shim over the essentially frictionless table, periodic electrical discharges, at a known time rate from the table to the disk, imprints upon the paper surface point-sized burn marks. The students propel the disks together, causing a collision, and then graphically determine the velocity and position of the disks from the marks embedded in the paper.

6) In this experiment, how can the speed of the disks be ascertained from the burning marks upon the paper?

   A. Measure the distance between any given 2 marks, and divide by spark time.
   B. Multiply the distances between any given 2 marks by the spark time.
   C. Add the spark time to the distance between marks.
   D. Record the sum of all distances between marks.

7) If the average measured distance between marks generated by a disk (i.e. disk A) is greater before a collision with another disk, what can one conclude?

   A. Disk A accelerated as a result of the collision.
   B. The collision resulted in a deceleration for Disk A.
   C. Friction decelerated disk A.
   D. The mass of Disk A decreased.

8) Assuming disks A and B collide inelastically as in the diagram below, what will the final momentum of the combined two disks be after the collision?

   $v = 10$ m/s
   $m = 5$ kg

   A ⟶ X
         ↑
      B $v = 3.75$ m/s
         $m = 20$ kg

   A. 45 kg·m/s
   B. 90 kg·m/s
   C. 135 kg·m/s
   D. 180 kg·m/s

9) The following graph shows the force exerted on a field hockey ball over time. The field hockey ball is initially stationary and has a mass of 150 g. Calculate the magnitude of the impulse of the ball.

   • Note that: Impulse is the product of the force applied by the time during which the force was applied to change the momentum.

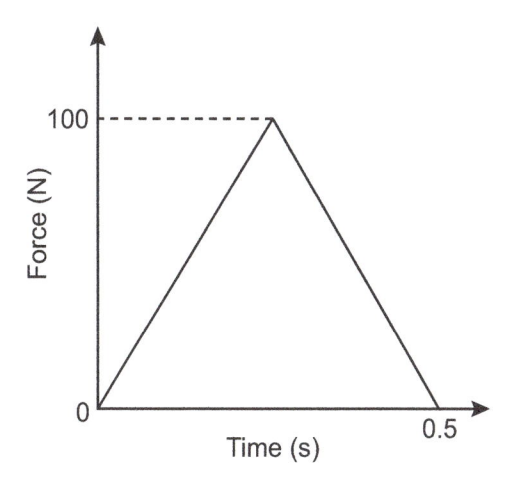

   [Graph: Force (N) vs Time (s), triangular shape peaking at 100 N, base from 0 to 0.5 s]

   A. 25 N·s
   B. 30 N·s
   C. 35 N·s
   D. 40 N·s

GOLD STANDARD GAMSAT-LEVEL PRACTICE QUESTIONS

10) Which of the following is a proper representation of the relation between torque (τ), length, mass, and time? M = mass, L = length, T = time

- A. $\tau = [M][L]/[T]^2$
- B. $\tau = [M][L]/[T]$
- C. $\tau = [M][L]^2/[T]^2$
- D. $\tau = [M][L]^2/[T]$

11) An 8-metre uniform bar whose weight W is 100 newtons is held in equilibrium by two vertical forces, F_1, and F_2, as shown. Which of the following expressions for F_1 is correct?

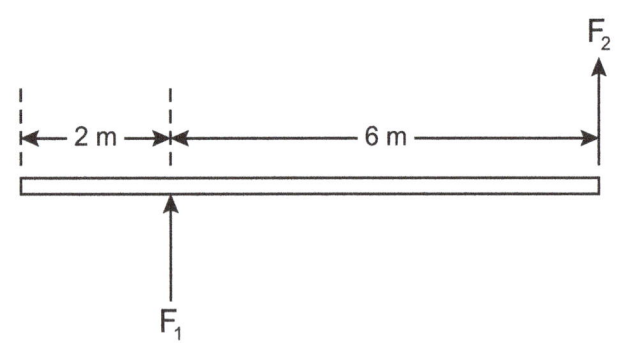

- A. $F_1 = 2F_2$
- B. $F_1 = W$
- C. $F_1 = W - 2F_2$
- D. $F_1 = W + 2F_2$

12) An assembly is composed of a 3-kg object attached to a 6-kg object by a weightless rod measuring 6 m in length. How far from the 3-kg object is the centre of gravity of the assembly?

- A. 2 m
- B. 4 m
- C. 6 m
- D. 8 m

13) Three children of masses 20 kg, 40 kg, and 60 kg want to balance themselves on an 8-metre long seesaw, pivoted at its centre. The 60-kg child sits 1 m from the left end. The 40-kg child sits at the right end. Where must the 20-kg child sit?

- A. 3 m from the right end
- B. 3 m from the left end
- C. 1 m from the right end
- D. 2 m from the right end

14) The biceps muscle holds the forearm and any load held by the hand, if present. There are forces at the elbow joint where the humerus meets the radius. The human forearm can be considered as a set of levers as illustrated below.

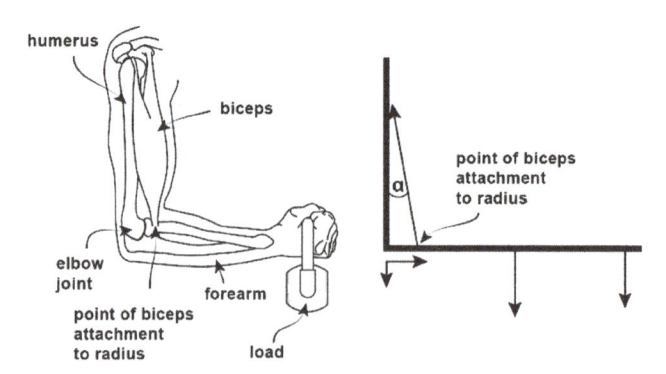

Consider that the arm is in rotational and translational equilibrium, as the load held in the hand increases, what would be the expected change in the vertical and horizontal components of the forces at the elbow, respectively?

- A. Decreased, increased
- B. Increased, does not change
- C. Increased, increased
- D. Decreased, does not change

15) A mass of 100 kg is placed on a uniform bar at a point 0.5 m to the left of a fulcrum. Where must a 75 kg mass be placed relative to the fulcrum in order to establish a state of equilibrium given that the bar was in equilibrium before any weights were applied?

   A. 0.66 m to the right of the fulcrum
   B. 0.66 m to the left of the fulcrum
   C. 0.38 m to the right of the fulcrum
   D. 0.38 m to the left of the fulcrum

16) In a freak accident, an explosion causes an F-16 jet to divide in half into two equal parts while in flight. If the explosion causes one half (part A) to come to a complete stop whereas the second half (part B) continues on along the same trajectory, at what speed will part B be traveling subsequent to the explosion? Assume the jet weighed 2000 kg and was originally traveling at a speed of 360 km/hr.

   A. 360 km/h
   B. 180 km/h
   C. 540 km/h
   D. 720 km/h

17) Torque is a turning force which is calculated by: force (F) multiplied by a distance (x). In the case of a piston engine, F is the downwards force pushing the piston vertically and rotating the crankshaft after the engine's ignition. The distance x is the horizontal distance between the crankpin and the crankshaft at a specific angle into the engine cycle.

   There are 4 different types of torques that are of particular interest in high-performance vehicles: torque ripple, peak torque, maximum torque, and direct control torque (cont. torque). See Figure 1.

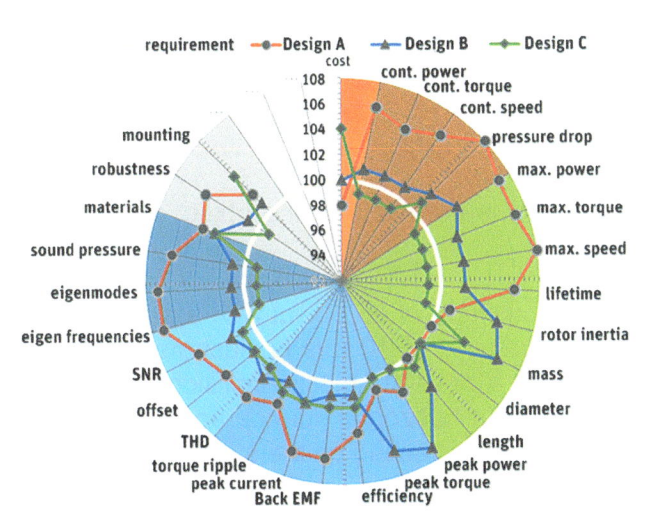

Figure 1: A radar chart illustrating three high-performance car design concepts and how well they meet established requirements.
(ANSYS Advantage; XI, issue 3, 2017)

According to Figure 1, with respect to torque, which of the following statements is most accurate?

   A. All 3 designs exceed the requirement for all 4 torque parameters.
   B. Only 2 designs exceed the requirement for all 4 torque parameters.
   C. Only 1 design exceeds the requirement for all 4 torque parameters.
   D. None of the designs exceed the requirement for all 4 torque parameters.

GAMSAT-Prep.com
GOLD STANDARD PHYSICS

Questions 18–19

The impulse *I* experienced by an object equals the change in momentum of the object, and is related to the acting force *F* and the change in time *t* as follows:

$$I = F \cdot \Delta t = m \cdot \Delta v$$

where m is the mass of the object and *v* is the velocity.

The movement of an object with a mass of 2 kg and a velocity of 10 m/s is illustrated in Figure 1 during a perfectly elastic collision. The object moves on a horizontal surface and there are no external forces acting on the system.

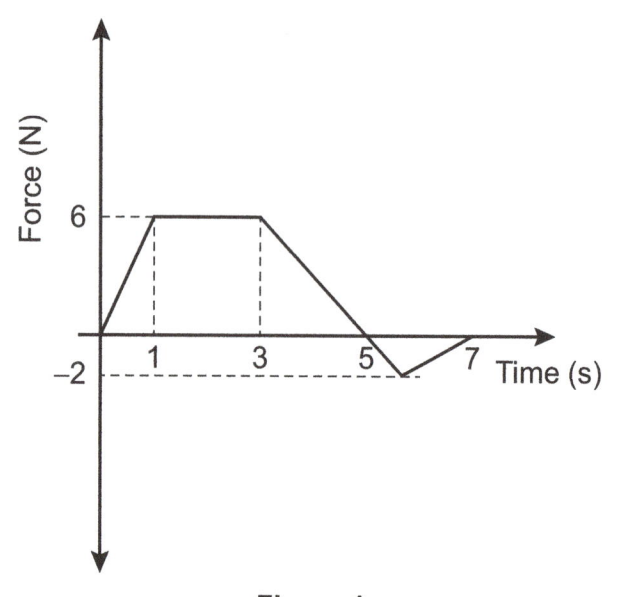

Figure 1

18) Approximate the velocity of the object at time = 7 s.
   A. 10 m/s
   B. 14.5 m/s
   C. 19.5 m/s
   D. 29.5 m/s

19) In the collision illustrated in Figure 1, which of the following can be asserted?
   A. Kinetic energy of the system alone is conserved.
   B. Only momentum is conserved.
   C. Both kinetic and momentum are conserved.
   D. Neither kinetic nor momentum is conserved.

20) Bed scales are ideal instruments to weigh patients who are bed-ridden. Often hospital staff must put the pair of legs at the head of the bed on the scale separately from the pair of legs at the foot of the bed. This procedure was followed for a particular patient and the scale read 190 kg and 170 kg, respectively. The centre of mass of the patient is 0.75 m from the head of the bed. The bed is uniform and 2 metres long. Which of the following best represents the mass of the patient?
   A. Less than 60 kg
   B. 65 kg
   C. 70 kg
   D. Between 75 kg and 85 kg

High-level Importance

PHY-58 CHAPTER 4: EQUILIBRIUM

GAMSAT MASTERS SERIES

⚠ SPOILER ALERT

Gold Standard has cross-referenced the content in this chapter to examples from ACER's official GAMSAT practice materials. It is for you to decide when you want to explore these questions since you may want to preserve some of ACER's materials for timed mock-exam practice.

Examples – Easy torque (bed-ridden patient): Q10-13 of 3; challenging torque (forces on the spine): Q44-47 of 2; momentum, impulse and a famous graph: 89-91 of 4; direct knowledge about elastic vs inelastic collisions as well as conservation of energy/momentum: Q91 of 4. Note that "Q" is followed by the question number, and, for example, "of 1" refers to booklet number 1 which is referenced in the Spoiler Alert table at the end of Chapter 1. The 10 full-length HEAPS GAMSAT practice tests (by Gold Standard and MediRed), exams 1 through 10, contain specific cross-references to this chapter within the worked solutions. Note that the torque forces implicated in the arm is a rare question included in this book from HEAPS-1 (Q22); the question with the 3 children is from HEAPS-8.

High-level Importance

Chapter Checklist

- ☐ Access your online account to view answers, worked solutions and discussion boards.
- ☐ Reassess your 'learning objectives' for this chapter: Go back to the first page of this chapter and re-evaluate the top 3 boxes and the Introduction.
  - ☐ Please be sure that you have completed the *Need for Speed* exercises at the beginning of this chapter.
- ☐ Complete a maximum of 1 page of notes using symbols/abbreviations to represent the entire chapter based on your learning objectives. These are your Gold Notes.
- ☐ Consider your multimedia options based on your optimal way of learning:
  - ☐ Download the free Gold Standard GAMSAT app for your Android device or iPhone.
  - ☐ Create your own, tangible study cards or try the free app: Anki.
  - ☐ Record your voice reading your Gold Notes onto your smartphone (MP3s) and listen during exercise, transportation, etc.
  - ☐ Try out the Gold Standard GAMSAT online videos at gamsat-prep.com, or you can try other options on YouTube like Khan Academy or Crash Course Physics.
- ☐ Reassess your schedule for your full-length GAMSAT practice tests: ACER and/or HEAPS exams. Ensure that you have scheduled one full day to complete a practice test and 1-2 days for a thorough assessment of worked solutions while adding to your abbreviated Gold Notes.
- ☐ Reassess your progress in scheduling and/or evaluating stress reduction techniques such as regular exercise (sports), yoga, meditation and/or mindfulness exercises (*see* YouTube for suggestions).

High-level Importance

GOLD NOTES

WORK AND ENERGY
Chapter 5

Memorise
* Define, equation, units: work
* Equations and units: potential energy, kinetic energy, power

Understand
* Path independence of work done in a g field
* Work-Energy Theorem
* Conservation of Energy; conservative forces
* Solving Conservation of Energy problems

Importance
Medium level: 5% of GAMSAT Physics questions released by ACER are related to content in this chapter (in our estimation).
* Note that approximately 75% of the questions in GAMSAT Physics are related to just 6 chapters: 1, 4, 6, 9, 11 and 12.

GAMSAT-Prep.com

Introduction

Work and energy are used to describe how bodies or masses interact with the environment or other bodies or masses. Conservation of energy, work and power describe the forms of energy and the changes between these forms.

Multimedia Resources at GAMSAT-Prep.com

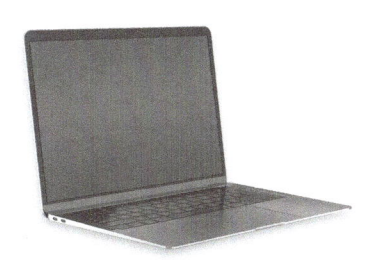

Open Discussion Boards   Foundational Videos   Flashcards   Special Guest

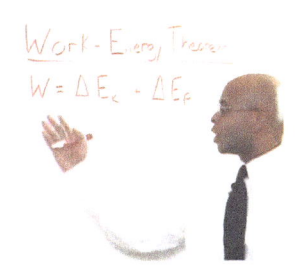

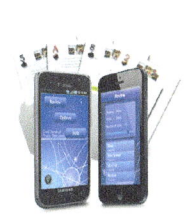

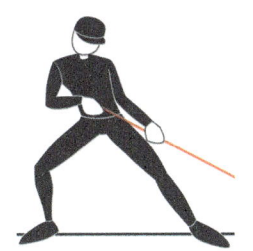

THE PHYSICAL SCIENCES   PHY-61

* The real GAMSAT may have advanced-level information presented (i.e. in a passage) but previous knowledge of said information is not required to answer the questions that would follow. Practice questions at the end of this chapter, as well as ACER and GS (HEAPS) practice GAMSATs can help you clarify this point.

GAMSAT-Prep.com
GOLD STANDARD PHYSICS

5.0 GAMSAT has a *Need for Speed*!

Section Number	GAMSAT Physics *Need for Speed* Exercises
5.1	How is work related to force?
	What is the SI unit for work and how does that unit relate to metres?
	What is the SI unit for kinetic and potential energy?
5.3	How is kinetic energy related to velocity?
5.4	How is potential energy related to the gravitational constant *G*?
	How is potential energy related to height?
5.5	How is the total mechanical energy related to kinetic and potential energy?
5.5.1	A 6.8×10^3 kg frictionless roller-coaster car starts at rest 30 metres above ground level. Determine the speed of the car at (a) 20 m above ground level; (b) at ground level. (scratch paper permitted!)
5.7	How does power relate to work?
	What is the SI unit of power and how does it relate to joules?

5.1 Work

The work of a force *F* on an object is the product of the force by the distance travelled by the object where the force is in the direction of the displacement: $W = F \times d$.

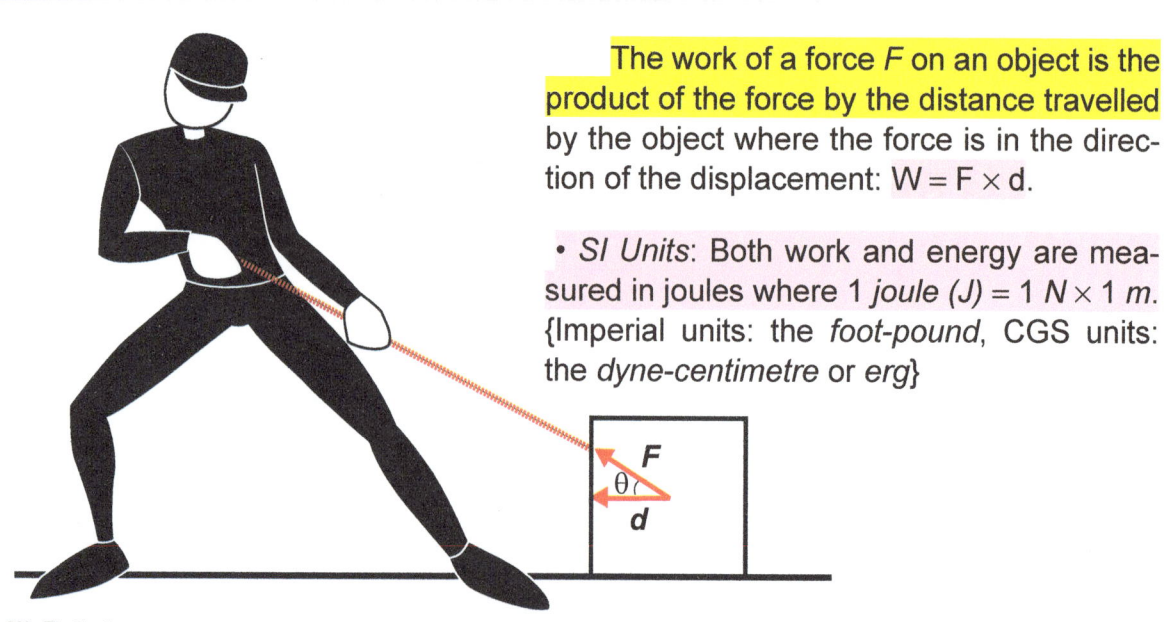

• *SI Units*: Both work and energy are measured in joules where 1 *joule (J)* = 1 *N* × 1 *m*. {Imperial units: the *foot-pound*, CGS units: the *dyne-centimetre* or *erg*}

Figure III.B.5.1: Work. The displacement depends on the final and initial positions of the object (PHY 1.2). The angle θ is necessary to determine the component of a constant force F in the same direction of the displacement. Note that if F acts perpendicular to the displacement then the work $W = F\,d\,cos(90°) = 0$.

5.2 Energy

We usually speak of mechanical, electrical, chemical, potential, kinetic, sound, atomic and nuclear energy, to name a few. In fact, these different kinds of energy are different forms or manifestations of the same energy. Energy is a scalar. It is defined as a physical quantity <u>capable of producing work</u>.

5.3 Kinetic Energy

1) *Definition of kinetic energy*

Kinetic energy (E_k) is the energy of motion which can produce work. It is proportional to the mass of the object and its velocity:

$$E_k = 1/2 \, mv^2.$$

Note that mass is always positive, and velocity squared guarantees a positive result. Thus, for a given mass, kinetic energy is always positive.

2) *The Work-Energy Theorem*

A net force is the sum of interior and exterior forces acting upon the system. The variation of the kinetic energy of a system is equal to the work of the net force applied to the system:

$$W \text{ (of the resultant force)} = \Delta E_k.$$

Consequently, if the speed of a particle is constant, $\Delta E_k = 0$, then the work done by the resultant force must be zero. For example, in uniform circular motion, the speed of the particle remains constant thus the centripetal force does no work on the particle. A force at right angles to the direction of motion merely changes the direction of the velocity but not its magnitude (we will explore this further in a cyclotron unit at the end of Chapter 9).

5.4 Potential Energy

Potential energy (E_p) is referred to as potential because it is accumulated by the system that contained it. It varies with the configuration of the system, i.e., when distances between particles of the system vary, the interactions between these particles vary. The variation of the potential energy is equal to the work performed by the interior forces caused by the interaction between the particles of the system. The following are examples of potential energy:

a) potential energy (= <u>e</u>lectric <u>p</u>otential = E_p) derived from the Coulomb force (r is the distance between point charges q_1 and q_2, PHY 9.1.4):

$$E_p = k \, q_1 q_2 / r$$

b) gravitational potential energy derived from the universal attraction force (G is the gravitational constant; r is the distance between the COG of masses m_1 and m_2):

$$E_p = G\, m_1 m_2 / r$$

c) potential energy derived from the gravitational force (h is the height):

$$E_p = mgh$$

d) potential energy derived from the elastic force (i.e. a compressed spring):

$$E_p = kx^2/2 .$$

{k = the spring constant, x = displacement, cf. PHY 7.2.1}

5.5 Conservation of Energy

a) Definition

The total mechanical energy (E_T) of a system is equal to the sum of its kinetic energy and its potential energy:

$$E_T = E_k + E_p.$$

b) Theorem of mechanical energy

The variation of the mechanical energy of a system is equal to the work of exterior forces acting on the system.

c) Consequence

An isolated system, i.e., which is not being acted upon by any exterior force, keeps a constant mechanical energy. The kinetic energy and the potential energy may vary separately but their sum remains constant. This makes conservation of energy a very simple way to solve many different types of GAMSAT Physics problems.

5.5.1 Conservation of Energy Problem (SI units)

A 6.8×10^3 kg frictionless roller-coaster car starts at rest 30 metres above ground level. Determine the speed of the car at **(a)** 20 m above ground level; **(b)** at ground level. {Consider using some scratch paper for your calculations.}

$$E_T = E_k + E_p = 1/2\, mv^2 + mgh$$

Initially v = 0 since the car starts at rest, h = 30 m, and the constant g ≈ 10 m/s², thus

$$E_T = 0 + m(10)(30) = 300m \text{ joules.}$$

Situation **(a)** where h = 20 m:

$$E_T = 300m = 1/2\, mv^2 + mgh$$

m cancels, multiply through by 2, solve for *v*:

$$300m = 1/2mv^2 + mgh$$
$$300 = 1/2v^2 + gh$$
$$2(300) = v^2 + (2)gh$$
$$v^2 = 2(300) - (2)gh$$
$$v = \sqrt{2(300) - 2(10)20} = \sqrt{2(100)}$$
$$= \sqrt{2}(10) = 14 \text{ m/s}$$

Situation **(b)** at ground level $h = 0$:

$$E_T = 300m = 1/2mv^2 + 0$$

m cancels, multiply through by 2, solve for *v*:

$$300m = 1/2mv^2$$
$$300 = 1/2v^2$$
$$600 = v^2$$
$$v = \sqrt{600} = \sqrt{6(100)} = 10\sqrt{6} = 24 \text{ m/s}$$

- Note: the mass of the roller coaster is irrelevant!
- Note: you must be able to quickly estimate square roots (GM 1.5.6; PHY 1.1.2, 2.6.1).

5.6 Conservative Forces

The three definitions of a conservative force are: **i)** after a round trip the kinetic energy of a particle on which a force acts must return to its initial value; **ii)** after a round trip the work done on a particle by a force must be zero; **iii)** the work done by the force on a particle depends on the initial and final positions of the particle and not on the path taken. {Note that we introduced the idea of conservation in PHY 4.3.1.}

Examples: Friction disobeys all three of the preceding criteria thus it is a non-conservative force (PHY 3.2). The force $F_s = -kx$ (Hooke's Law, PHY 7.2.1) of an ideal spring on a frictionless surface is a conservative force. Gravity is a conservative force. If you throw a ball vertically upward, it will return with the same kinetic energy it had when it left your hand (*neglect air resistance*). Note that the definition of a conservative force does not need to be commited to memory for GAMSAT purposes. But the idea that some forces restore energy and others do not, can be helpful for occasional GAMSAT problem-solving and rare direct questions.

5.7 Power

The power *P* applied during the work *W* performed by a force *F* is equal to the work divided by the time necessary to do the work. In other words, power is the rate of doing work:

$$P = \Delta W / \Delta t.$$

- The SI unit for power is the *watt* (W) which equals one *joule per second* (J/s).

- Power can also be expressed as the product of a force on an object and the object's velocity: $P = Fv$.

CHAPTER 5: Work and Energy

GOLD STANDARD FOUNDATIONAL GAMSAT PRACTICE QUESTIONS

1) All of the following have the same SI unit EXCEPT one. Which one is the EXCEPTION?
   A. Work
   B. Power
   C. Mechanical energy
   D. Potential energy derived from the spring force

2) All of the following represent the same SI unit EXCEPT one. Which one is the EXCEPTION?
   A. Joule per second
   B. Newton metre per second
   C. Watt
   D. Kilogram metre squared per second squared

3) Which of the following is a scalar quantity that is always positive or zero?
   A. Linear momentum
   B. Angular momentum
   C. Work
   D. Kinetic energy

4) Two objects are in motion, one has ½ the velocity of the other but twice the mass. External forces bring each mass to rest. Choose the correct statement.
   A. Twice as much work is done on the smaller mass.
   B. Twice as much work is done on the larger mass.
   C. The same amount of work is done on both masses.
   D. The work cannot be determined without knowing the displacement.

5) An object with mass m is launched horizontally from a cliff with a velocity of v_o from a height h.

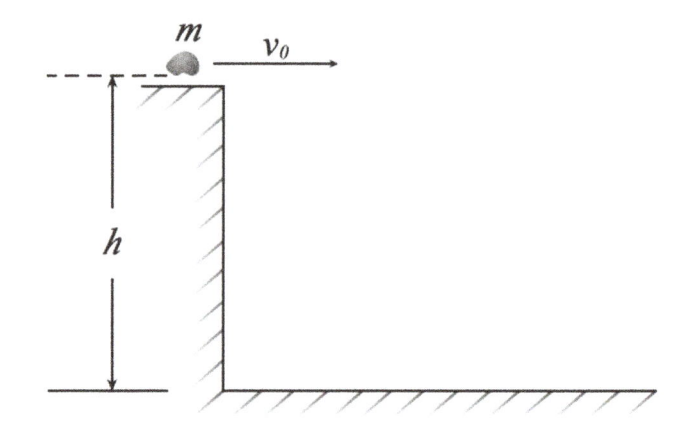

   Which of the following is consistent with the kinetic energy of the object just before it hits the ground?
   A. $1/2\ mv_o^2$
   B. mgh
   C. $1/2\ mv_o^2 - mgh$
   D. $1/2\ mv_o^2 + mgh$

6) A teenager lifts a 5-kg box 1 metre in 2 seconds, then her friend does the same thing but it takes 4 seconds, which of the following is true about the work done on the box?
   A. It is the same in both cases.
   B. The teenager did 3 times the work as her friend.
   C. The teenager did 9 times the work as her friend.
   D. The teenager did 1/3rd the work as her friend.

7) If a muscle is capable of doing 8 J of work in 0.3 seconds, what average power is it capable of?

   A. 8 watts
   B. 16 watts
   C. 24 watts
   D. 32 watts

8) Pressure is the force applied perpendicular to the surface of an object per unit area over which that force is distributed. Identify the equation which is dimensionally correct.

   A. Pressure = momentum/volume
   B. Pressure = force/volume
   C. Pressure = energy/volume
   D. Pressure = energy/area

9) Which of the following physical quantities would be the result of multiplying megawatts by the amount of time?

   A. Power
   B. Energy
   C. Current
   D. Charge

10) A force is applied to an object resulting in its displacement. The event is summarised in Figure 1.

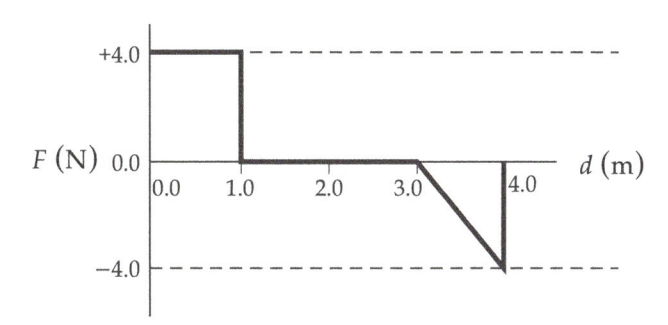

Figure 1

For the time interval 0–4 seconds, what is the work done on the object by the force?

   A. 1 J
   B. 2 J
   C. 4 J
   D. 6 J

GOLD STANDARD GAMSAT-LEVEL PRACTICE QUESTIONS

11) A child is holding a ball and then throws it straight upwards. Which of the following energy (*E*) vs. height (*h*) graphs best represents the changes in kinetic energy and gravitational potential energy of the ball?

— Kinetic energy
--- Gravitational potential energy

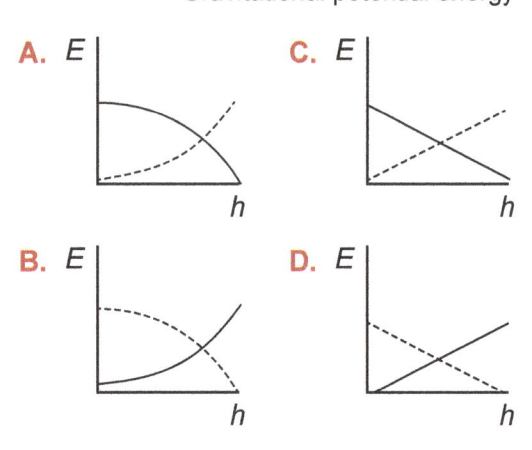

A. *E* vs *h*

B. *E* vs *h*

C. *E* vs *h*

D. *E* vs *h*

12) Starting from the same height, two small objects of equal mass m slide down the two frictionless inclined planes A and B as shown in Figure 1. The object sliding down plane A reaches the bottom of the plane with a final velocity V_A, and the object sliding down plane B achieves a final velocity V_B. What is the magnitude of the ratio V_B/V_A?

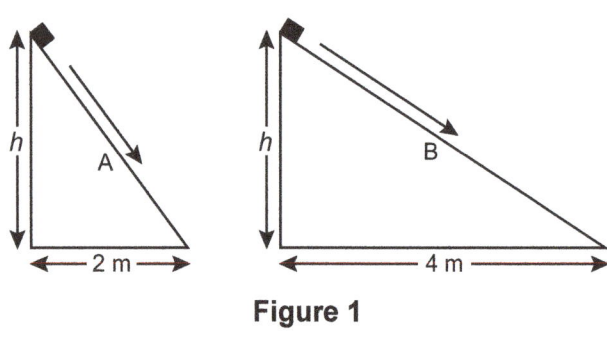

Figure 1

A. 0.5
B. 1
C. 2
D. 4

Questions 13–14

Consider the following diagram of extended and flexed positions, respectively, of a person doing press-ups.

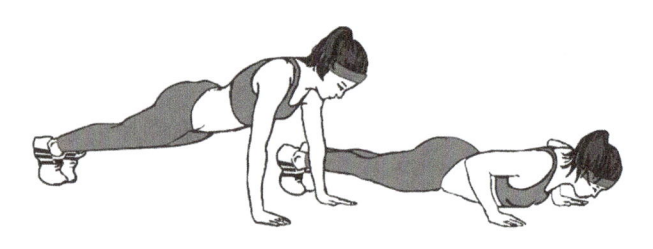

Figure 1

Note that: Her mass is 50 kg; the distance from her feet to her centre of gravity is 0.90 m; the distance from her feet to her hands is 1.50 m; the gravitational acceleration (*g*) of a free-falling object can be estimated as 10 m s^{-2}.

The following questions are based on her movement from the flexed to the extended position which she accomplishes at constant velocity.

13) What maximum force should each hand exert on the floor for the woman in Figure 1 to complete one press-up?

A. 150 N
B. 250 N
C. 300 N
D. 500 N

14) For each press-up, her centre of mass rises 24 cm. What is her useful power output if she does 25 press-ups in one minute?

A. 2 W
B. 25 W
C. 50 W
D. 100 W

15) A child is riding a tricycle with a combined mass of 22 kg travelling with a velocity of 1 m/s. The distance from the ground to the top of the child's head is 0.5 m. If the child increases the velocity of the tricycle to 3 m/s, determine what would happen to the kinetic energy.

One or more of the following equations may be of help, where m is the mass, v is the velocity, g is the gravitational constant (approximately 10 m/s^2), and h is the height:

- Momentum $M = mv$
- Kinetic energy $KE = \frac{1}{2}mv^2$
- Potential energy $PE = mgh$

A. The kinetic energy would decrease by a factor of 9.
B. The kinetic energy would decrease by a factor of 3.
C. The kinetic energy would increase by a factor of 3.
D. The kinetic energy would increase by a factor of 9.

16) A student pushed a box of 15-kg mass to the top of a 10-m long ramp inclined at 30° to the horizon. The student weighed 620 N, pushed with a 45-N force parallel to the ramp, and took 3 minutes to reach the top of the ramp.

Suppose that the box fell from the top of the ramp to the ground. Which of the following represents the velocity of the box at impact?

Note that: sin(30°) = 0.5; cos(30°) = 0.87

A. 3 m/s
B. 6.5 m/s
C. 10 m/s
D. 15.5 m/s

17) Power is the rate of work. Work is force times distance.

The dimension of a physical quantity can be expressed as a product of the basic physical dimensions of mass (M), length (L) and time (T). For example, the dimension of the physical quantity speed or velocity (m/s) is length/time (= L/T).

A physiotherapist tells her patient that muscle times speed equals power. What dimensions are implied for "muscle"?

A. MLT^{-2}
B. MLT
C. MLT^2
D. ML^2T^{-2}

18) Consider an object being lifted vertically each of the distances shown below at constant speed, in the time periods provided.

Case 1: 4 m; 4 seconds
Case 2: 8 m; 2 seconds

In which case is the average power employed greater?

A. Case 1
B. Case 2
C. It is the same in both cases.
D. That determination cannot be made based on the information provided.

GAMSAT-Prep.com
GOLD STANDARD PHYSICS

Questions 19–20

A graph is sometimes used to assess certain characteristics of electronic equipment with rotating parts. Figure 1 relates power, rotating speed, and torque. Two of the values were known for the appliances labelled (A) and (B) thus the third value could be determined from Figure 1.

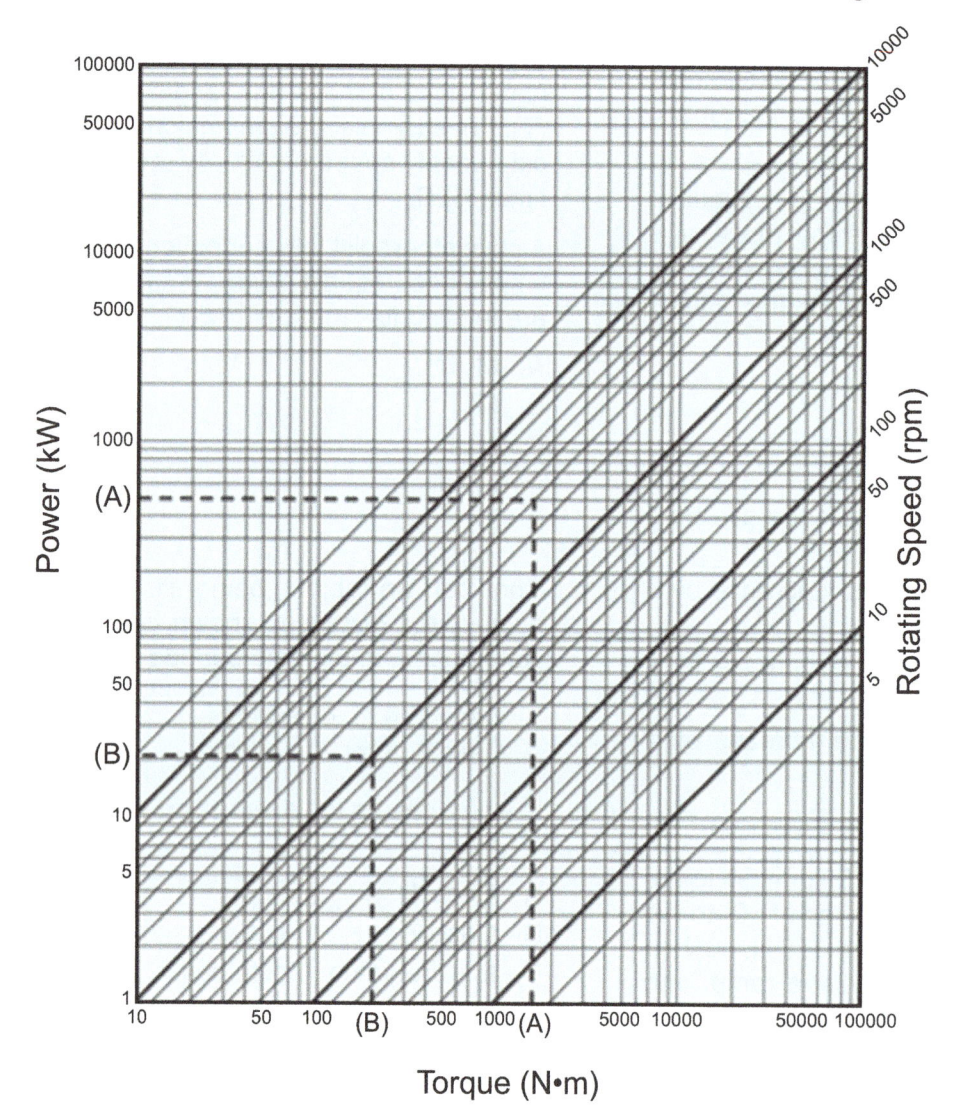

Figure 1: Graph depicting the relationship between power, rotary speed, and torque.
(Relabelled after Kyowa Electronic, 2020)

19) Based on Figure 1, which of the following statements is correct?

　A. The power for (A) is approximately twice the power for (B).
　B. The difference in power between (A) and (B) is approximately 480 watts.
　C. The difference in power between (A) and (B) is approximately 4.8×10^6 watts.
　D. Neither **A**, nor **B**, nor **C** is correct.

20) Based on Figure 1, which of the following best expresses the relationship between the power P (W), the rotating speed R (rpm), and the torque T (N·m)?

　A. $P = RT$
　B. $P = 2\pi RT$
　C. $P = 2\pi RT/60$
　D. $P = 2\pi RT/600$

GAMSAT MASTERS SERIES

⚠ SPOILER ALERT

Gold Standard has cross-referenced the content in this chapter to examples from ACER's official GAMSAT practice materials. It is for you to decide when you want to explore these questions since you may want to preserve some of ACER's materials for timed mock-exam practice.

Examples – Mechanical energy, conservation of energy (be careful with the COG!): Q7-9 of 2; direct knowledge question about elastic vs inelastic collisions and conservation of energy/momentum: Q91 of 4. Note that "Q" is followed by the question number, and, for example, "of 1" refers to booklet number 1 which is referenced in the Spoiler Alert table at the end of Chapter 1. The 10 full-length HEAPS GAMSAT practice tests (by Gold Standard and MediRed), exams 1 through 10, contain specific cross-references to this chapter within the worked solutions. Note that the unit with press-ups is a rare visitor from HEAPS-1 (Americans, Canadians: *push-ups*!).

High-level Importance

Chapter Checklist

- ☐ Access your online account to view answers, worked solutions and discussion boards.
- ☐ Reassess your 'learning objectives' for this chapter: Go back to the first page of this chapter and re-evaluate the top 3 boxes and the Introduction.
  - ☐ Please be sure that you have completed the *Need for Speed* exercises at the beginning of this chapter.
- ☐ Complete a maximum of 1 page of notes using symbols/abbreviations to represent the entire chapter based on your learning objectives. These are your Gold Notes.
- ☐ Consider your multimedia options based on your optimal way of learning:
  - ☐ Download the free Gold Standard GAMSAT app for your Android device or iPhone.
  - ☐ Create your own, tangible study cards or try the free app: Anki.
  - ☐ Record your voice reading your Gold Notes onto your smartphone (MP3s) and listen during exercise, transportation, etc.
  - ☐ Try out the Gold Standard GAMSAT online videos at gamsat-prep.com, or you can try other options on YouTube like Khan Academy or Crash Course Physics.
- ☐ Reassess your schedule for your full-length GAMSAT practice tests: ACER and/or HEAPS exams. Ensure that you have scheduled one full day to complete a practice test and 1-2 days for a thorough assessment of worked solutions while adding to your abbreviated Gold Notes.
- ☐ Reassess your progress in scheduling and/or evaluating stress reduction techniques such as regular exercise (sports), yoga, meditation and/or mindfulness exercises (*see* YouTube for suggestions).

High-level Importance

GOLD NOTES

FLUIDS AND SOLIDS
Chapter 6

Memorise
* Equation: density
* Density of water
* Equations for pressure, pressure change

Understand
* Buoyancy force, SG and height immersed
* Streamline, turbulent flow; continuity/ Bernouilli's equation
* Fluid viscosity, Archimedes' principle, surface tension; vapor press., atmospheric press.
* Elastic properties of solids; effect of temperature

Importance
High level: 12% of GAMSAT Physics questions released by ACER are related to content in this chapter (in our estimation).
* Note that approximately **75%** of the questions in GAMSAT Physics are related to just 6 chapters: 1, 4, 6, 9, 11 and 12.

GAMSAT-Prep.com

Introduction

A fluid is a substance that flows (*deforms*) under shear stress. This includes all gases and liquids. It is important to understand the properties without movement (hydrostatic pressure, Archimedes' principle) and with movement (continuity, Bernoulli's). On the other hand, a solid *resists* being deformed or submitting to changes in volume. A basic understanding of this *elastic* property of solids is helpful.

Multimedia Resources at GAMSAT-Prep.com

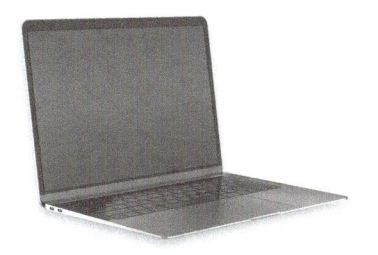

Open Discussion Boards   Foundational Videos   Flashcards   Special Guest

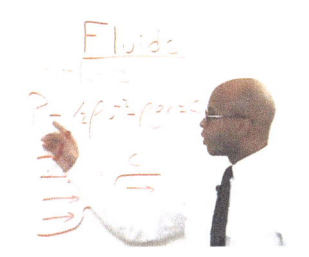

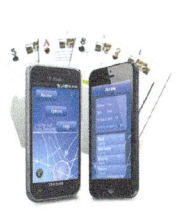

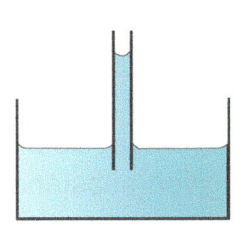

THE PHYSICAL SCIENCES PHY-73

* The real GAMSAT may have advanced-level information presented (i.e. in a passage) but previous knowledge of said information is not required to answer the questions that would follow. Practice questions at the end of this chapter, as well as ACER and GS (HEAPS) practice GAMSATs can help you clarify this point.

GAMSAT-Prep.com
GOLD STANDARD PHYSICS

6.0 GAMSAT has a *Need for Speed*!

High-level Importance

Section Number	GAMSAT Physics *Need for Speed* Exercises
6.1.1	What is density?
	What is specific gravity?
6.1.2	How is pressure related to force?
	What is the SI unit for pressure and how does it relate to newtons?
	How is the change of pressure in a fluid related to the depth?
	How does the buoyant force relate to volume, and to the weight of fluid displaced?
	If an object has a specific gravity of 9/10 and it is placed in water, what percent of the height of the object will be below the surface of the water?

6.1 Fluids

6.1.1 Density, Specific Gravity

The *density* of an object is defined as the ratio of its mass to its volume.

$$\text{density} = \text{mass} / \text{volume}$$

This definition holds for solids, fluids and gases. From the definition, it is easy to see that solids are more dense than liquids which are in turn more dense than gases. This is true because for a given mass, the average distance between molecules of a given substance is bigger in the liquid state than in the solid state. Put simply, the substance occupies a bigger volume in the liquid state than in the solid state and a much bigger volume in gaseous state than in the liquid state.

At a given temperature, the *specific gravity* (SG) is defined as:

$$SG = \frac{\text{density of a substance}}{\text{density of water}}$$

The density of water is about 1 g/ml (= 1 g/cm^3 = 10^3 kg/m^3) over most common temperatures. So in most instances the specific gravity of a substance is the same as its density.

Note that the dimension of density is mass per unit volume, whereas the specific gravity is dimensionless. Density is one of the key properties of fluids (liquids or gases) and the other is pressure.

CHAPTER 6: FLUIDS AND SOLIDS

6.1.2 Hydrostatic Pressure, Buoyancy, Archimedes' Principle

Pressure (P) is defined as the force (F) per unit area (A):

$$P = F/A.$$

The force F is the normal (*perpendicular*) force to the area. The SI unit for pressure is the *pascal* (1 Pa = 1 N/m^2). Other units are: 1.00 atm = 1.01 × 10^5 Pa = 1.01 bar = 760 mmHg = 760 torr = 14.7 lb/in^2.

Pressure is also formulated as potential energy per unit volume (V) as follows:

$$P = \frac{F}{A} = \frac{mg}{A} = \frac{(mg/A)}{(h/h)} = \frac{mgh}{V} = \rho g h$$

where ρ = density and h = depth below surface; if the depth is changing, we can write:

$$\Delta P = \rho g \Delta h.$$

We will now examine **6 key rules** of incompressible fluids (liquids) that are not moving (*statics*).

1) In a fluid confined by solid boundaries, pressure acts perpendicular to the boundary – it is a <u>normal force</u>, sometimes called a *surface force*.

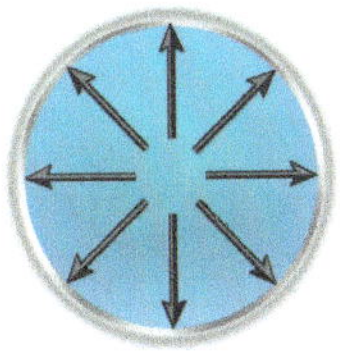

pipe or tube 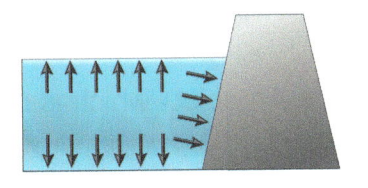   dam

2) At any particular depth, the pressure of the fluid is the same in all directions.

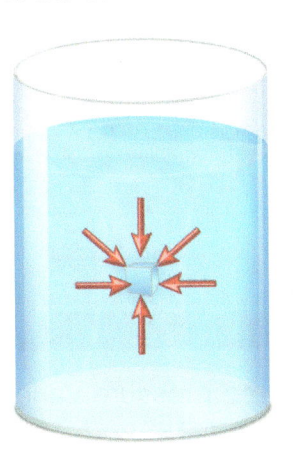

3) The fluid or *hydrostatic pressure* depends on the density and the depth of the fluid. So it is easy to calculate the change in pressure in an open container, swimming pool, the ocean, etc.:

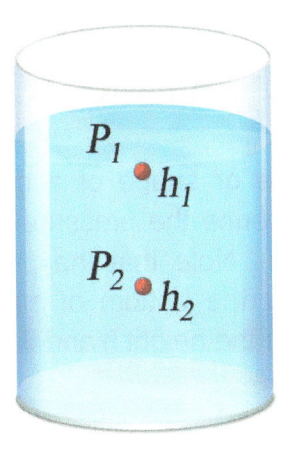

P_1 = atmospheric pressure
h_1 = surface = a depth of 0
$P_2 - P_1 = \Delta P$
$h_2 - h_1 = \Delta h$
$\Delta P = \rho g \Delta h$

High-level Importance

Vertical plane surfaces

We can now combine rules 1, 2 and 3 about fluids to examine a special case which is that of a vertical plane surface like a vertical wall that is underwater.

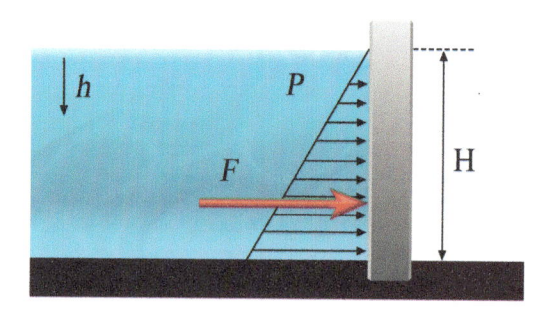

Of course pressure varies linearly with depth because $\Delta P = \rho g \Delta h$.

If the height of the vertical rectangular wall is H and the width W, with the help of calculus (which is *not* on the GAMSAT!), the equation for the force on the wall, or vertical plane, at any depth can be determined to be:

$$F = 1/2 \, \rho g W H^2$$

4) The size or shape of a container does not influence the pressure (= *hydrostatic paradox*). Note that the pressure is the same at the bottom of all 3 containers because the height h and fluid density are the same.

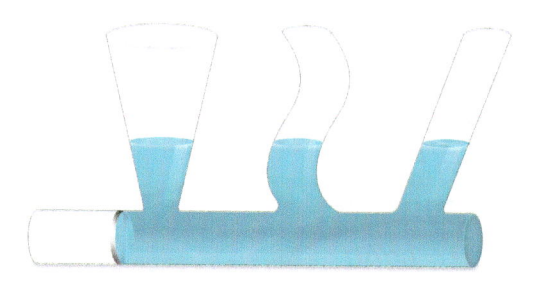

5) Pascal's Principle: If an external pressure is applied to a confined fluid, the pressure at every point within the fluid increases by that amount. This is the basis for hydraulic systems (e.g., lifts, brakes, shock absorbers, etc.). Key points: (1) the pressure of the system is constant throughout and (2) by definition, P = F/A, so we get:

$$F_1/A_1 = F_2/A_2$$

Hydraulic systems, like the brakes in a car, can multiply the force applied. For example, if a 50 N force is applied by the left piston in the diagram and if the right piston has an area five times greater, then the force out at F_2 is 250 N (thus the force vector F_2 is 5 times longer).

$$F_2 = A_2(F_1/A_1) = 5A_1(F_1/A_1) = 5(F_1)$$

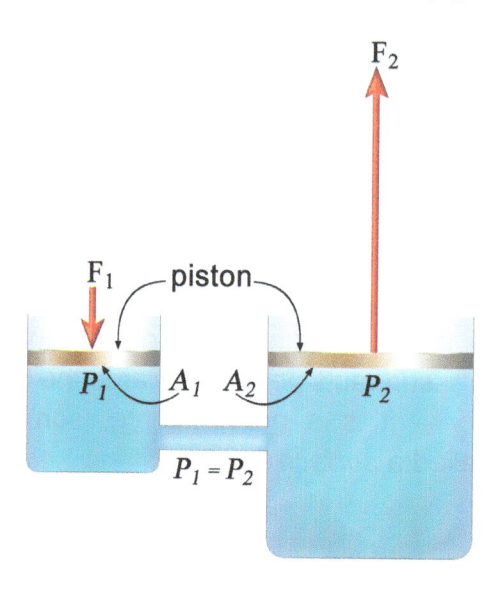

6) An object which is completely or partially submerged in a fluid experiences an upward force equal to the weight of the fluid displaced (*Archimedes' principle*).

PHY-76   CHAPTER 6: FLUIDS AND SOLIDS

This buoyant force F_b is :

$$F_b = V\rho g = mg$$

where ρ is the density of the fluid displaced. An object that floats must displace at most its own weight.

Archimedes' principle can be used to calculate specific gravity. And in turn, specific gravity is equivalent to the fraction of the height of a buoyant object below the surface of the fluid. Thus if SG = 0.90, then 90% of the height of the object would be immersed in water. Therefore, less dense objects float.

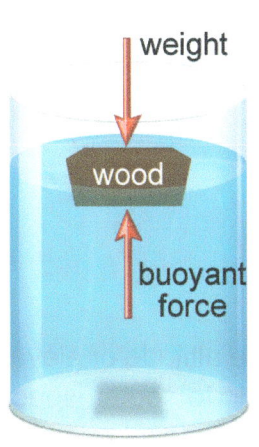

6.1.2.1 Atmospheric Pressure

Atmospheric pressure is the force per unit area exerted against a surface by the weight of the air above that surface. If the number of air molecules above a surface increases, there are more molecules to exert a force on that surface and thus, the pressure increases. On the other hand, a reduction in the number of air molecules above a surface will result in a decrease in pressure. Atmospheric pressure is measured with a "barometer", which is why atmospheric pressure is also referred to as *barometric* pressure.

Atmospheric pressure is often measured with a mercury (Hg) barometer, and a height of approximately 760 millimetres (30 in) of mercury represents atmospheric pressure at sea level (760 mmHg).

Unit	Definition or Relationship
SI Unit: 1 pascal (Pa)	1 kg m^{-1} s^{-2} = 1 N/m^2
1 bar	1 × 10^5 Pa
1 atmosphere (atm)	101,325 Pa = 101.3 kPa
1 torr	1 / 760 atm
760 mmHg	1 atm
14.7 pounds per sq. in. (psi)	1 atm

Units of Pressure

GAMSAT-Prep.com
GOLD STANDARD PHYSICS

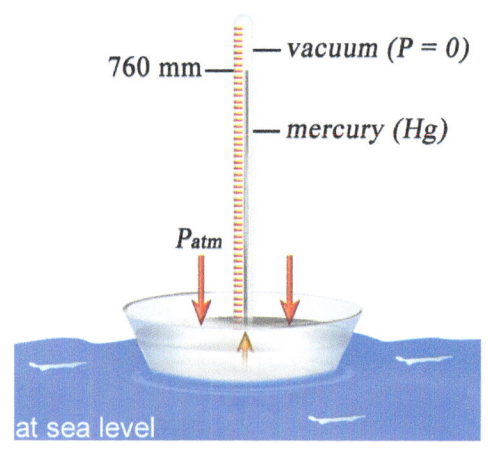

High-level Importance

When the altitude or elevation increases, we get closer to "outer space" so there is less overlying atmospheric mass from gases, so that pressure decreases with increasing elevation.

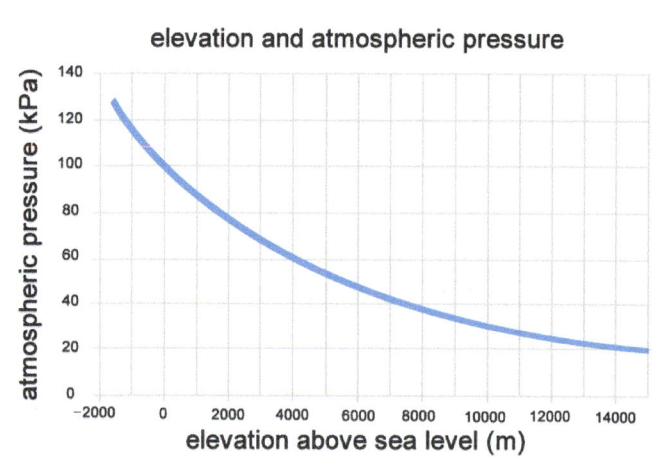

Figure III.B.6.0: Atmospheric pressure decreases with elevation. Mount Everest is about 8,800 metres (m) and a 747 can cruise at an altitude of 10,000 m but requires increased cabin pressure to prevent passengers from having altitude sickness and low oxygen (hypoxia). Note that this is a classic exponential decay curve.

6.1.2.2 Gauge Pressure

When you measure the pressure in your tyres, you are measuring the pressure difference between the tyres and atmospheric pressure, which is the *gauge* (or *gage*) pressure.

Absolute pressure is the pressure of a fluid relative to the pressure in a vacuum. The absolute pressure is then the sum of the gauge pressure, which is what you measure, and the atmospheric pressure.

$$P_{abs} = P_{atm} + P_{gauge}$$

Pressure can be measured in devices in which one or more columns of a liquid (i.e. mercury or water) are used to determine the pressure difference between two points (i.e. U-tube manometer, inclined-tube manometer).

Of course, electronic instruments for measurement are used more frequently.

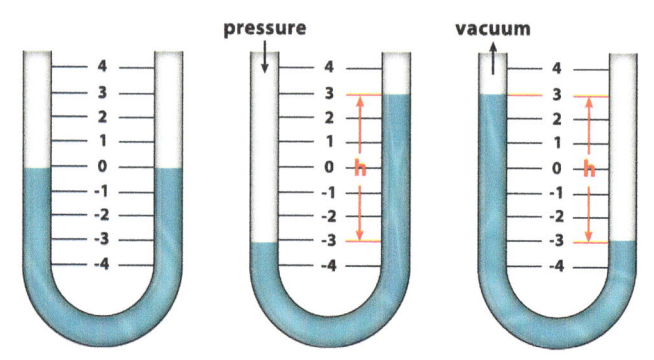

Figure III.B.6.0.0: When the U-tube has both ends open to the same pressure, the height of the liquid will be the same in each leg. If positive pressure is applied to one leg, it will force a difference in height h. When a vacuum (= *no pressure*) is applied to one leg, the liquid rises in that leg and falls in the other. The difference in pressure can be calculated: $\Delta P = \rho g \Delta h$ (PHY 6.1.2).

PHY-78   CHAPTER 6: FLUIDS AND SOLIDS

6.1.3 Fluids in Motion, Continuity Equation, Bernoulli's Equation

Fluids in motion are described by two equations, the continuity equation and Bernoulli's equation. Fluids are assumed to have streamline (= *laminar*) flow which means that the motion of every particle in the fluid follows the same path as the particle that preceded it. Turbulent flow occurs when that definition cannot be applied, resulting in molecular collisions, irregularly shaped whirlpools (*see image in PHY 6.1.4*), energy is then dissipated and frictional drag is increased. The rate (R) of streamline flow, as can be imagined as the movement of water in a stream or relatively calm river, is given by:

$$R = \text{(volume past a point)/time} = Avt/t = Av$$

volume = (cross-sectional area) (length) = (A) (vt) = Avt

length = distance = (velocity) (time) = vt

cross-sectional area of a tube = area of a circle = πr^2 where π can be estimated as 3.14 and *r* is the radius of the circle.

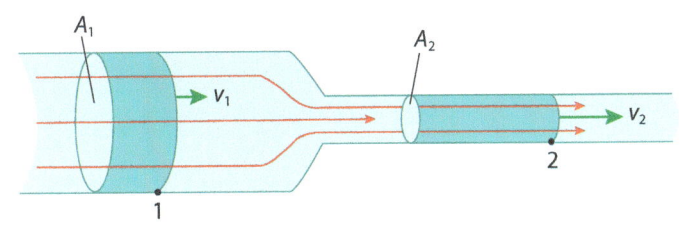

Figure III.B.6.0.1: Application of the continuity equation. When a tube narrows, the same volume occupies a greater length. For the same volume to pass points 1 and 2 in a given time, the speed must be greater at point 2.

- The equation can also be written as the **continuity equation**:

$$A_1 v_1 = A_2 v_2 = constant$$

where subscripts 1 and 2 refer to different points in the line of flow. The continuity equation can be used for an incompressible fluid flowing in an enclosed tube. For a compressible fluid:

$$\rho_1 A_1 v_1 = \rho_2 A_2 v_2 = constant$$

- **Bernoulli's equation** is an application of the law of conservation of energy and is:

$$P + \rho g h + \tfrac{1}{2} \rho v^2 = constant$$

It follows:

$$P_1 + \rho g h_1 + \tfrac{1}{2} \rho v_1^2 = P_2 + \rho g h_2 + \tfrac{1}{2} \rho v_2^2$$

where subscripts 1 and 2 refer to different points in the flow.

A commonly encountered consequence of Bernoulli's equation is that where the height is relatively constant and the velocity of a fluid is high, the pressure is low, and vice versa.

{Various applications of the preceding equations will be explored in the practice questions at the end of this chapter.}

6.1.4 Fluid Viscosity and Determining Turbulence

Viscosity is analogous to friction between moving solids. It may, therefore be viewed as the resistance to flow of layers of fluid (as in streamline or laminar flow) past each other. This also means that viscosity, as in friction, results in dissipation of mechanical energy. As one layer flows over another, its motion is transmitted to the second layer and causes this layer to be set in motion. Since a mass m of the second layer is set in motion and some of the energy of the first layer is lost, there is a transfer of momentum between the layers.

The greater the transfer of this momentum from one layer to another, the more energy that is lost and the slower the layers move.

The viscosity (η) is the measure of the efficiency of transfer of this momentum. Therefore the higher the viscosity coefficient, the greater the transfer of momentum and loss of mechanical energy, and thus loss of velocity. The reverse situation holds for a low viscosity coefficient.

Consequently, a high viscosity coefficient substance flows slowly (e.g. molasses), and a low viscosity coefficient substance flows relatively fast (e.g. water or, especially helium). Note that the transfer of momentum to adjacent layers is in essence, the exertion of a force upon these layers to set them in motion.

Whether flow is streamline or turbulent depends on a combination of factors already discussed. A convenient measure is Reynolds Number (R):

$$R = vd\rho / \eta$$

v = velocity of flow
d = diameter of the tube
ρ = density of the fluid
η = viscosity coefficient

In general, if R < 2000 the flow is streamline; if R > 2000 the flow is turbulent. Note that as v, d or ρ increases or η decreases, the flow becomes more turbulent.

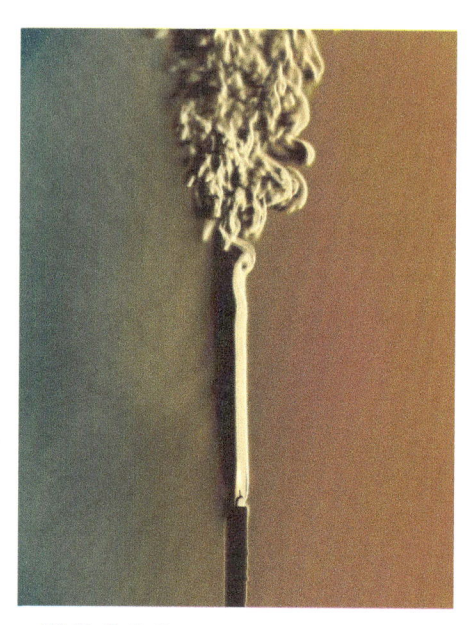

Figure III.B.6.0.2: The plume from this candle flame goes from laminar to turbulent in the upper 1/3 of the image. The Reynolds number can be used to predict where this transition takes place (Schlieren photograph of an ordinary candle in still air by Dr. Gary Settles).

6.1.5 Surface Tension

Molecules of a liquid exert attractive forces toward each other (cohesive forces), and exert attractive forces toward the surface they touch (adhesive forces). If a liquid is in a gravity-free space without a surface, it will form a sphere (smallest area relative to volume).

If the liquid is lining an object, the liquid surface will contract (due to cohesive forces) to the lowest possible surface area. The forces between the molecules on this surface will create a membrane-like effect. Due to the contraction, a potential energy (PE) will present in the surface.

This PE is directly proportional to the surface area (A). An exact relation is formed as follows:

$$PE = \gamma A$$

γ = surface tension = PE/A = joules/m²

An alternative formulation for the surface tension (γ) is:

$$\gamma = F/l$$

F = force of contraction of surface
l = length along surface

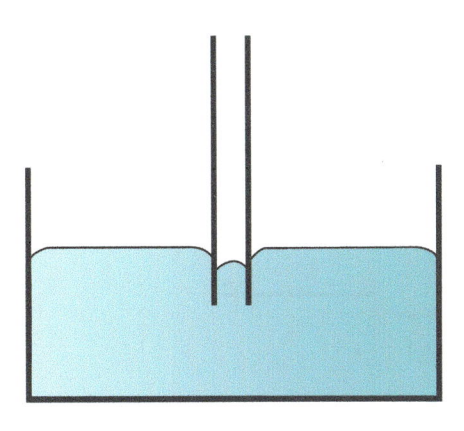

(a) cohesive > adhesive

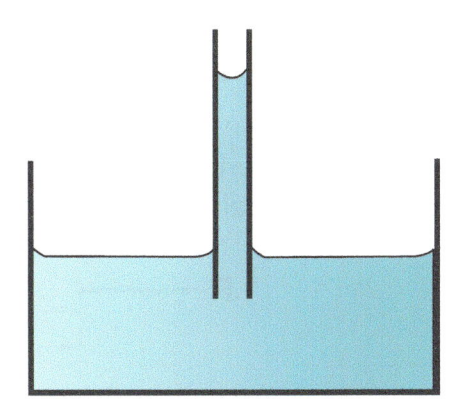

(b) adhesive > cohesive

Figure III.B.6.1: Effects of adhesive and cohesive forces. The distance the liquid rises or falls in the tube is directly proportional to the surface tension γ and inversely proportional to the liquid density and radius of the tube. Examples of 2 liquids consistent with the illustrations include: (a) mercury; (b) water.

Because of the contraction, a small object which would ordinarily sink in the liquid may float on the surface membrane. For example, a small insect like a "water strider."

The liquid will rise or fall on a wall or in a capillary tube if the adhesive forces are greater than cohesive or vice versa (see Figure III.B.6.1).

6.2 Solids

6.2.1 Elastic Properties of Solids

When a force acts on a solid, the solid is deformed. If the solid returns to its original shape, the solid is elastic. The effect of a force depends on the area over which it acts. Stress is defined as the ratio of the force to the area over which it acts. Strain is defined as the relative change in dimensions or shape of the object caused by the stress. This is embodied in the definition of the modulus of elasticity (ME) as:

$$ME = \frac{stress}{strain}$$

Some different types of stresses are tensile stress (equal and opposite forces directed away from each other), compressive stress (equal and opposite forces directed towards each other), and shearing stress (equal and opposite forces which do not have the same line of action). There are two commonly used moduli of elasticity:

1) Young's Modulus (Y) for compressive or tensile stress:

$$Y = \frac{longitudinal\ stress}{longitudinal\ strain}$$

$$Y = \frac{(F/A)}{(\Delta l/l)} = \frac{F \times l}{A \Delta l}$$

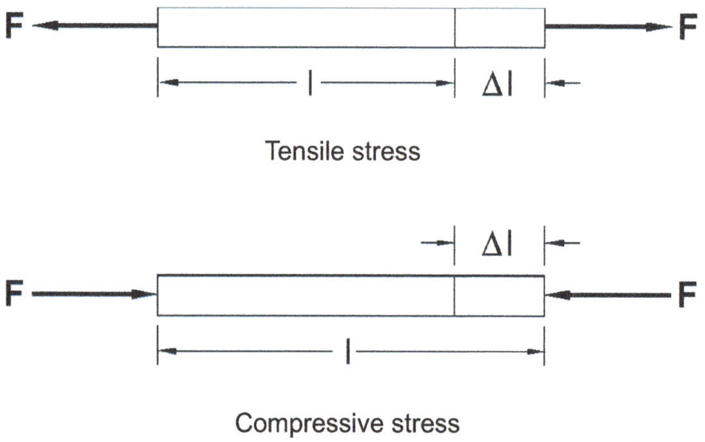

Tensile stress

Compressive stress

Figure III.B.6.2: Compressive and Tensile Stress.

2) Shear modulus (S) or the modulus of rigidity is:

S = shearing stress / shearing strain

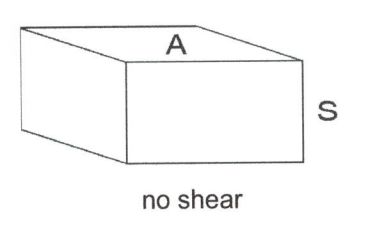

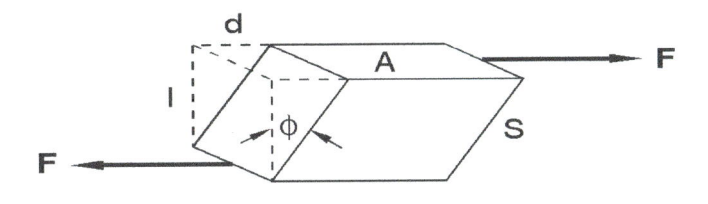

$$S = (F/A) / \tan\phi$$

Figure III.B.6.3: Shear Stress. A is the area tangential to the force F.

6.3 The Effect of Temperature on Solids and Liquids

When substances gain or lose heat they usually undergo expansion or contraction.

Expansion or contraction can be by linear dimension, by area or by volume.

Table III.B.6.1: Substance thermal expansion.

Type	Final	Original	Change caused by heat
(1) Linear	L $L = L_0 + \alpha \Delta T L_0$ $L = L_0(1 + \alpha \Delta T)$ α = coefficient of linear thermal expansion ΔT = change in temperature	L_0	$\alpha \Delta T L_0$
(2) Area	A $A = A_0 + \gamma \Delta T A_0$ $A = A_0(1 + \gamma \Delta T)$ γ = coefficient of area thermal expansion = 2α	A_0	$\gamma \Delta T A_0$
(3) Volume	V $V = V_0 + \beta \Delta T V_0$ $V = V_0(1 + \beta \Delta T)$ β = coefficient of volume thermal expansion = 3α	V_0	$\beta \Delta T V_0$

GOLD STANDARD PHYSICS

CHAPTER 6: Fluids and Solids

GOLD STANDARD FOUNDATIONAL GAMSAT PRACTICE QUESTIONS

1) The dimension of a physical quantity can be expressed as a product of the basic physical dimensions of mass (M), length (L) and time (T). What are the dimensions for density?

   A. M
   B. ML^3
   C. ML^{-3}
   D. M/L^{-3}

2) Which of the following is an expression for pressure?

   A. (mass • velocity) / (volume)
   B. (mass • velocity) / (area • time)
   C. (mass • acceleration) / (volume)
   D. (mass • acceleration) / (area • time)

3) Water droplets on skin tend to resemble spheres as opposed to other shapes so as to:

   A. minimise surface tension.
   B. maximise the area to volume ratio.
   C. minimise cohesive forces.
   D. maximise adhesive forces.

GOLD STANDARD GAMSAT-LEVEL PRACTICE QUESTIONS

Questions 4–7

Archimedes, one of the great mathematicians of all time, is famous for the story of how he managed to determine whether the king's crown was really made of gold. The mathematical law that he derived which enabled him to accomplish this challenge, states that any fluid applies a buoyant force to an object which is partially or completely immersed in it, the magnitude of which is equal to the weight of fluid the object displaces.

Equation I

$$F_b = W_{fluid}$$

where F_b = magnitude of the buoyant force and W_{fluid} = weight of fluid displaced. Once the maximum buoyant force possible is greater than or equal to the weight of the object, the object will float.

Consider the situation where a square block of pine wood is being immersed in water.

Density of water = 1.00×10^3 kg m^{-3}
Density of pine = 500 kg m^{-3}
Gravitational acceleration = 9.8 m s^{-2}
Length of one side of the block = 4.0 m

4) What is the maximum possible buoyant force that can be obtained when the block is held underwater?

   A. 6.27×10^5 N
   B. 1.57×10^5 N
   C. 8.62×10^4 N
   D. 2.16×10^4 N

5) Given that the block of pine wood floats, how much of its height is out of the water?

   A. 0.5 m
   B. 1.0 m
   C. 2.0 m
   D. 4.0 m

6) The block is replaced by one with identical dimensions but greater density. Which of the following is true?

   A. The height of the block above the water is the same as before.
   B. The height of the block above the water is greater than before.
   C. The height of the block above the water is less than before.
   D. The height of the block above the water will depend on the temperature of the block.

7) Another block of identical dimensions to the first is held half-immersed in the water. When released, it submerged to a greater degree but remained afloat. When the block was initially released, which of the following must have been true?

   A. Weight of fluid displaced > weight of block
   B. Density of fluid < density of block
   C. Buoyant force < maximum buoyant force
   D. Maximum buoyant force = half the weight of the block

8) A student observes that when an ice cube floats in a glass of water, part of the ice cube projects above the surface of the water. When the ice cube melts, the level of the water surface will:

   A. go down slightly.
   B. go up slightly.
   C. remain the same.
   D. change depending on the weight of the ice cube.

9) If F is the viscous force associated with an area A between adjoining layers of fluid and v is the change in relative flow velocity in a distance d perpendicular to the flow, then the coefficient of viscosity, η, is defined by

$$\eta = (F/A)/(v/d)$$

The cgs system is the centimetre–gram–second system of units. The cgs unit for viscosity is "poise" and for force is the "dyne." Which of the following is correct?

   A. poise = g•cm-sec
   B. poise = g•sec
   C. poise = dyne•sec/cm^2
   D. poise = dyne•cm/sec

Questions 10–11

10) The following equation is used to relate force and fluid viscosity η:

$$F = -2\pi r l \frac{v}{R} \eta$$

where F is force, r is radius, l is length, v is speed, R is distance and η is the viscosity. What are the dimensions of viscosity in the fundamental quantities of mass (M), length (L) and time (T)?

   A. $M \cdot L^3 \cdot T^{-3}$
   B. $M \cdot L^{-1} \cdot T^{-1}$
   C. $M \cdot L^2 \cdot T^{-1}$
   D. $M \cdot L^{-2} \cdot T^{-2}$

11) In the fundamental quantities described in the previous question, which of the following is equivalent to L^3?

   A. (joules)/(pascals)
   B. (joules)(pascals)
   C. (volume)(joules)(pascals)
   D. (volume)(joules)/(pascals)

GAMSAT-Prep.com
GOLD STANDARD PHYSICS

Questions 12–15

The viscosity of a fluid, that is, a gas, a pure liquid or a solution, is an index of its resistance to flow. The viscosity of a fluid in a cylindrical tube of radius R and length L is given by:

$$n = \pi \Delta P R^4 t / (8VL) \qquad \text{Equation I}$$

where n = viscosity of fluid, ΔP = change in pressure, t = time, V = volume of fluid and V/t = rate of flow of fluid. This equation can be applied to the study of blood flow in our bodies. The heart pumps blood through the various vessels in our bodies to supply all of its tissues. At rest, the rate of blood flow is about 80 cm³ s⁻¹ and this is maintained in all blood vessels. However, the radii of the blood vessels decrease the further away blood moves from the heart. Therefore, in order to maintain the rate of blood flow, a pressure drop occurs as one moves from one blood vessel to another of smaller radius.

A great number of physiological conditions can be explained using Equation I, for example, hypertension.

12) What would be the pressure drop per cm of the blood in the first blood vessel leaving the heart if the blood vessel is of unit radius and the body is at rest?

$$n_{blood} = 0.04 \text{ dyn s cm}^{-3}$$

- A. $25.6/\pi$ dyn cm⁻³
- B. $16000/\pi$ dyn cm⁻³
- C. $\pi/25.6$ dyn cm⁻³
- D. $\pi/16000$ dyn cm⁻³

13) Which of the following has the greatest effect on the viscosity of a fluid per unit change in its value?

- A. Volume of the fluid
- B. Length of the tube
- C. Pressure of the fluid
- D. Radius of the tube

14) Ohm's law relates voltage to the product of current and resistance. The equation for the rate of flow of a fluid (Equation I) has often been compared to Ohm's law. Given that P can be likened to the voltage and flow rate can be likened to the current, which of the following can be likened to resistance?

- A. πR^4
- B. $\pi R^4/(8Ln)$
- C. $8Ln/(\pi R^4)$
- D. $8Ln$

15) Hypertension involves the decrease in the radius of certain blood vessels. If the radius of a blood vessel is halved, by what factor must the pressure increase to maintain the normal rate of blood flow, all other factors being constant?

- A. 2
- B. 4
- C. 8
- D. 16

Questions 16–20

The four forces that act on a plane are lift, weight, air resistance (*drag*), and thrust, the last of which is produced by the plane's engine.

Impact pressure produces 30% of the lift. It results from the fact that wings are given a *dihedral* angle where the distance from the tip of the wing to the ground is greater than that from the root of the wing to the ground.

The other 70% of lift can be accounted for by the Bernoulli effect. A cross-section of an airplane's wing reveals greater surface area above the wing compared to a flatter, lower surface. In the "equal transit-time" theory of lift, the air - moving in streamline flow - must move more rapidly over the top of the wing.

CHAPTER 6: FLUIDS AND SOLIDS

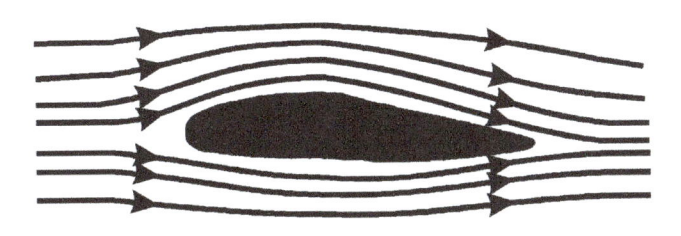

Bernoulli's equation, $P + \frac{1}{2}\rho v^2 + \rho gh = $ constant, is often modified when discussing an airplane's wing. The "ρgh" component is usually left out since the difference in distance from the top of the wing to the ground compared to the bottom of the wing to the ground is usually negligible.

Note that:
- Streamline flow is governed by the continuity equation where $A_1 v_1 = A_2 v_2$.
- For Bernoulli's and/or the continuity equation: P is pressure, ρ is density, v is velocity, g is gravity, h is the height and A is the cross-sectional area.

16) Newton's third law states that for every action there must be an equal and opposite reaction. This is applicable to lift and the dihedral angle because:

   A. the fast moving air above the wing increases the pressure.
   B. drag must be as low as possible to improve forward motion.
   C. there is a large pressure difference between the wings.
   D. the wing deflects the air downward and the air in turn deflects the wing upward.

17) Based on the "equal transit-time" theory of lift, compared to the wing's upper surface, the air moving along the undersurface has:

   A. greater velocity, greater pressure.
   B. greater velocity, lower pressure.
   C. lower velocity, greater pressure.
   D. lower velocity, lower pressure.

18) The following represents an incompressible fluid in laminar flow through pipes. Where is the pressure highest?

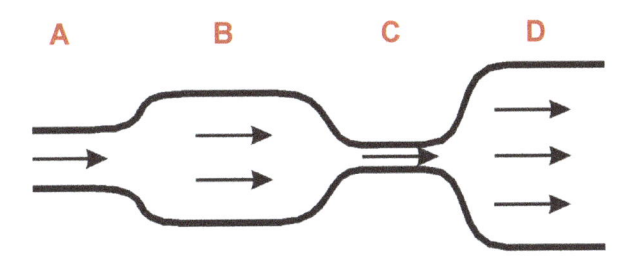

19) Flow is defined as volume per unit time. Concerning the preceding diagram, what can be determined regarding the flow?

   A. It is highest at C.
   B. It is highest at D.
   C. It cannot be determined.
   D. It is constant throughout.

20) Bernoulli's equation and the continuity equation, not only apply to an airplane's wing or an incompressible fluid moving through a pipe, they also approximate blood circulating through blood vessels such as arteries. Atherosclerosis and thrombosis can partially occlude an artery as material adheres to the arterial walls over a small portion of its length. What happens to the pressure and the velocity of blood in the partially occluded region as compared to just prior to the partial occlusion?

   A. Velocity decreases, pressure decreases
   B. Velocity decreases, pressure increases
   C. Velocity increases, pressure increases
   D. Velocity increases, pressure decreases

GAMSAT-Prep.com
GOLD STANDARD PHYSICS

High-level Importance

> ## ⚠ SPOILER ALERT
>
> Gold Standard has cross-referenced the content in this chapter to examples from ACER's official GAMSAT practice materials. It is for you to decide when you want to explore these questions since you may want to preserve some of ACER's materials for timed mock-exam practice.
>
> **Examples** – Determining the dimensions of volume and other parameters given the equation of state Q99-101 of 3; Archimedes principle and specific gravity: Q29-32 of 4; incompressible fluid flow and a dam (PHY 6.1.2): Q66-68 of 4. Note that "Q" is followed by the question number, and, for example, "of 1" refers to booklet number 1 which is referenced in the Spoiler Alert table at the end of Chapter 1. The 10 full-length HEAPS GAMSAT practice tests (by Gold Standard and MediRed), exams 1 through 10, contain specific cross-references to this chapter within the worked solutions. Note that the Archimedes' unit, the airplane's wing unit (with the discredited "equal transit-time" theory of lift!), and the viscosity dimensional analysis unit are visitors from HEAPS-6.

Chapter Checklist

- ☐ Access your online account to view answers, worked solutions and discussion boards.
- ☐ Reassess your 'learning objectives' for this chapter: Go back to the first page of this chapter and re-evaluate the top 3 boxes and the Introduction.
    - ☐ Please be sure that you have completed the *Need for Speed* exercises at the beginning of this chapter.
- ☐ Complete a maximum of 1 page of notes using symbols/abbreviations to represent the entire chapter based on your learning objectives. These are your Gold Notes.
- ☐ Consider your multimedia options based on your optimal way of learning:
    - ☐ Download the free Gold Standard GAMSAT app for your Android device or iPhone.
    - ☐ Create your own, tangible study cards or try the free app: Anki.
    - ☐ Record your voice reading your Gold Notes onto your smartphone (MP3s) and listen during exercise, transportation, etc.
    - ☐ Try out the Gold Standard GAMSAT online videos at gamsat-prep.com, or you can try other options on YouTube like Khan Academy or Crash Course Physics.
- ☐ Reassess your schedule for your full-length GAMSAT practice tests: ACER and/or HEAPS exams. Ensure that you have scheduled one full day to complete a practice test and 1-2 days for a thorough assessment of worked solutions while adding to your abbreviated Gold Notes.
- ☐ Reassess your progress in scheduling and/or evaluating stress reduction techniques such as regular exercise (sports), yoga, meditation and/or mindfulness exercises (*see* YouTube for suggestions).

WAVE CHARACTERISTICS AND PERIODIC MOTION
Chapter 7

Memorise
* Define: wavelength, frequency, velocity, amplitude
* Define: intensity, constructive/destructive interference

Understand
* SHM, transverse vs. longitudinal waves, phase
* Resonance, nodes, antinodes, pipes (standing waves)
* Periodic motion: force, acceleration, velocity, displacement, period
* The simple pendulum: theory and calculations

Importance
Medium level: **6%** of GAMSAT Physics questions released by ACER are related to content in this chapter (in our estimation).
* Note that approximately **75%** of the questions in GAMSAT Physics are related to just 6 chapters: 1, 4, 6, 9, 11 and 12.

GAMSAT-Prep.com

Introduction

Wave characteristics and periodic motion describe the motion of systems that vibrate. Topics include transverse and longitudinal waves, interference, resonance, Hooke's law and simple harmonic motion (SHM). If an equation related to this chapter is required to answer an exam question, even something as simple as the relationship between period and frequency, ACER will normally provide the equation and define the terms. It is for this reason that there are no *Need for Speed* exercises for this chapter but, of course, you will have the full range of practice questions at the end of this chapter.

Multimedia Resources at GAMSAT-Prep.com

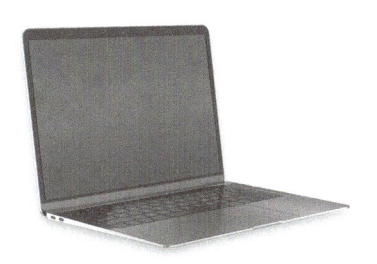

Open Discussion Boards   Foundational Videos   Flashcards   Special Guest

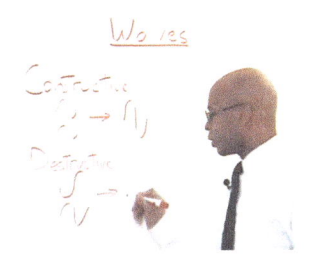

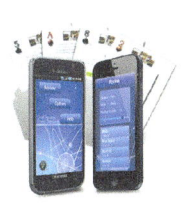

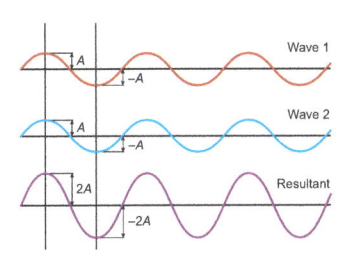

THE PHYSICAL SCIENCES   PHY-89

* The real GAMSAT may have advanced-level information presented (i.e. in a passage) but previous knowledge of said information is not required to answer the questions that would follow. Practice questions at the end of this chapter, as well as ACER and GS (HEAPS) practice GAMSATs can help you clarify this point.

7.1 Wave Characteristics

7.1.1 Transverse and Longitudinal Motion

A wave is a disturbance in a medium such that each particle in the medium vibrates about an equilibrium point in a simple harmonic (*periodic* = from time to time, regular intervals) motion. If the direction of vibration is perpendicular to the direction of propagation of the wave, it is called a <u>transverse wave</u> (e.g. light or an oscillating string under tension). A fair analogy would be a bug caught on an ideal water wave: Its motion is up and down even as the wave carries to the shore.

If the direction of vibration is in the same direction as the propagation of the wave, it is called a <u>longitudinal wave</u> (e.g. sound). Longitudinal waves are characterised by condensations (regions of crowding of particles) and rarefactions (regions where particles are far apart) along the wave in the medium. If you have been to a concert or a big party, you may have witnessed the movement of a large speaker's cone (or diaphragm) literally pushing sound (most visible for bass) forward into the air.

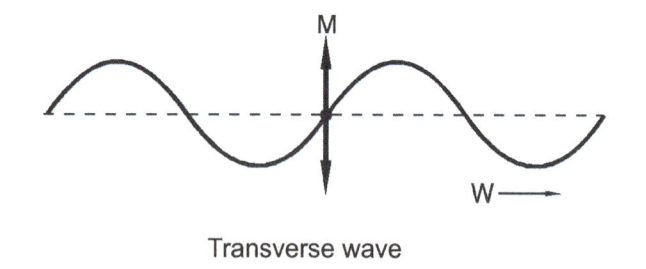

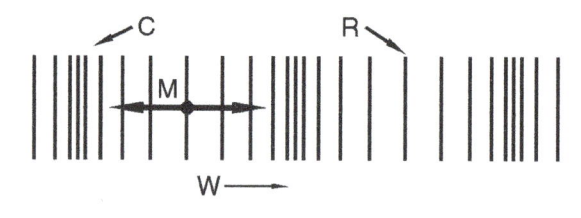

Transverse wave

Longitudinal wave

Figure III.B.7.1: Transverse and longitudinal waves.
W = wave propagation, R = rarefaction, C = condensation, M = motion of particle.

7.1.2 Wavelength, Frequency, Velocity, Amplitude, Intensity

The wavelength (λ) is the distance measured in metres (SI unit) from crest to crest (or valley to valley) of a transverse wave (crest = top; valley = bottom). It may also be defined as the distance between two particles with the same displacement and direction of displacement. In a longitudinal wave, the wavelength is the distance from one rarefaction (or condensation) to another (*see* Figure III.B.7.1). The *amplitude* (A) is the maximum displacement of a particle in one direction from its equilibrium point. The *intensity* (I) of a wave is the square of the amplitude. For sound, loudness is related to both amplitude and intensity.

Frequency (*f*) is the number of cycles per unit time (per second = s^{-1} = hertz = Hz =

SI unit). *Period* (*T*) is the duration of one cycle, it is the inverse of the frequency: $T = 1/f$. The *velocity* (*v*) of a wave is the velocity of the propagation of the disturbance that forms the wave through the medium.

The velocity is inversely proportional to the inertia of the medium. In other words, the less that the material resists the movement of particles, the faster the particles can move. The velocity can be calculated according to the following equation (dimensionally: m/s = m × s^{-1}):

$$v = \lambda f$$

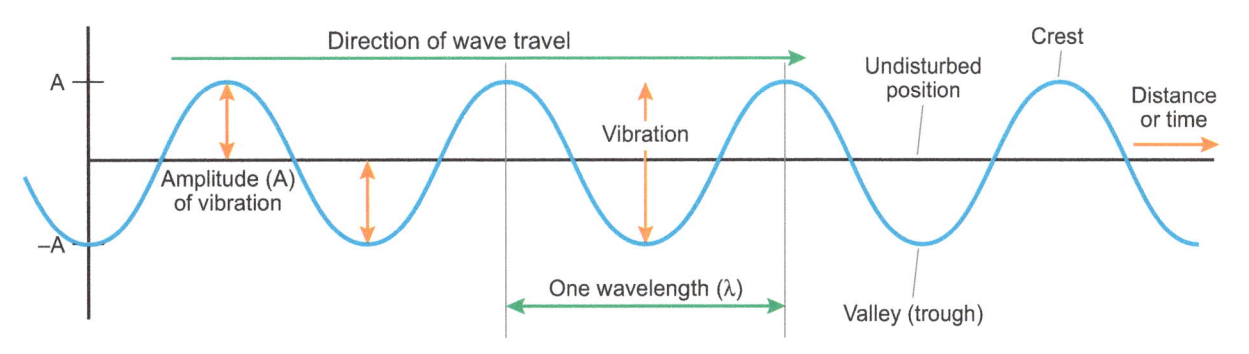

Figure III.B.7.2: Characteristics of waves.

7.1.3 Superposition of Waves, Phase, Interference, Addition

The superposition principle states that the effect of two or more waves on the displacement of a particle is independent. The final displacement of the particle is the resultant effect of all the waves added algebraically, thus the amplitude may increase or decrease. The *phase* of a particle under vibration is its displacement at the time of origin (t = 0).

Interference is the summation of the displacements of different waves in a medium. Constructive interference is when the waves add to a larger resultant wave than either original. Destructive interference is when the waves add to a smaller resultant wave than either original wave (*see* Figures III.B.7.3/7.4).

Because it is additive, the theoretical consequences for constructive interference are as would be expected: a bigger wave, a louder sound, a brighter light. However, the theoretical consequences of maximal (*complete*) destructive interference are simply stupefying: 2 water waves creating still water, 2 loud sounds creating silence, 2 bright lights creating darkness. You can see why destructive interference is used in stealth technologies.

GAMSAT-Prep.com
GOLD STANDARD PHYSICS

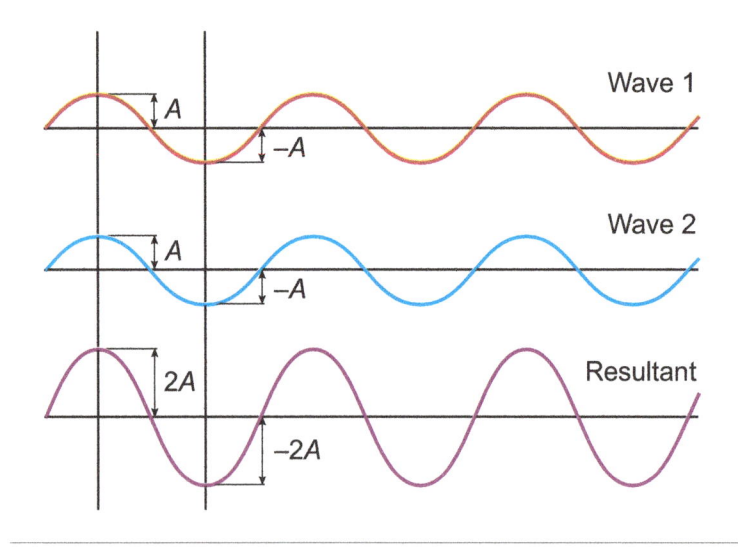

Figure III.B.7.3: Maximal constructive interference: Two identical waves (same amplitude, frequency and phase) produce a single wave with twice the amplitude, but the same wavelength.

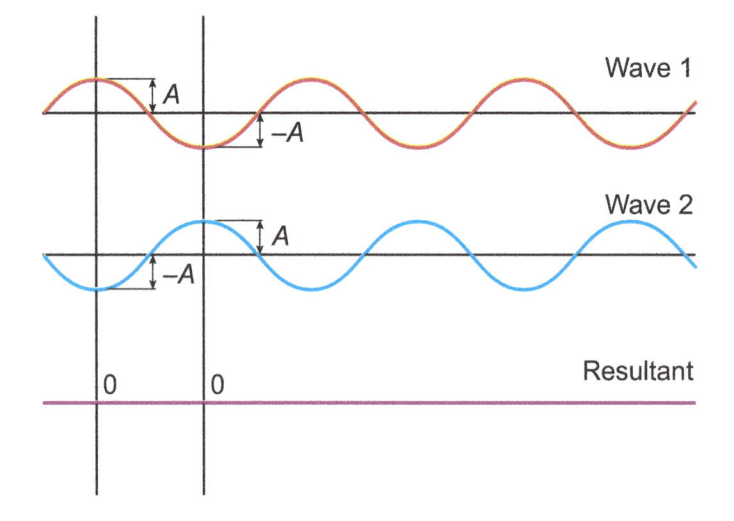

Figure III.B.7.4: Maximal destructive interference: Two identical waves (same amplitude and frequency but out of phase) produce zero amplitude, or complete cancellation.

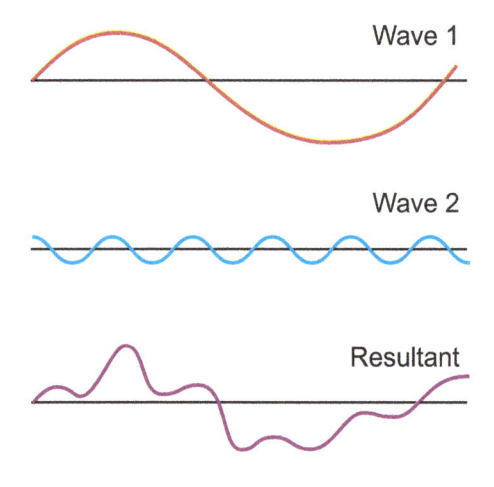

Figure III.B.7.5: Superposition (*one being added to the other*) of two non-identical waves (different amplitudes and frequencies) showing elements of both constructive and destructive interference. The result, for sound, is an alternation of loudness which is known to musicians tuning instruments as a *beat* (frequency).

PHY-92   CHAPTER 7: WAVE CHARACTERISTICS AND PERIODIC MOTION

GAMSAT MASTERS SERIES

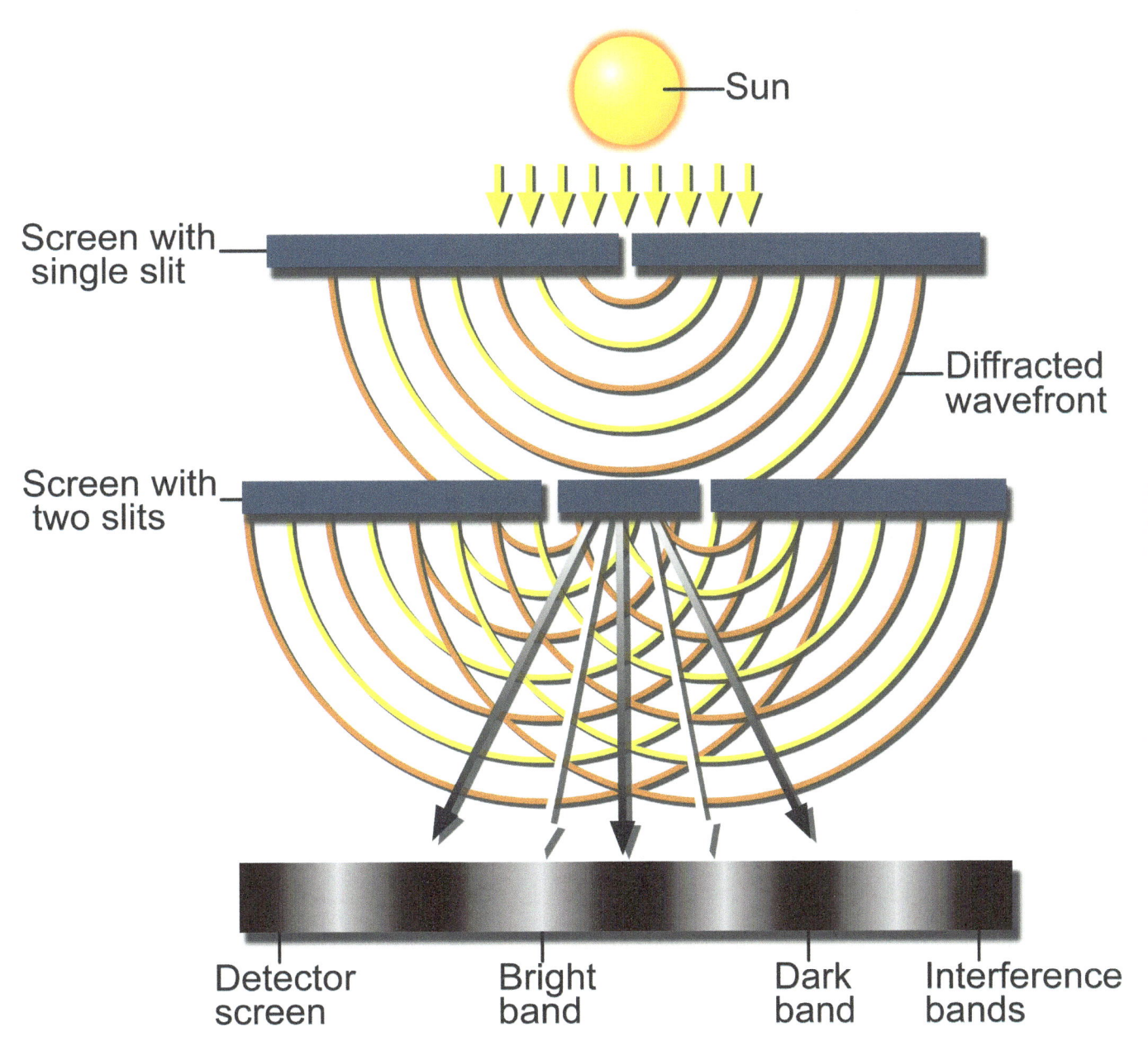

Figure III.B.7.5.1: An example of constructive and destructive interference (light): Thomas Young's double-slit experiment. Young's experiment demonstrates both the wave and particle natures of light. A light source illuminates a thin plate with two parallel slits cut in it, and the light passing through the slits strikes a screen behind them. The wave nature of light causes the light waves passing through both slits to interfere, creating an interference pattern of bright and dark bands on the screen. However, at the screen, the light is always found to be absorbed as though it were made of discrete particles (photons). The double-slit experiment can also be performed (using a different apparatus) with particles of matter such as electrons with the same results. Again, this provides an additional circumstance demonstrating particle-wave duality (PHY 11.1). Note that *diffraction* is the apparent bending of a wave around a small obstacle. We see diffracted light waves through each of the slits above.

THE PHYSICAL SCIENCES   PHY-93

7.1.4 Resonance

Forced vibrations occur when a series of waves impinge upon an object and cause it to vibrate. Natural frequencies are the intrinsic frequencies of vibration of a system. If the forced vibration causes the object to vibrate at one of its natural frequencies, the body will vibrate at maximal amplitude. This phenomenon is called *resonance*. Since energy and power are proportional to the amplitude squared, they also are at their maximum.

The 'classic' example of resonance is the opera singer singing a note which is resonant to a wine glass, and by sustaining that note, the glass shatters.

7.1.5 Standing Waves, Pipes and Strings

Standing waves result when waves are reflected off a stationary object back into the oncoming waves of the medium and superposition results. *Nodes* are points where there is no particle displacement, which are similar to points of maximal destructive interference.

Nodes occur at fixed end points (points that cannot vibrate). Antinodes are points that undergo maximal displacements and are similar to points of maximal constructive interference. Antinodes occur at open or free end points (*see Figure III.B.7.6*).

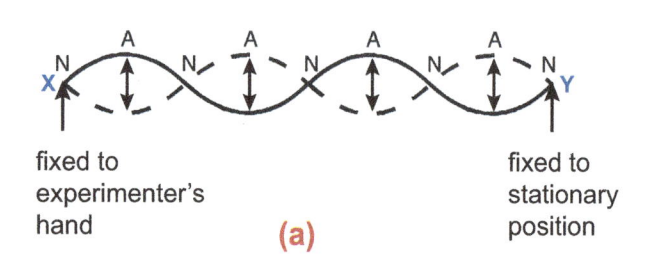

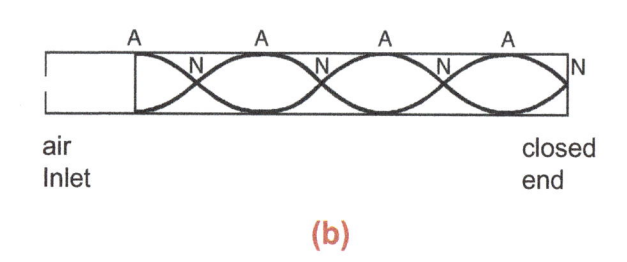

Figure III.B.7.6: Standing waves.
(a) String: Standing waves produced by an experimenter wiggling a string or rubber tube at point **X** towards a fixed point **Y** at the correct frequency; for example, a string could be fixed to a wall at point **Y**. (b) Pipe: Standing wave produced in a pipe with a closed end point; for example, in a closed organ pipe where sound originates in a vibrating air column (A = *antinode* and N = *node*).

7.2 Periodic Motion

GAMSAT MASTERS SERIES

7.2.1 Hooke's Law

The particles that are undergoing displacement when a wave passes through a medium undergo motion called simple harmonic motion (SHM) and are acted upon by a force described by Hooke's Law. SHM is caused by an inconstant force (called a *restoring force*) and as a result has an inconstant acceleration. The force is proportional to the displacement (*distance from the equilibrium point*) but opposite in direction,

$$F = -kx \text{ (Hooke's Law)}$$

where k = the spring constant, x = displacement from the equilibrium. The work W can be determined according to $W = \frac{1}{2}kx^2$.

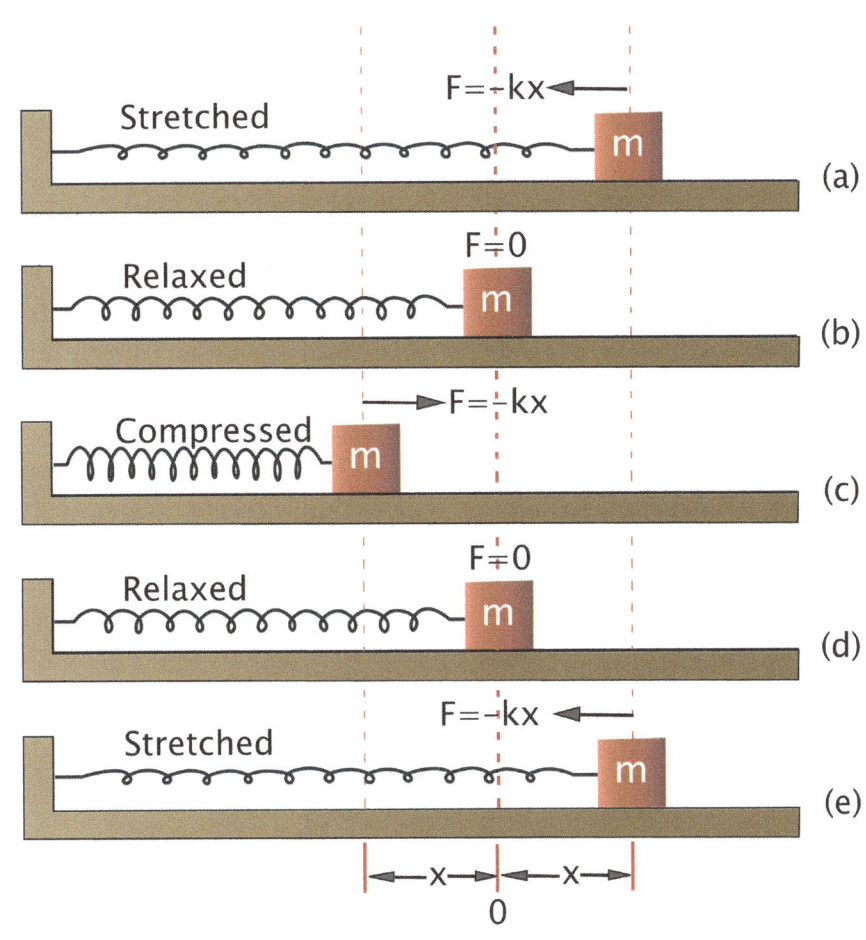

Figure III.B.7.7: Simple harmonic motion. A block of mass m exhibiting SHM. The force F exerted by the spring on the block is shown in each case. Notice that the restoring force F is always pointing in the opposite direction to the direction of the displacement x. Because these two vectors are always opposite to each other, there is a negative sign built into the equation $F = -kx$.

Notice that the equation for the work done by the spring is identical to the potential energy of a spring (PHY 5.4). This is because when an external force stretches the spring, this work is stored in the force field, which is said to be stored as potential energy. If the external force is removed, the force field acts on the body to perform the work as it moves the body back to the initial position, reducing the stretch of the spring. For example, an archer applies human force over a distance (= work; PHY 5.1) to pull an arrow back in the bow, elastic potential energy is now stored in the stretched bow, when the arrow leaves the bow, the potential energy turns into kinetic energy.

Examples of objects that have elastic potential energy include stretched or compressed elastic bands, springs, bungee cords, shock absorbers (cars, trucks, bicycles), trampolines, etc.

The work done in compressing or stretching a spring can be determined by taking the area under a Force vs. Displacement graph for the spring (the latter is because work is force times displacement; PHY 5.1).

7.2.2 Features of SHM and Hooke's Law

1) Force and acceleration are always in the same direction.
2) Force and acceleration are always in the opposite direction of the displacement (*this is why there is a negative sign in the equation for force*).
3) Force and acceleration have their maximal value at +A and –A; they are zero at the equilibrium point (*the amplitude* A *equals the maximum displacement* x).
4) Velocity direction has no constant relation to displacement and acceleration.
5) Velocity is maximum at equilibrium, and zero at A and –A.
6) The period T can be calculated from the mass m of an oscillating particle:

$$T = 2\pi\sqrt{m/k}$$

where k is the spring constant. The frequency f is simply $1/T$, where T is the period.

7.2.3 SHM Problem: The Simple Pendulum

A simple pendulum consists of a point mass m suspended by a light inextensible cord of length l. When pulled to one side of its equilibrium position, the pendulum swings under the influence of gravity producing a periodic, oscillatory motion (= *SHM*). Given that the angle θ with the vertical is small, thus sinθ ≈ θ, determine the general equation for the period T.

The tangential component of mg is the restoring force since it returns the mass to its equilibrium position. Thus the restoring force is:

$$F = -mg\sin\theta.$$

Recall sinθ ≈ θ, x = lθ, and for SHM F = –kx:

$$F = -mg\theta = -mgx/l = -(mg/l)x = -kx.$$

Hence mg/l = k, thus the equation for the period T becomes:

$$T = 2\pi\sqrt{\frac{m}{k}} = 2\pi\sqrt{\frac{m}{mg/l}} = 2\pi\sqrt{\frac{l}{g}}$$

==The equation for the period of a simple pendulum is therefore independent of the mass of the particle.==

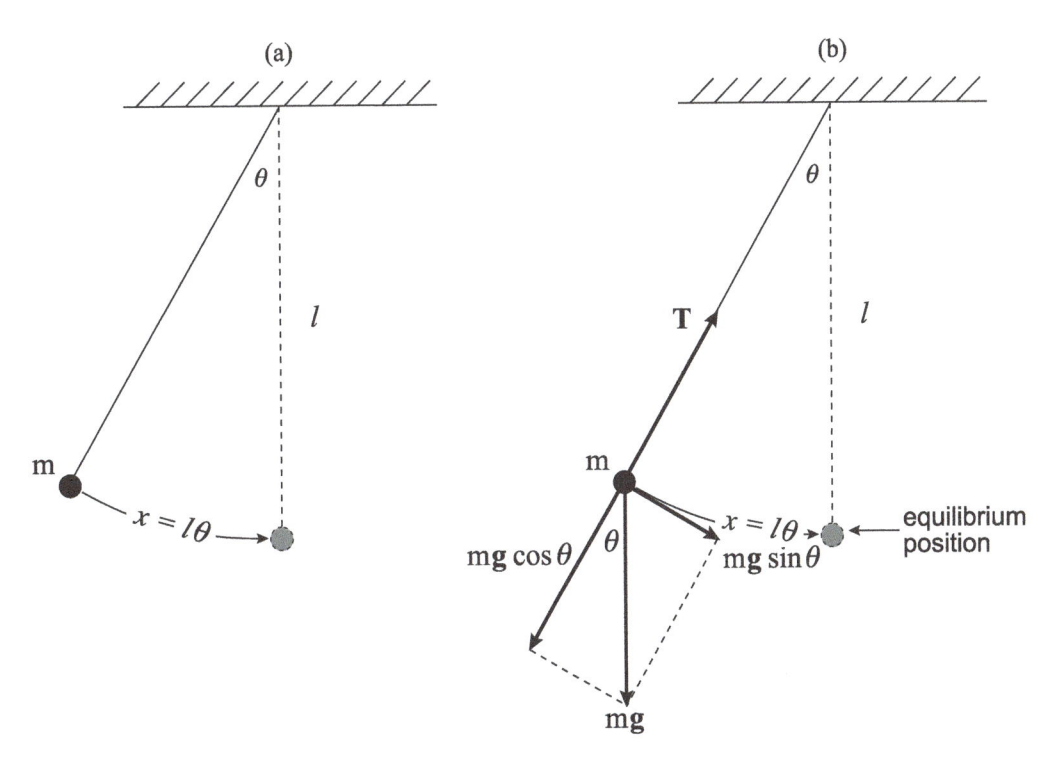

Figure III.B.7.8: The Simple Pendulum.
(a) The problem as it could be presented; the displacement x along the section of the circle (arc) is lθ. (b) The vector components that should be drawn to solve the problem. The forces acting on a simple pendulum are the tension **T** in the string and the weight mg of the mass. The magnitude of the radial component of mg is mgcosθ and the tangential component is mgsinθ.

> A rough approximation of SHM would be a grandfather clock or a child on a swing. However, note that the *length l* in the equation of a simple pendulum refers to the length of the cord to the bob's or child's centre of gravity (COG; PHY 2.1).

EXAMPLE 1

Please try the following practice questions before looking at the worked solutions. Prepare your scratch paper and write down the equation for the period of a simple pendulum.

$$T = 2\pi\sqrt{\frac{\ell}{g}}$$

If the length of the pendulum increases by 70%, by what percentage will the period increase?

A. 30%
B. 40%
C. 50%
D. 70%

If the length increases by 70%, that is the same as saying 1.70(ℓ), 1.70 is similar to 1.69 and since we know that the square root of 1.69 is 1.3 (because 13 squared is 169; GM 1.5.6), this means that the original value of ℓ has increased by 30%.

The following is the way to manipulate the equation so that, in the end, you can see by what factor the original equation is being affected:

$$T = 2\pi\sqrt{\frac{\ell}{g}}$$

$$T = 2\pi\sqrt{\frac{(1.69)\ell}{g}}$$

$$T = 1.30\left[2\pi\sqrt{\frac{\ell}{g}}\right]$$

Translation: the original equation is 1.30 times higher which means 30% greater. Answer: **A**.

EXAMPLE 2

If a pendulum is moved to an environment with 1/50th of Earth's gravity, what would be the change in the period?

A. It would be 15 times the original.
B. It would be 10 times the original.
C. It would be 7 times the original.
D. It would decrease the original by a factor of 50.

$$T = 2\pi\sqrt{\frac{\ell}{g}}$$

By observing that gravity will change and a square root is imminent (as well as the fact that the answer choices are not very 'tight' or close together), let's estimate 50 as 49 which has a simple square root (GM 1.5, 1.5.6):

$$T = 2\pi\sqrt{\frac{\ell}{g/49}}$$

==A denominator in a denominator is the same as a numerator== (in other words, if you divide by a fraction, it is the same as multiplying by the inverse; GM 1.4.2B):

$$T = 2\pi\sqrt{\frac{(49)\ell}{g}}$$

CHAPTER 7: WAVE CHARACTERISTICS AND PERIODIC MOTION

Of course, the square root of 49 is 7:

$$T = 7\left[2\pi\sqrt{\frac{\ell}{g}}\right]$$

Translation: the original equation is 7 times greater. Answer: **C**. Note that the actual square root of 50 is approximately 7.1 so our estimate is valid considering the answer choices. The preceding manipulations are commonly required for the real exam and so we will be doing some more after your mini-break!

> What do physicists enjoy doing the most at football games?
> The 'wave' :)

CHAPTER 7: Wave Characteristics and Periodic Motion

GOLD STANDARD FOUNDATIONAL GAMSAT PRACTICE QUESTIONS

1) What is the period of a pendulum that has a frequency of 150×10^{-2} Hz?

   A. 1/4 sec
   B. 1/2 sec
   C. 2/3 sec
   D. 1 sec

2) If the period is 2 minutes, what is the frequency?

   A. ½ Hz
   B. ½ mHz
   C. 8.3 mHz
   D. 8.3 kHz

3) Which of the following units is equivalent to metres per second?

   A. m/Hz
   B. Hz/s
   C. Hz·m
   D. Hz·s

4) The energy of a water wave seen at the beach is most closely related to its:

   A. amplitude.
   B. frequency.
   C. period.
   D. wavelength.

5) Consider the following diagram of two pulses of equal amplitude A approaching point P along a uniform string.

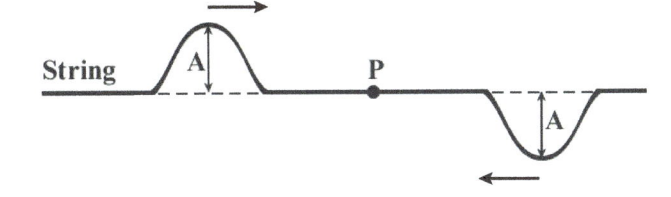

   What will the vertical displacement of the string at point P be when the 2 pulses meet?

   A. –A
   B. 0
   C. A
   D. 2A

THE PHYSICAL SCIENCES   PHY-99

GOLD STANDARD GAMSAT-LEVEL PRACTICE QUESTIONS

Questions 6–11

Pendula are useful for examining the nature of simple harmonic motion. A pendulum consists of a mass, or bob, attached to the end of a string or in this case, a rod of negligible mass. The other end or "top" of the rod is anchored to a solid surface from which it can swing free of friction. Simple harmonic motion results when the rod swings at angles of less than 15° from a perfectly vertical orientation.

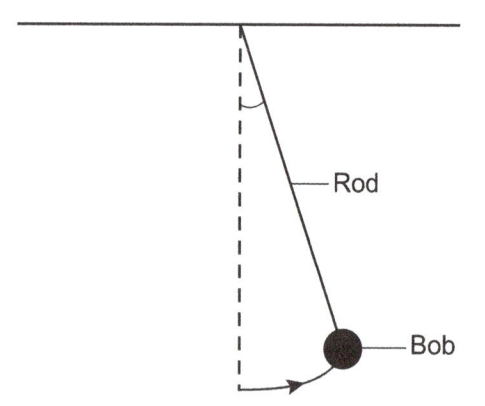

The period of a pendulum can be determined using the equation:

$$T = 2\pi \sqrt{l/g}$$

where "*l*" is the length of the rod of the pendulum, and "*g*" is the acceleration due to gravity. (Note: Assume air resistance is negligible, all angles from vertical are less than 15°, and $g = 9.8$ m/s²)

6) If the length of the rod were shortened by 1/4 of its original length, what effect would this have on the period of the pendulum?
   A. The period would decrease by 1/2.
   B. The period would decrease by 1/4.
   C. The period would stay the same.
   D. The period would increase by 1/4.

7) What is the approximate frequency of a pendulum whose rod length is 10 m?
   A. 2π Hz
   B. 4π Hz
   C. $1/(2\pi)$ Hz
   D. $1/(4\pi)$ Hz

8) Which of the following accurately describes the velocity of the pendulum's bob as it moves from a small angle of displacement to the lowest point of its arc?
   A. The velocity of the bob is negligible, due to the angular acceleration of the bob being zero.
   B. The velocity of the bob remains constant throughout the motion, due to a constant angular acceleration.
   C. The velocity of the bob increases.
   D. The velocity of the bob decreases.

9) If a pendulum's bob is replaced with one that weighs 2 times as much, how will this affect its period?
   A. The period will double in magnitude.
   B. The period will quadruple in magnitude.
   C. The period will remain approximately the same, but slightly higher in magnitude.
   D. The period will remain the same.

10) An airplane is carrying a pendulum and begins accelerating down a runway during takeoff. The bob of the pendulum:
    A. hangs downward and forward, because the net force on the bob must be nonzero.
    B. hangs downward and forward, because the net force on the bob must be zero.
    C. hangs downward and backward, because the net force on the bob must be nonzero.
    D. hangs downward and backward, because the net force on the bob must be zero.

11) Frequency is the inverse of the period.

Consider a child sitting on a swing in a park moving back and forth simulating simple harmonic motion. What would be expected to occur to the frequency of the swing's movement if the child stood up on the swing's seat?

A. It would increase.
B. It would decrease.
C. It would stay the same.
D. It would decrease and then increase in a process like a wave.

12) The Richter scale is a scale of numbers used to tell the power (or *magnitude*) of earthquakes. First, a seismogram is examined which is a record of an earthquake-induced motion at a measuring station as a function of time. In the original formulation, the maximum amplitude A and a certain correction factor (i.e., the distance from the earthquake, the S-P time from the seismogram) provides the earthquake magnitude level:

$$M_L = \log_{10} A(mm) + \text{(Distance correction factor)}$$

Table 1

Magnitude level	Category	Effects
less than 1.0 to 2.9	micro	generally, not felt by people, though recorded on local instruments
3.0–3.9	minor	felt by many people; no damage
4.0–4.9	light	felt by all; minor breakage of objects
5.0–5.9	moderate	some damage to weak structures
6.0–6.9	strong	moderate damage in populated areas
7.0–7.9	major	serious damage over large areas; loss of life
8.0 and higher	great	severe destruction and loss of life over large areas

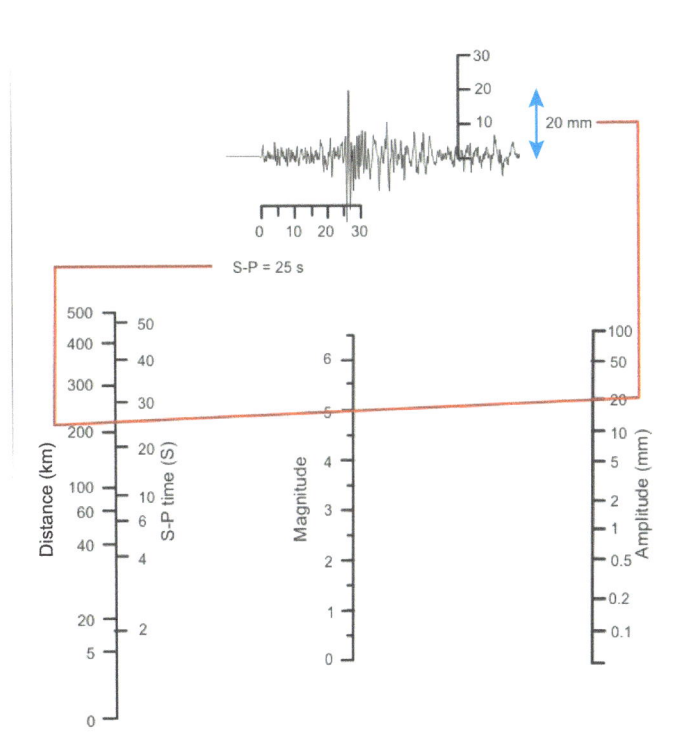

Figure 1: How to read the Richter Scale. The seismogram at the top of the image provides the amplitude (20 mm) and the correction factor of the S-P time (25 s) which, in this case, lines up with a magnitude 5.0 earthquake.

According to the information provided, if the seismogram presents an amplitude of 50 mm and the S-P time suggests that the distance to the earthquake is 40 km, what result would be expected from that earthquake?

A. No damage
B. Minor breakage of objects
C. Moderate damage in populated areas
D. Loss of life

Questions 13–15

Oscillatory motion occurs when a system repeats its motion in a given period of time. The period *T* refers to the time it takes for the system to complete the repetition. The period *T* is determined by the equation:

$$T = 2\pi\sqrt{\frac{L}{g}}$$

where *L* is the length of the string and *g* is the acceleration due to gravity (approximately 10 m/s² on Earth).

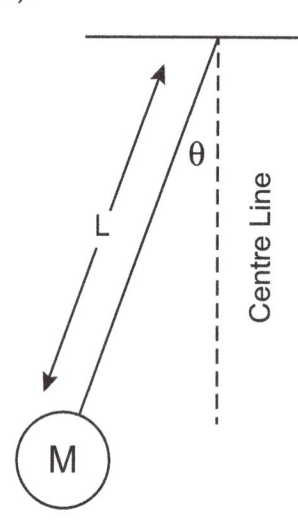

Figure 1

In an attempt to experimentally confirm this expression the following data was gathered using pendula where *L* varies.

Table 1

Length (cm)	Period (sec)
156.0	2.76
103.5	1.99
75.8	1.96
53.7	1.54
39.1	1.26

Another experiment was performed in an attempt to confirm the accepted formula for a simple oscillating spring. The formula is:

$$T = 2\pi\sqrt{\frac{m}{k}}$$

where *T* is the period, *m* is the mass attached to the spring, and *k* is the spring constant. (Note: It was assumed that the mass of the spring was negligible when compared to the mass *m*.) Various masses were hung on a spring to determine their effect on the period of oscillation.

Table 2

Mass (grams)	Period (sec)
129	.856
230	1.154
330	1.323
430	1.495
973	1.921
1000	2.175
1023	2.178

13) Suppose one of the pendula (*L* = 103.5 cm) is taken to the moon to be tested. What approximate difference in *T* would an experimenter observe? (Note: free-fall acceleration at the surface of the moon is 1.6 m/s²)

A. 1 s
B. 2 s
C. 3 s
D. 4 s

14) Compute the value of *k* for a spring with mass *m* = 1.0 kg.

A. 2.9 N/m
B. 8.3 N/m
C. 8354 N/m
D. 91.4 N/m

15) For a simple linear oscillator, experimenters tested what effect the position, x, of the spring from the floor has on its period of oscillation. Which of the following graphs best represents what their results were?

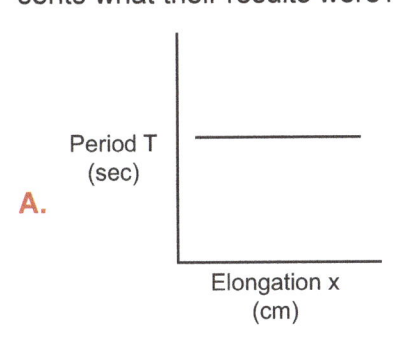

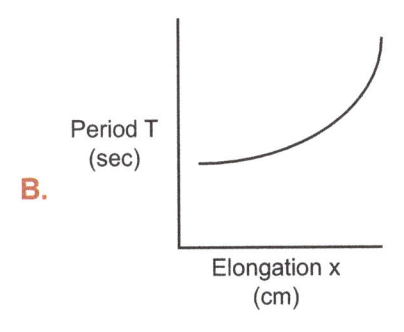

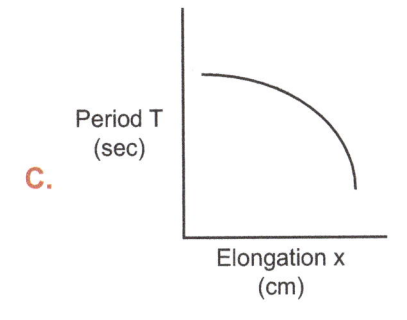

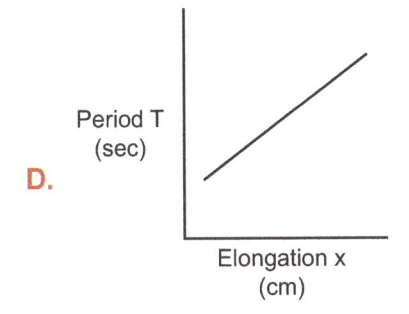

A. Period T (sec) vs Elongation x (cm) — horizontal line

B. Period T (sec) vs Elongation x (cm) — upward curving

C. Period T (sec) vs Elongation x (cm) — downward curving

D. Period T (sec) vs Elongation x (cm) — increasing straight line

16) Hooke's law is a law of Physics that states that the force (F) needed to extend or compress a spring by some distance (x) is related by the following form of the equation: $F_s = kx$, where k is a constant factor characteristic of the spring (i.e., its stiffness), and x is small compared to the total possible deformation of the spring.

A bungee cord is known to obey Hooke's law. An experimenter wished to determine to what extent it does and graphed the results. At which point, in Figure 1, did the bungee cord stop obeying Hooke's law?

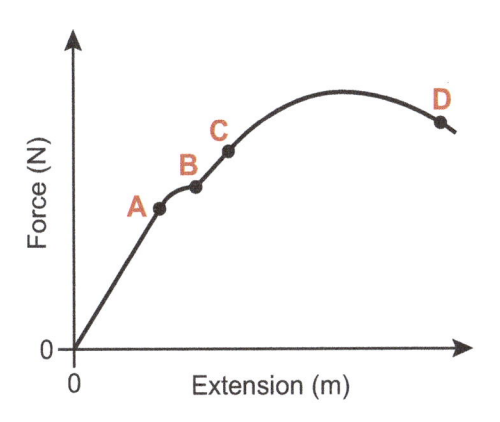

17) Extracorporeal shock wave lithotripsy (ESWL) is a treatment option that uses sound waves (ultrasound) to break up simple kidney stones. Consider two ESWL mechanical waves of the same frequency passing through the same kidney stone. The range of amplitudes possible when the two waves pass through the medium is between four and eight units. Which of the following best describes the possible amplitudes of the two waves?

A. 6 units and 2 units
B. 8 units and 4 units
C. 12 units and 4 units
D. 10 units and 2 units

GAMSAT-Prep.com
GOLD STANDARD PHYSICS

Questions 18–20

More than a century before Einstein revealed the particulate nature of light through the photoelectric effect, Thomas Young performed classic experiments which confirmed the wave nature of light. In one experiment, light was projected through very fine slits - of the order of the magnitude of the wavelength of light. As a result of its wavy nature, light appears to bend around the corners of the slits. Once past the slits, the light is free to engage in interference patterns with the light wave from the neighboring slit.

In this Young slit experiment, the interference patterns form an image which consists of a pattern of bright lines (constructive interference) and dark lines (destructive interference) projected on a screen. Figures 1 and 2 demonstrate the summation waves for maximal interference.

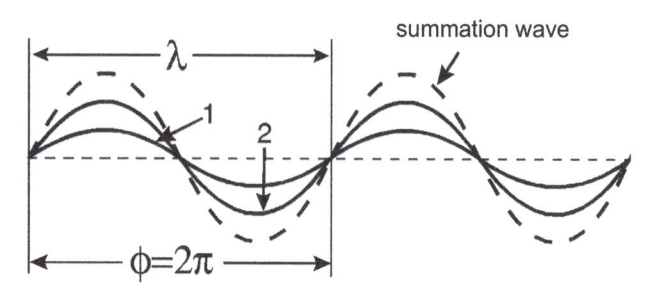

Figure 1: Maximal constructive interference.

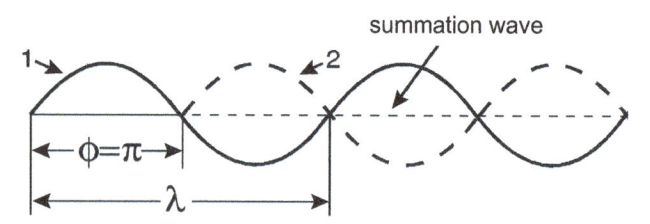

Figure 2: Maximal destructive interference.

The conditions for maximal constructive interference for the double-slit experiment where d is the distance between the slits, l is the distance from the screen to the slits, y_n is the distance on the screen from the central maximum interference pattern to the nth order maximum, can be calculated as the integral number n of wavelengths λ, where n can be 0, ±1, ±2,..., as follows:

Equation I

$$n\lambda = d y_n/l$$

The conditions for maximal destructive interference for the double-slit experiment is given by:

Equation II

$$(n + 1/2)\lambda = d y_n/l$$

18) In terms of the wave nature of sound and light, respectively, the summation wave in Figure 2 would produce:

   A. silence and darkness.
   B. increased amplitude, decreased brightness.
   C. decreased amplitude, increased brightness.
   D. unchanged sound, dark lines.

19) Under otherwise constant conditions, what would happen to the distance on a screen from the central maximum interference pattern to the nth order maximum if the distance between the slits was doubled?

   A. It would double.
   B. It would be halved.
   C. It would remain the same.
   D. It cannot be determined based on the information provided.

20) Based on the information in the passage, if the paths taken by two waves differ by $(9/2)\lambda$, then the interference pattern would be destructive and:

   A. $n = 9.5$.   C. $n = 4.5$.
   B. $n = 9$.   D. $n = 4$.

PHY-104   CHAPTER 7: WAVE CHARACTERISTICS AND PERIODIC MOTION

GAMSAT MASTERS SERIES

SPOILER ALERT ⚠️

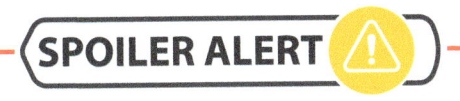

Gold Standard has cross-referenced the content in this chapter to examples from ACER's official GAMSAT practice materials. It is for you to decide when you want to explore these questions since you may want to preserve some of ACER's materials for timed mock-exam practice.

Examples – Period, wavelength and resonance (note that even f = 1/T and the units are defined in the passage): Q5-7 of 5; energy and intensity (PHY 7.1.4) of a wave: Q88-89 of 5. Note that "Q" is followed by the question number, and, for example, "of 1" refers to booklet number 1 which is referenced in the Spoiler Alert table at the end of Chapter 1. The 10 full-length HEAPS GAMSAT practice tests (by Gold Standard and MediRed), exams 1 through 10, contain specific cross-references to this chapter within the worked solutions. Note that the oscillatory motion unit is from HEAPS-3 and the extracorporeal shock wave lithotripsy unit (smash those kidney stones!) is from HEAPS-9.

High-level Importance

Chapter Checklist

- ☐ Access your online account to view answers, worked solutions and discussion boards.
- ☐ Reassess your 'learning objectives' for this chapter: Go back to the first page of this chapter and re-evaluate the top 3 boxes and the Introduction.
- ☐ Complete a maximum of 1 page of notes using symbols/abbreviations to represent the entire chapter based on your learning objectives. These are your Gold Notes.
- ☐ Consider your multimedia options based on your optimal way of learning:
  - ☐ Download the free Gold Standard GAMSAT app for your Android device or iPhone.
  - ☐ Create your own, tangible study cards or try the free app: Anki.
  - ☐ Record your voice reading your Gold Notes onto your smartphone (MP3s) and listen during exercise, transportation, etc.
  - ☐ Try out the Gold Standard GAMSAT online videos at gamsat-prep.com, or you can try other options on YouTube like Khan Academy or Crash Course Physics.
- ☐ Reassess your schedule for your full-length GAMSAT practice tests: ACER and/or HEAPS exams. Ensure that you have scheduled one full day to complete a practice test and 1-2 days for a thorough assessment of worked solutions while adding to your abbreviated Gold Notes.
- ☐ Reassess your progress in scheduling and/or evaluating stress reduction techniques such as regular exercise (sports), yoga, meditation and/or mindfulness exercises (*see* YouTube for suggestions).

THE PHYSICAL SCIENCES   PHY-105

High-level Importance

GOLD NOTES

SOUND
Chapter 8

Memorise
* Sensory vs. physical correspondence of hearing

Understand
* Relative velocity of sound in solids, liquids and gases
* The relation of intensity to P, area, f, amplitude
* Calculation of the intensity level
* Rules of logarithms
* Doppler effect and calculations
* Audiograms (graphs; *see* GAMSAT-level practice questions)

Importance
Low level: **1%** of GAMSAT Physics questions released by ACER are related to content in this chapter (in our estimation).
* Note that approximately **75%** of the questions in GAMSAT Physics are related to just 6 chapters: 1, 4, 6, 9, 11 and 12.

GAMSAT-Prep.com

Introduction

Sound waves are longitudinal waves which can only be transmitted in a material, elastic medium. Speed, intensity, resonance (Chapter 7) and the Doppler effect help to describe the behavior of sound in different media. If the equations for sound intensity or the Doppler effect are required for the GAMSAT, they will be provided by ACER. Reminder: The 'Importance level' refers to assumed knowledge and is NOT related to the practice questions. The questions at the end of this chapter use reasoning, logs, equation manipulation and graph analysis which are all skills that will benefit you even when the questions are not based on the content of this chapter.

Multimedia Resources at GAMSAT-Prep.com

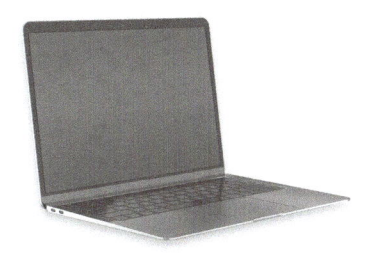

Open Discussion Boards   Foundational Videos   Flashcards   Special Guest

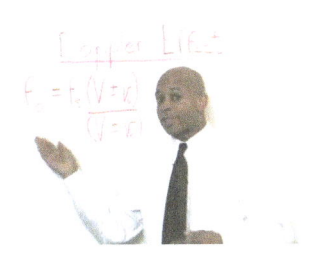

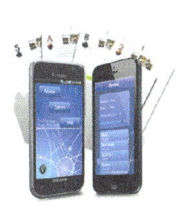

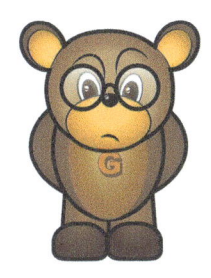

THE PHYSICAL SCIENCES   PHY-107

* The real GAMSAT may have advanced-level information presented (i.e. in a passage) but previous knowledge of said information is not required to answer the questions that would follow. Practice questions at the end of this chapter, as well as ACER and GS (HEAPS) practice GAMSATs can help you clarify this point.

8.1 Production of Sound

Sound is a longitudinal mechanical wave which travels through an elastic medium. **Sound is thus produced by vibrating matter.** There is no sound in a *vacuum* because it contains no matter (note: we have placed a table in PHY 11.6 comparing light and sound).

Compressions (condensations) are regions where particles of matter are close together; they are also high pressure regions. Rarefactions are regions where particles are sparse, they are low pressure regions of sound waves (PHY 7.1.1).

8.2 Relative Velocity of Sound in Solids, Liquids, and Gases

The velocity of sound is proportional to the square root of the elastic restoring force and inversely proportional to the square root of the inertia of the particles (e.g., density is a measure of inertia). Thus as a rule, the velocity of sound is higher in liquids as compared to gases, and highest in solids.

Furthermore, an increase in temperature increases the velocity of sound; conversely, a decrease in temperature decreases the velocity of sound in that medium.

8.3 Intensity, Pitch

Hearing is subjective but its characteristics are closely tied to physical characteristics of sound.

The quality depends on the number and relative intensity of the overtones of the waveform. Frequency, and therefore pitch are perceived by the ear from 20 to 20,000 Hz (hertz = cycles/second = s^{-1}). Frequencies below 20 Hz are called infrasonic. Frequencies above 20,000 Hz are called ultrasonic.

Sensory	Physical
loudness	intensity
pitch	frequency
quality	waveform

Table III.B.8.1:
Sensory and physical correspondence of hearing.

Sound intensity (I) is the rate of energy (power) propagation through space:

$I = $ (power/area) which is proportional to $(f^2 A^2)$

where f = frequency, A = amplitude.

The loudness varies with the frequency. The ears are most sensitive (hears sounds of lowest intensity) at approximately 2000 to 4000 Hz. I_0 is taken to be 10^{-12} watts/cm², is barely audible and is assigned a value of 0 dB (zero *decibels*). Then intensity level (I) of a sound wave in dB is,

$$dB = 10 \log_{10}(I/I_0)$$

where dB = the sound level, I = the intensity at a given level, I_0 = the threshold intensity. {To calculate a change in the sound level or volume ΔV in units of dB, given two values for sound intensity, the given equation can be modified thus: $\Delta V = 10\log(I_{new}/I_{old})$}

Examples of some values of dB's are: whisper (20), normal conversation (60), subway car (100), pain threshold (120), and jet engine (160). Continual exposure to sound greater than 90 dB can lead to hearing impairment.

8.3.1 Calculation of the Intensity Level

What is the loudness or intensity level of Mr. Yell Alot's voice when he generates a sound wave ten million times as intense as I_0?

$I = (10\ 000\ 000)I_0 = (10^7)I_0$

Now we can substitute for I given the equation for dBs in the previous section (PHY 8.3), and then I_0 will cancel.

Thus: $dB = 10 \log_{10}(10^7 I_0/I_0)$
$= 10 \log_{10} 10^7$
$= 70 \log_{10} 10 = 70$

{*See* GM 3.7 for rules of logarithms. Also, re-examine log curves (GM 3.8) – <u>especially the audiogram</u> with GAMSAT-level MCQs, Fig. IV.3.6 (*note that there are 2 more audiogram-based units at the end of Chapter 8*). Logs are common amongst ACER's GAMSAT materials.}

8.4 Beats

When sound of different frequencies are heard together, they interfere. Constructive interference results in beats (PHY 7.1.3). The number of beats per second is the absolute value of the difference of the frequencies ($|f_1 - f_2|$).

Hence, the new frequency heard includes the original frequencies and the absolute difference between them.

8.5 Doppler Effect

The classic example of the Doppler effect is a train blowing its horn as it passes by. As it approaches, the sound waves compress and rise in pitch for the stationary listener, as the train recedes from the same listener, the waves decompress and the pitch goes down. Of course, the signal (train horn) remains a steady pitch for the folks on the train.

Thus the Doppler effect is the effect upon the observed frequency (*pitch*) caused by the relative motion of the observer (*o*) and the source (*s*). If the distance is decreasing between them, there is a shift to higher frequencies and shorter wavelengths (to higher pitch for sound and toward blue-violet for light, PHY 8.3 and 9.2.4). If the distance is increasing between them, there is a shift to longer wavelengths and lower frequencies (to lower pitch for sound and toward red for light). The summary equation of the above in terms of frequency (f) is:

$$f_o = f_s(V \pm v_o)/(V \pm v_s)$$

V = speed of the wave, v = speed of the observer (*o*) or the source (*s*).

Choose the sign such that the frequency varies consistently with the relative motion of the source and the observer. In other words, when the distance between the source and observer is *decreasing* use $+v_o$ and $-v_s$; if the distance is *increasing* use $-v_o$ and $+v_s$.

Source receding:

$$f_{observed} = \left[\frac{V}{V+V_{source}}\right] f_{source}$$

Source approaching:

$$f_{observed} = \left[\frac{V}{V-V_{source}}\right] f_{source}$$

Hears the sound of a longer wavelength, lower frequency, lower pitch.

Stationary source of frequency f_{source}

All observers hear the same frequency.

Moving source

Hears the sound of a shorter wavelength, higher frequency, higher pitch.

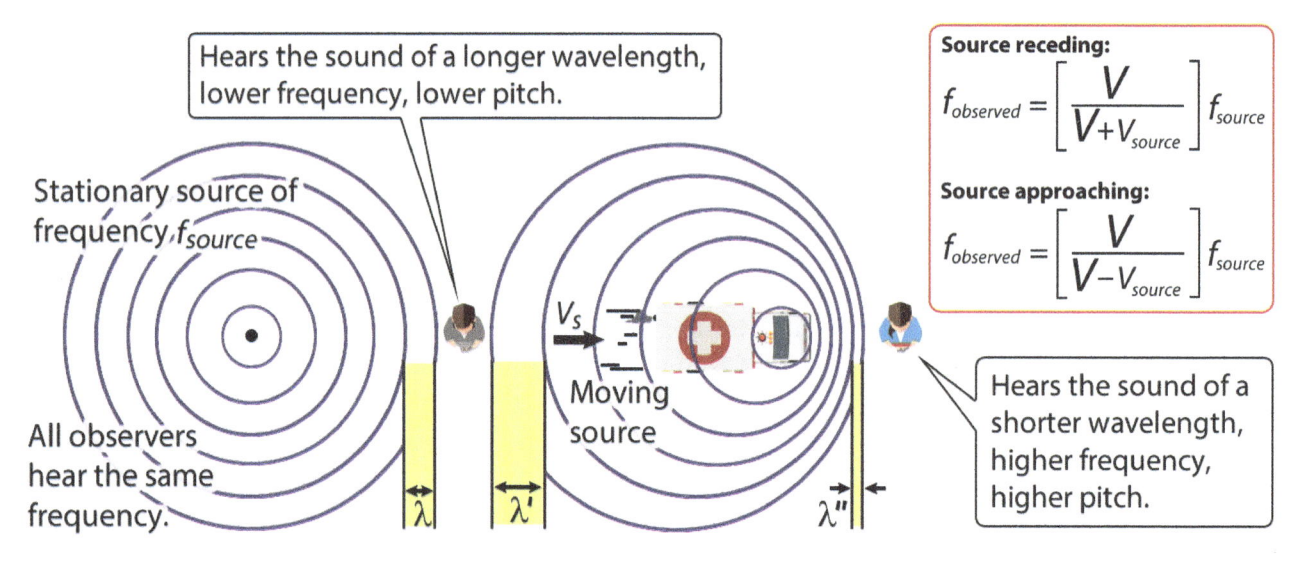

Figure III.B.8.1: The Doppler effect (AKA, the Doppler shift). When you hear the high pitch of a siren of an approaching emergency vehicle or ambulance, and notice that its pitch drops suddenly as it passes you: That is the Doppler effect. This occurs because the movement of the source alters the wavelength and the received frequency of the sound, even though the source frequency and wave velocity are unchanged.

Essentially, the approaching source moves closer during the period of the sound wave so the effective wavelength is shortened, giving a higher pitch since the velocity of the wave is unchanged. Similarly, the pitch of the receding sound source will be lowered. Note that the observers in the image are stationary so in each case $v_o = 0$. Note that the Doppler effect occurs due to relative motion between the source and observer - either of which could be moving or stationary. (Image adapted from HyperPhysics, Georgia State University)

8.5.1 Doppler Effect Problem (SI units)

A car drives towards a bus stop with its car stereo playing opera. The opera singer sings the note middle C (= 262 Hz) loudly; however, the people waiting at the bus stop hear C sharp (= 277 Hz). Given that the speed of sound V in air is 331 m/s, how fast is the car moving?

{Remember the sign convention: since the distance between the source (the car) and the observer (people at the bus stop) is <u>decreasing</u> we use $+v_o$ and $-v_s$}

- the car (the *source* of the frequency) f_s = 262 Hz, v_s = unknown.

- the bus stop (where the *observers* are stationary) f_o = 277 Hz, v_o = 0 m/s.

$$f_o = f_s(V + v_o)/(V - v_s)$$

Thus

$$V - v_s = f_s(V + v_o)/f_o$$

Hence

$$v_s = -f_s(V + v_o)/f_o + V$$

Substitute

$$v_s = -262(331 + 0)/277 + 331 = 17.9 \text{ m/s}.$$

- Note that the answer contains three significant figures.

- If there is any step that you cannot do, go to gamsat-prep.com/forum, GAMSAT Physics, question 8.5.1, and post which step you find is disagreeable.

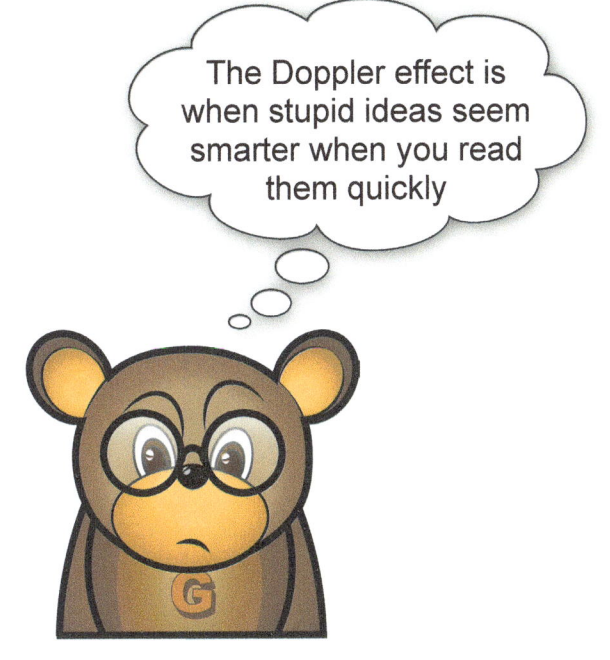

GAMSAT-Prep.com
GOLD STANDARD PHYSICS

CHAPTER 8: Sound

GOLD STANDARD FOUNDATIONAL GAMSAT PRACTICE QUESTIONS

1) An old-fashioned clock with bells can be seen and heard ringing. When it is placed in a container devoid of air particles (*a vacuum*), it can be seen ringing but it cannot be heard. Which of the following best describes this phenomenon?

   A. Sound waves have a greater period than light waves.
   B. Sound waves have a greater amplitude than light waves.
   C. Sound waves cannot travel through a vacuum but light waves can.
   D. The described phenomenon cannot occur unless the container itself is somehow blocking the sound of the clock.

2) The energy of a wave E is related to the frequency of a wave f by Planck's constant h, $E = hf$.

   The data below illustrates the range of frequencies that four different ultrasound devices can generate. Which ultrasound device is able to generate the greatest amount of kinetic energy?

Wave Emitting Machine	Frequency Range (Hz)
1	$8.0 \times 10^4 - 6.4 \times 10^4$
2	$3.2 \times 10^3 - 2.9 \times 10^4$
3	$1.2 \times 10^2 - 7.4 \times 10^5$
4	$2.0 \times 10^4 - 0.6 \times 10^6$

   A. Device 1
   B. Device 2
   C. Device 3
   D. Device 4

3) When a source of sound waves, whose frequency is in the auditory range, is moving toward a stationary observer, which of the following is true?

   A. The observer hears a frequency of sound which is higher than the frequency of sound emitted from the source.
   B. The observer hears a frequency of sound which is lower than the frequency of sound emitted from the source.
   C. The observer hears a frequency of sound which is the same as the frequency of sound emitted from the source.
   D. Cannot be determined from the information given.

4) A sound wave which originates from a stationary observer is reflected off an object approaching with velocity v. The reflected wave, relative to original wave, has:

   A. decreased frequency and increased velocity.
   B. same frequency and same velocity.
   C. same frequency and increased velocity.
   D. increased frequency and same velocity.

5) An ultrasound is a medical test that uses high-frequency sound waves to capture live images from the inside of your body. The scanning device emits a wave and that is reflected back to the same device for detection and interpretation. If an ultrasonic wave with a frequency of 3.0×10^4 Hz is detected 4×10^{-5} seconds after entering the body, how deep is the surface it is detecting? (Note: ultrasonic waves travel at approximately 1.5×10^3 m/s in the body)

   A. 0.03 m
   B. 0.04 m
   C. 0.06 m
   D. 0.08 m

GAMSAT MASTERS SERIES

GOLD STANDARD GAMSAT-LEVEL PRACTICE QUESTIONS

Questions 6–7

Sound pressure or acoustic pressure is the local pressure deviation from the ambient atmospheric pressure, caused by a sound wave. Sound pressure can be measured by the pascal (Pa) or in decibels (dB).

The hearing range - the difference between the highest and lowest frequency - of different organisms can be plotted including data points within the range by using graphs called 'audiograms'. Audiograms show the audible threshold for measured, standardised frequencies.

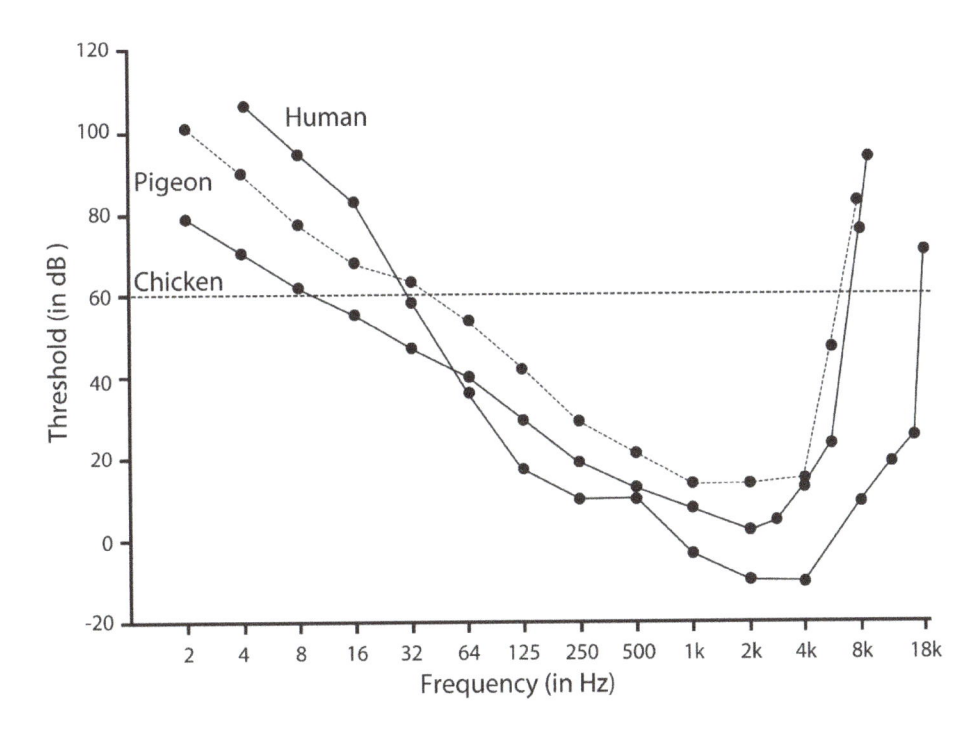

Figure 1: Audiogram of chickens compared with the audiograms of humans (Jackson et al. 1999) and pigeons (Heffner et al. 2013). The horizontal dashed line at 60 dB represents the mean threshold of the 3 organisms.

High-level Importance

6) Which of the following is most consistent with the hearing ranges shown in Figure 1?

   A. The 3 ranges are identical.
   B. The 3 ranges are the same within an acceptable range of error.
   C. The range for chicken and human is similar.
   D. Both the range for pigeon and the range for chicken are each less than half of the range for human.

7) According to Figure 1, which organisms would be able to detect a sound with a sound intensity of 50 dB and a frequency of 64 Hz?

   A. Human only
   B. Pigeon only
   C. Chicken and human only
   D. Human, pigeon and chicken

THE PHYSICAL SCIENCES   PHY-113

GAMSAT-Prep.com
GOLD STANDARD PHYSICS

Questions 8–10

The phon is a unit of loudness. Human sensitivity to sound is variable across different frequencies (Hz); therefore, although two different tones may have the identical sound intensity (watts/m^2), they may be psycho-acoustically *perceived* as differing in loudness. The purpose of the phon is to provide a standard measurement for perceived intensity, as opposed to the actual intensity of the sound.

The decibel (symbol: dB) is a relative unit on a logarithmic scale. The human perception of the intensity of sound approximates the log base 10 of intensity rather than a linear relationship, making the dB scale a useful measure. Consider Figure 1.

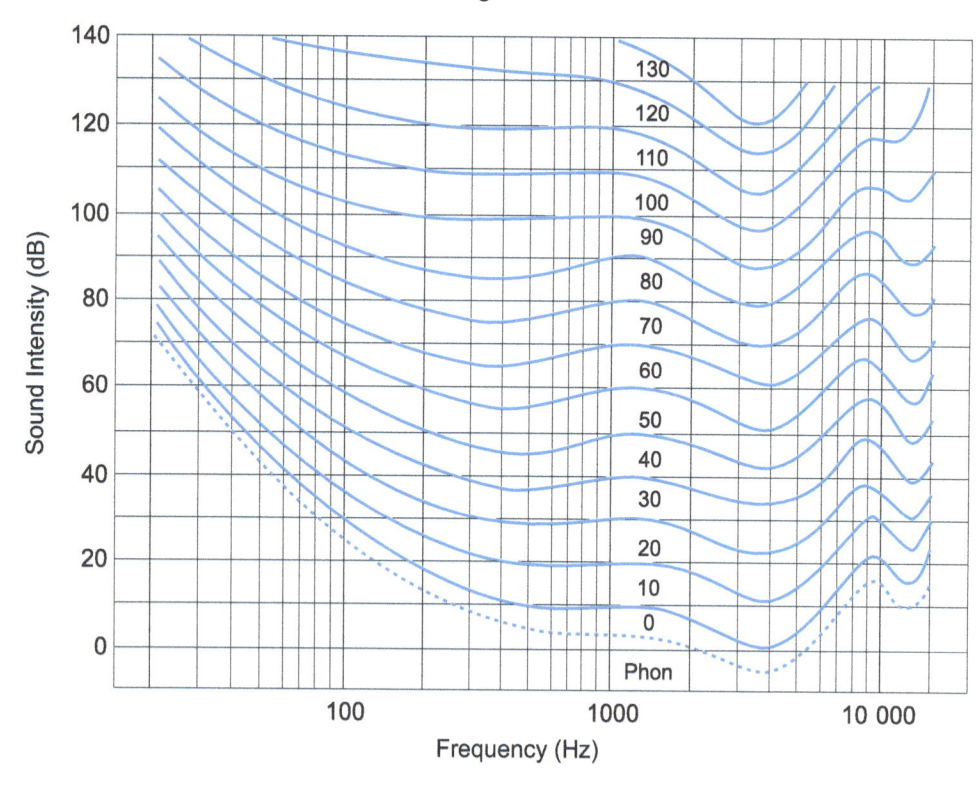

Figure 1: Phon contour curves for the human perception of loudness. The clinical threshold of hearing at 1000 Hz measured at approximately 4 dB is the reference that establishes phon = 0 (indicated by the dotted line). (axes relabelled from A7N8X, Wikimedia Commons)

8) At a phon value of 70, the ears are most sensitive (i.e. able to hear sounds of lowest intensity) closest to which of the following frequencies?

   A. 500 Hz
   B. 2 kHz
   C. 4 kHz
   D. 6 kHz

9) At 60 phon, the greatest drop in sound intensity (W/m^2) occurs between which of the following ranges in frequencies?

   A. 30–50 Hz
   B. 50–100 Hz
   C. 100–400 Hz
   D. 100–3000 Hz

10) According to Figure 1, which of the following is the loudest sound that a person would perceive?

    A. 65 dB, 50 Hz
    B. 58 dB, 9 kHz
    C. 42 dB, 20 kHz
    D. 40 dB, 1 kHz

11) In a liquid, the speed of sound is inversely proportional to the square root of the density of the liquid. If a liquid X has a density equal to twice the density of liquid Y, what is the ratio of the velocity of the wave in X to the velocity of the wave in Y?

    A. $1 : \sqrt{2}$
    B. 1 : 2
    C. 2 : 1
    D. $\sqrt{2} : 1$

Questions 12–13

Sound intensity level is usually measured in decibels, dB. The decibel is defined as 1 dB = 10 log(I/I$_o$), where I is the intensity of the sound to be measured, and I$_o$ is an arbitrary reference level.

12) If one jet airplane produces a sound level of 100 decibels, what sound level is produced by two jets? (Log 2 = 0.30)

   A. 103 decibels
   B. 200 decibels
   C. 230 decibels
   D. 300 decibels

13) If the intensity of a sound is said to increase by 20 dB, how many times does the sound intensity increase?

   A. 1000 times
   B. 100 times
   C. 20 times
   D. 10 times

Questions 14–16

Every time a police car rushes by with its siren roaring, the physics phenomenon called the *Doppler effect* is illustrated. An observer at rest will probably notice that the pitch of the sound becomes higher as the vehicle races towards him and lower as it speeds away. As the patrol car approaches the observer, a larger number of wave fronts reach the observer every second, which consequently increases the frequency or pitch of the sound heard. Conversely, as the patrol car recedes, the observer perceives a decrease in frequency.

The Doppler effect is not only limited to mechanical waves; light emitted by a moving source also exhibits the Doppler effect. As the light source moves toward the observer, the frequency of its emitted radiation appears to increase, this is known as *blueshift*. In contrast, the radiation emitted by a source that moves away has decreasing frequency, this is known as *redshift*.

Sound intensity (I) is the rate of energy (power) propagation through space. The loudness varies with the frequency. The ears are most sensitive (hears sounds of lowest intensity) at approximately 2000 to 4000 Hz. I$_o$ is taken to be 10^{-12} watts/m^2, is barely audible and is assigned a value of 0 dB (zero decibels). Then intensity level (I) of a sound wave in dB is,

$$dB = 10 \log_{10}(I/I_o)$$

where dB = the sound level, I = the intensity at a given level, I$_o$ = the threshold intensity.

Note that: Wavelength is inversely proportional to the frequency of a wave.

14) The requirement for experiencing the Doppler effect is:

   A. a relative motion between source and observer.
   B. a relative acceleration between source and observer.
   C. a medium to propagate light.
   D. an observer at rest in an inertial frame of reference.

15) Light is said to be redshifted when:

   A. its wavelength increases.
   B. its frequency increases.
   C. its wavelength decreases.
   D. its wavelength and frequency both decrease.

16) The humming sound of a traffic light happens to be quite clear once your car comes to a stop. If you detect its level to be 20 dB, what is its intensity?

   A. 10^{-10} watts/m^2
   B. 10^{-12} watts/m^2
   C. 10^{-14} watts/m^2
   D. 10^{-20} watts/m^2

GAMSAT-Prep.com
GOLD STANDARD PHYSICS

High-level Importance

> ## ⚠ SPOILER ALERT
>
> Gold Standard has cross-referenced the content in this chapter to examples from ACER's official GAMSAT practice materials. It is for you to decide when you want to explore these questions since you may want to preserve some of ACER's materials for timed mock-exam practice.
>
> **Examples** – Log calculation (dB): Q52 of 2; hearing, decibels (dB) and graph analysis: Q108-110 of 4; frequency of sounds and resonance: Q5-7 of 5 (however, we did not count these latter 3 questions in terms of Importance because there was no assumed knowledge based on Chapter 8); small changes at the top end of a log scale can have the biggest impact: Q104-105 of 3 (also not counted, not Chapter 8-specific). Note that "Q" is followed by the question number, and, for example, "of 1" refers to booklet number 1 which is referenced in the Spoiler Alert table at the end of Chapter 1. The 10 full-length HEAPS GAMSAT practice tests (by Gold Standard and MediRed), exams 1 through 10, contain specific cross-references to this chapter within the worked solutions. Note that the square root proportion question is from HEAPS-3 and the Doppler effect unit is from HEAPS-8.

Chapter Checklist

- ☐ Access your online account to view answers, worked solutions and discussion boards.
- ☐ Reassess your 'learning objectives' for this chapter: Go back to the first page of this chapter and re-evaluate the top 3 boxes and the Introduction.
- ☐ Complete a maximum of 1 page of notes using symbols/abbreviations to represent the entire chapter based on your learning objectives. These are your Gold Notes.
- ☐ Consider your multimedia options based on your optimal way of learning:
    - ☐ Download the free Gold Standard GAMSAT app for your Android device or iPhone.
    - ☐ Create your own, tangible study cards or try the free app: Anki.
    - ☐ Record your voice reading your Gold Notes onto your smartphone (MP3s) and listen during exercise, transportation, etc.
    - ☐ Try out the Gold Standard GAMSAT online videos at gamsat-prep.com, or you can try other options on YouTube like Khan Academy or Crash Course Physics.
- ☐ Reassess your schedule for your full-length GAMSAT practice tests: ACER and/or HEAPS exams. Ensure that you have scheduled one full day to complete a practice test and 1-2 days for a thorough assessment of worked solutions while adding to your abbreviated Gold Notes.
- ☐ Reassess your progress in scheduling and/or evaluating stress reduction techniques such as regular exercise (sports), yoga, meditation and/or mindfulness exercises (*see* YouTube for suggestions).

ELECTROSTATICS AND ELECTROMAGNETISM
Chapter 9

Memorise
* Equations: for charge Q, Coulomb's law, electric field
* Equation relating energy, planck's constant, frequency

Understand
* Conservation of charge, use of Coulomb's law
* Graphs/theory: electric field/potential lines, magnetic induction
* Potential difference, electric dipoles
* Laplace's law, the right-hand rule, magnetic field
* Direction of F in magn. field; electromagnetism

Importance
High level: 10% of GAMSAT Physics questions released by ACER are related to content in this chapter (in our estimation).
* Note that approximately **75%** of the questions in GAMSAT Physics are related to just 6 chapters: 1, 4, 6, 9, 11 and 12.

GAMSAT-Prep.com

Introduction

Electricity refers to either stationary or moving electric charges. The electric charge is a sub-atomic particle, the *electron*, which carries a charge designated as negative. Thus, the various manifestations of electricity are the result of the accumulation or motion of electrons.

Electrostatics (*statics* = at rest) refers to the science of stationary or slowly moving charges. Such charges can interact and behave in ways described by charge, electric force, electric field and potential difference. When a charge is in motion, it creates a magnetic field. Electromagnetism describes the relationship between electric charges and magnetism. The electromagnetic spectrum includes light and X-rays.

Multimedia Resources at GAMSAT-Prep.com

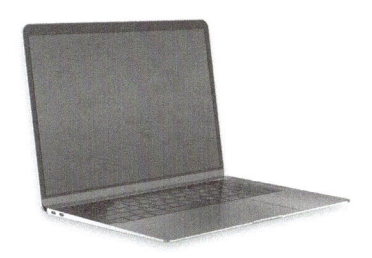

Open Discussion Boards   Foundational Videos   Flashcards   Special Guest

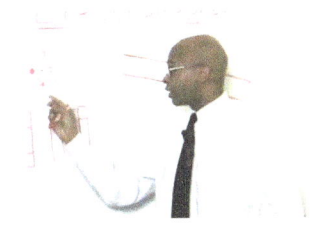

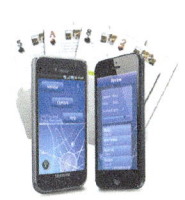

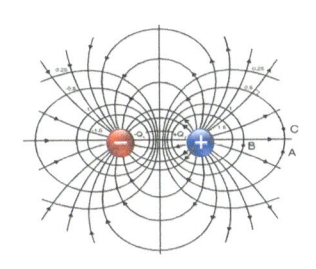

* The real GAMSAT may have advanced-level information presented (i.e. in a passage) but previous knowledge of said information is not required to answer the questions that would follow. Practice questions at the end of this chapter, as well as ACER and GS (HEAPS) practice GAMSATs can help you clarify this point.

GAMSAT-Prep.com
GOLD STANDARD PHYSICS

9.0 GAMSAT has a *Need for Speed*!

High-level Importance

Section Number	GAMSAT Physics *Need for Speed* Exercises
9.1.1	How would you calculate the total charge Q if you are given the number of particles n and the charge e on each particle? (N.B. dimensional analysis!)
9.1.2	Write the equation known as "Coulomb's law."
9.1.3	For the images below, draw arrow heads on the lines to indicate the direction of movement of a test charge (i.e. the direction of the electric field lines). For the image on the right: Extend the velocity vector of the electron coming from the "Electron gun" as it passes through the electric field as indicated.
9.2.2	What kind of field does a moving electric charge generate that a stationary charge cannot?
9.2.4	What are the colours of the rainbow, in order, from highest to lowest wavelength?

9.1 Electrostatics

9.1.1 Charge, Conductors, Insulators

By friction of matter we create between substances repulsive or attractive electric forces. These forces are due to two kinds of electric charges, distinguished by positive (+) and negative (−) signs. Each has a charge of 1.6×10^{-19} coulombs (= C = an SI derived

PHY-118   CHAPTER 9: ELECTROSTATICS AND ELECTROMAGNETISM

unit; GM 2.1.3, Table 3) but differ in sign. The electron is the negative charge carrier, and the proton is the positive charge carrier. Substances with an excess of electrons have a net negative charge. Substances with a deficiency of electrons have a net positive charge. The total amount of charge Q of matter depends on the number of particles n and the charge e on each particle, thus $Q = ne$.

The conservation of charge states that a net charge cannot be created but that charge can be transfered from one object to another. One way of charging substances is by rubbing them (i.e., by contact).

For example, glass rubbed on fur becomes positive, and rubber rubbed on fur becomes negative.

Objects can also be charged by induction which occurs when one charged object is brought near to another uncharged object causing a charge redistribution in the latter to give net-charge regions. Conductors transmit charge readily. Insulators resist the flow of charge.

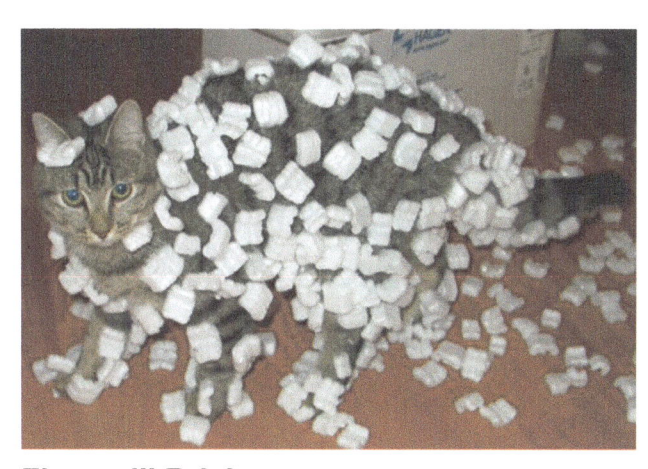

Figure III.B.9.0a: Styrofoam peanuts clinging to a cat's fur. The static electricity that builds up on the fur causes a separation of charge (*polarisation*) of the molecules of the styrofoam due to electrostatic induction, resulting in a slight attraction of the very light styrofoam to the charged fur. (Sean McGrath, Black Rainbow 999; Wikimedia Commons)

9.1.2 Coulomb's Law, Electric Force

Charges exert forces upon each other. Like charges repel each other, and unlike charges attract. For any two stationary charges q_1 and q_2 the force F is given by Coulomb's law:

$$F = k\frac{q_1 q_2}{r^2} = \frac{1}{4\pi\varepsilon_o}\left(\frac{q_1 q_2}{r^2}\right)$$

where k = Coulomb's constant = 9.0×10^9 N-m²/C², ε_o = permittivity constant = 8.85×10^{-12} C²/N-m², and r = the distance between the charges. Note that the relationship of force and distance follows an inverse square law. Thus if the distance r is doubled [$(2r)^2 = 4r^2$], the new force is quartered ($F_{new} = F/4$). {Compare with the Law of Gravity: PHY 2.4.}

GAMSAT-Prep.com
GOLD STANDARD PHYSICS

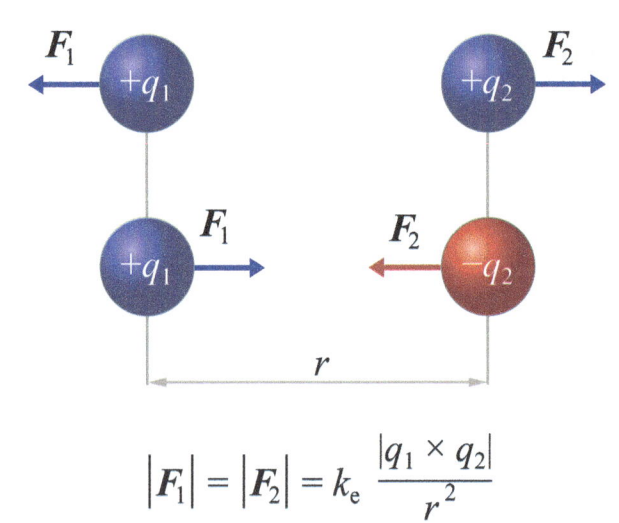

High-level Importance

$$|F_1| = |F_2| = k_e \frac{|q_1 \times q_2|}{r^2}$$

Figure III.B.9.0b: Electrostatics. The magnitude of the electrostatic force F between 2 point charges q_1 and q_2 is directly proportional to the product of the magnitudes of the charges and inversely proportional to the square of the distance between them (Coulomb's law). Opposites attract, like charges repel. (Dna-Dennis; Wikimedia Commons)

9.1.3 Electric Field, Electric Field Lines

A charge generates an electric field (E) in the space around it. Fields (*force fields*) are vectors. A field is generated by an object and it is that region of space around the object that will exert a force on a second object brought into that field. The field exists independently of that second object and is not altered by its presence. The force exerted on the second object depends upon that object and the field. The electric field *E* is given by:

$$E = F/q = k\, Q/r^2$$

where *E* and *F* are vectors, Q = the charge generating the field, and q = the charge placed in the field.

Charges exert forces upon each other through fields. The direction of a field is the direction a positive charge would move if placed in it. *Electric field lines* are imaginary lines which are in the same direction as *E* at that point. The direction is away from positive charges and toward negative charges, or put another way, the electric field is directed toward the decreasing potentials.

If an electric potential is applied between two plates in a vacuum (*in vacuo: a space devoid of matter*), and an electron is introduced, the electron will experience an attractive force to the positive plate (*see Figure III.B.9.2*).

The force will cause the electron to accelerate towards the positive plate in a straight line. It suffers no collisions because the area between the plates is *in vacuo*.

PHY-120   CHAPTER 9: ELECTROSTATICS AND ELECTROMAGNETISM

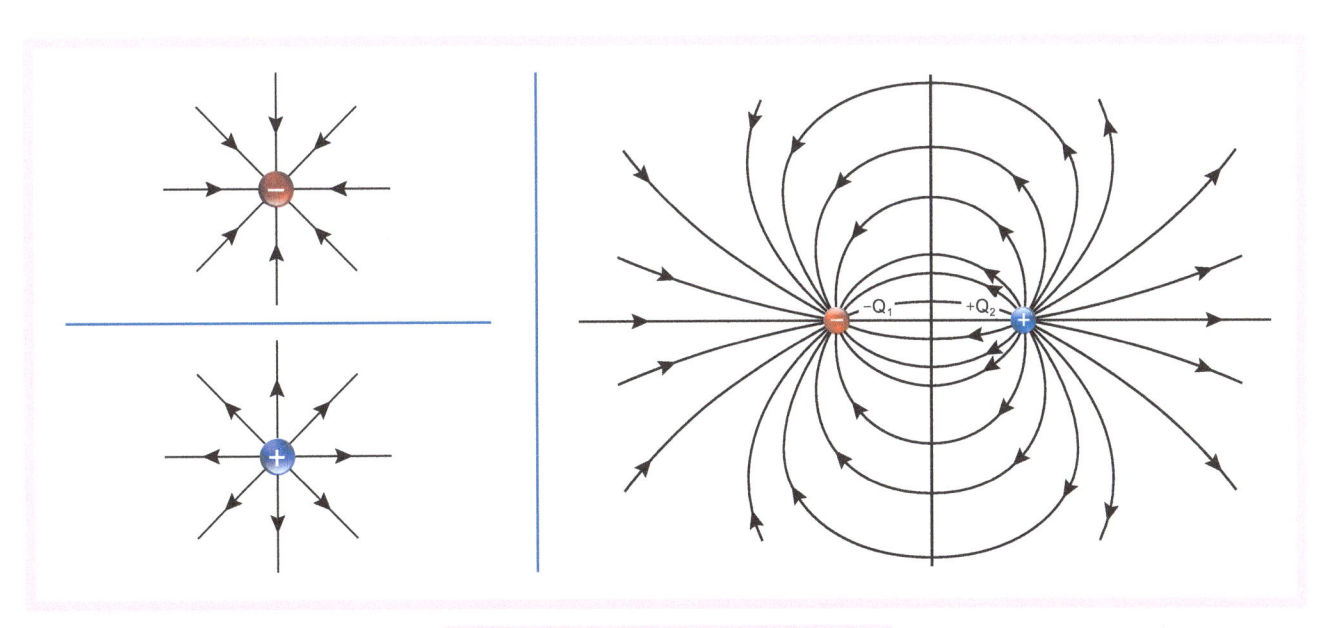

Figure III.B.9.1: Electric field lines.
The electric field is generated by the charges –Q_1 and +Q_2. The arrowheads show the direction of the electric field.

If the electron is given some motion, and the electric field is applied perpendicular to the motion, interesting things happen (see Figure III.B.9.3). For example, a beam of electrons is emitted from a device called an electron gun. These electrons are moving in the x-direction.

As the electrons pass between the plates they are accelerated in the y-direction, as explained before, but their velocity in the x-direction is unaltered. The electron beam is thus deflected as shown.

By varying the potential applied to the plates, the angle of deflection can be controlled. This effect is the basis of the cathode ray oscilloscope.

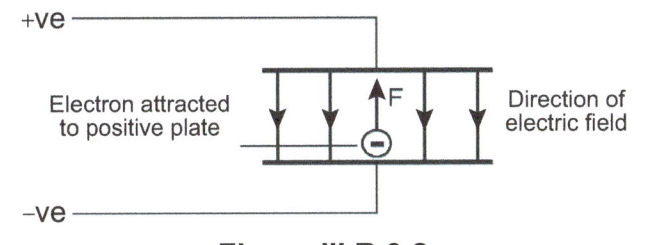

Figure III.B.9.2:
Electric field between parallel plates.

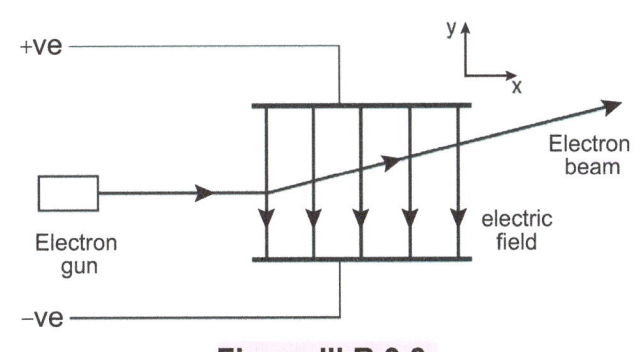

Figure III.B.9.3:
Electrostatic deflection of an electron beam.

9.1.4 Potential Energy, Absolute Potential

The *potential energy* (E_p) of a charged object in a field equals the work done on that object to bring it from infinity to a distance (r) from the charge setting up the electric field,

$$E_p = work = Fr = (qE)r = kQq/r$$

where Q = the charge setting up field, and q = the charge brought in to a distance r.

When a +q moves against E, its E_p increases. When a −q moves against the electric field E, its E_p decreases. If two positive or negative charges were brought together, work would have to be done to the system (and E_p would increase), and vice versa for charges of opposite charges.

The *absolute potential* (V) is a scalar, and it is defined at each distance (r) from a charge (Q) generating an electric field. It represents the negative of the work per unit charge in bringing a +q from infinity to r:

- $V = E_p/q = kQ/r$ in volts where 1 volt = 1 joule/coulomb.

9.1.5 Equipotential Lines, Potential Difference, Electric Dipoles

Equipotential lines are lines (and surfaces) of equal V and are *perpendicular* to electric field lines. Work can only be done when moving between surfaces of unequal V and is, therefore, independent of the path taken. <u>No work is done</u> when a charge (q) is moved along an <u>equal potential</u> (*equipotential*) surface (or line), because the component of force is zero along it. Potential (V) is defined in terms of positive charges such that V is positive when due to a +Q and negative when due a −Q. Potential (V) is added algebraically at a point (because it is a scalar).

See Figure III.B.9.4:

1) V_1, V_2 are two potentials perpendicular to the electric field E and the force F;

2) $V_2 - V_1$ is the potential difference (PD);

3) charge (q) moved from A ($V_1 = 0.5$) to B ($V_2 = 1$) has work (W) done on it:

$$W = q(V_2 - V_1) = q(PD)$$

4) charge (q) moved from A to C has no work done on it because this is along an equipotential surface (V = 0.5) and the non-zero component of force (F) is perpendicular to it;

5) the lines of F are along the lines of E.

The *potential difference* (PD) is the difference in V between two points, or it is the work per unit positive charge done by electric forces moving a small test charge from the point of higher potential to the point of lower potential:

$$PD = V_a - V_b = \text{volts} = \text{work/charge}$$

$$\text{work} = q(V_a - V_b) = q(PD).$$

An *electric dipole* consists of two charges separated by some finite distance (d). Usually the charges are equal and opposite. The laws of forces, fields, etc., apply to dipoles. A dipole is characterised by its *dipole moment* which is the product of the charge (q) and d.

Dipoles tend to line up with the electric field (*see* Figure III.B.9.5). Motion of dipoles against an electric field requires energy as previously discussed.

If you consider a single isolated point charge and the circular equipotential line produced, in 3D, it is a sphere where each point on the surface of the sphere has the same potential because it is the same distance from the charge. This imaginary 3D shape is called a *gaussian* surface.

$$\boxed{\text{dipole moment} = (charge)(distance) = qd}$$

Figure III.B.9.4: Equipotential lines. The circle-like curves around each charge $-Q_1$ and $+Q_2$ are the equipotential lines corresponding to each charge. The numbers represent the electric potential value (i.e. in millivolts) of the respective equipotential lines. Note the electric field lines as in Figure III.B.9.1.

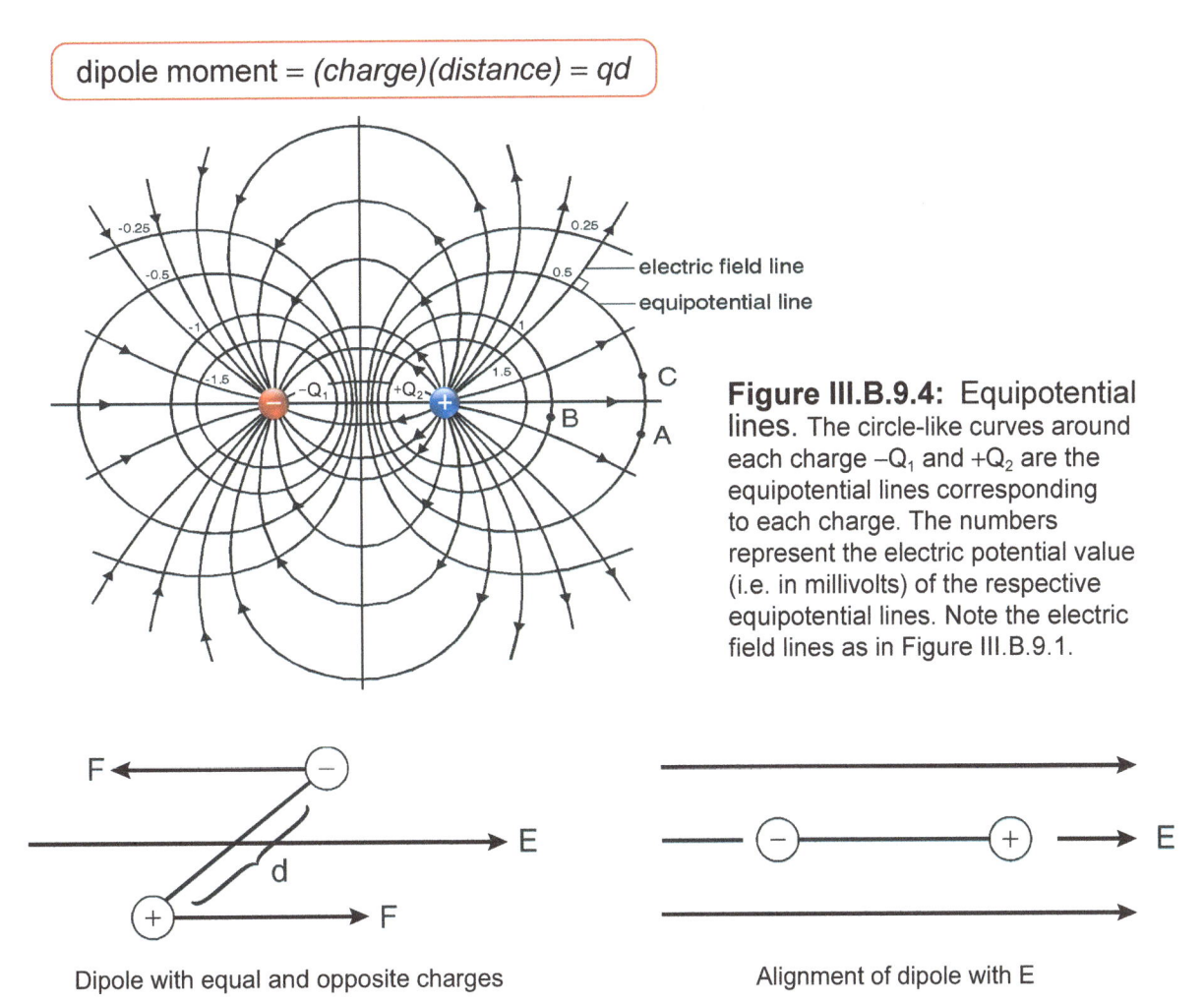

Dipole with equal and opposite charges

Alignment of dipole with E

Figure III.B.9.5: Dipole and electric field. E = electric field, F = forces exerted by E on the dipole

9.2 Electromagnetism

9.2.1 Notion of Electromagnetic Induction

You may have played with magnets as a child or, more recently, used a magnet to hold notes on a refrigerator door. Some materials (and perhaps some people!) have a natural magnetism. The basis of that magnetism involves quantum mechanics. We will now move to a more GAMSAT-testable topic: induced magnetism and related vectors…

Coulomb's Law in electrostatics (PHY 9.1.2) gives the nature of the forces acting upon electric charges at rest, but when those charges are moving, new forces appear. These new forces are not of the same nature as the electrostatic forces, and they act differently on the electric charges. They are called *electromagnetic forces*.

9.2.2 Magnetic Field Vector

Experiments have shown that two straight conductors (e.g. copper wires) traversed by electric currents of intensities I and I' in the same direction are acted upon by an attractive force proportional to the product of the intensities and inversely proportional to the distance between the two conductors. It can be demonstrated that when the electric current in one of the conductors disappears, the force also disappears.

Therefore, the force is due to the motion of the electric charges in both conductors.

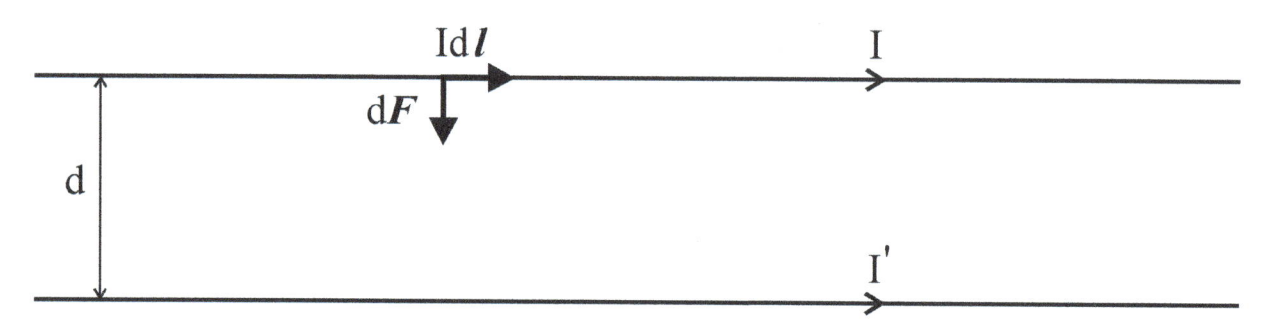

Figure III.B.9.6: Magnetic field.
Two conductors a distance d apart; the current element Idl and the perpendicular force dF associated with the magnetic field vector B are both shown.

We can express this phenomenon by introducing a new physical quantity: the magnetic field vector B, also created by magnets.

The SI unit for B is the tesla where 1 T = 1 N/(A·m) = 10^4 gauss.

Thus, two effects have been shown by the preceding experiment:

1) a moving charge produces a magnetic field (i.e. *induces* a magnetic field).

2) under certain circumstances, a magnetic field may exert a force on a nearby moving charge.

9.2.3 The Lorentz Force

A test particle with charge q moving at a velocity v in a magnetic induction field B is acted upon by a force F given by the following formula:

$$F = q\,(v \times B)$$

which is a "*cross product.*"

The force element *dF* is perpendicular to the magnetic field vector, and also perpendicular to the displacement velocity vector of the charge (see Figure III.B.9.6).

In order to determine the direction of a cross (= *vector*) product we can use the right-hand rule. If c = a × b then the right hand is held so that the curled fingers follow the rotation of a to b, the extended right thumb will point in the direction of c (*dF* in the preceding example; F in the image to the right).

Student's trick: "Grab the Wire!" Examine Fig. III.B.9.6b. With your right-hand open and thumb extended, your fingers point in the direction of the force *F* and your thumb points in the direction of the current *I*. As you begin to grab the wire, the initial direction of the tips of your fingers move perpendicular to both *F* and *I*. Now the tips of your fingers make a circular motion around the wire (*note the colour green in the image*). Those fingers have just described the direction of the magnetic field vector *B*!

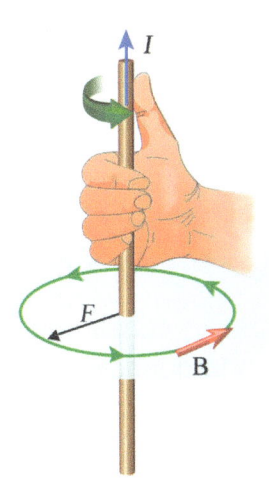

Figure III.B.9.6b: Right-hand rule.

9.2.4 Electromagnetic Spectrum, Radio, Infrared, X-rays

An electromagnetic field is described as having at every point of the field, two perpendicular vectors: *the electric field* vector *E* and the magnetic field vector *B* (these 2 fields are on display in PHY 11.2). You can see a summary of the complete electromagnetic spectrum in this section: Figure III.B.9.7.

Radar (= *radio detection* and ranging) is an example of a radio wave.

Visible light can be broken down into colours remembered by the mnemonic (*from highest to lowest wavelength*), Roy G. BIV: Red, Orange, Yellow, Green, Blue, Indigo, Violet. {*The reason this is highlighted will be revealed in Spoiler Alert!*}

The separation of white light into these colours can occur as a result of refraction through a prism (Figure III.B.9.7) or through water (i.e. mist or rain resulting in a rainbow).

Planck developed the relation between energy (*E*) and the frequency *f* of the electromagnetic radiation,

$$E = hf$$

where *h* = Planck's constant. Thus a high frequency or a short wavelength corresponds to high energy, and vice versa.

The speed of light (= *electromagnetic radiation*), given by c, can be measured from the wavelength λ and the frequency f of an electromagnetic wave in a vacuum (= *in vacuo* = no pressure/no particles approximated by outer space). Recall that v = λf (PHY 7.1.2), and so we have the special case for the speed of light,

$$c = \lambda f$$

The result is the constant $c = 3 \times 10^8$ m/s which, if required to answer a question during the GAMSAT, would be given in the passage or question stem. The speed at which light propagates through transparent materials, such as glass, water or air, is less than c, given by the refractive index n of the material (n = c/v; PHY 11.4). The change in c in different materials (refraction) is responsible for the colours of a rainbow.

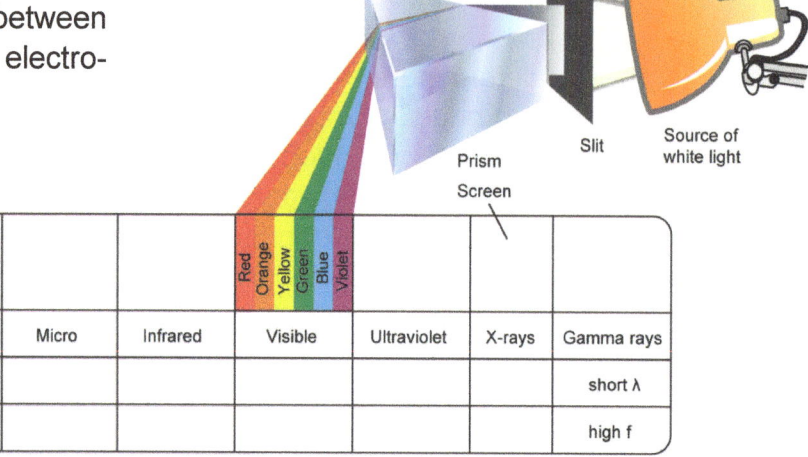

Radio	Micro	Infrared	Visible	Ultraviolet	X-rays	Gamma rays
long λ			R O Y G B V			short λ
low f						high f

Figure III.B.9.7: The complete electromagnetic spectrum.

CHAPTER 9: Electrostatics and Electromagnetism

GOLD STANDARD FOUNDATIONAL GAMSAT PRACTICE QUESTIONS

1) A piece of fur is rubbed on a rubber rod resulting in the rod having a negative charge. Which of the following is consistent with the event described?

   A. The fur remains neutral.
   B. Protons are removed from the rod.
   C. Electrons are added to the rod.
   D. The fur is also charged negatively.

2) A repelling force must occur between two charged objects when the charges are of:

   A. unequal magnitude.
   B. equal magnitude.
   C. like signs.
   D. unlike signs.

3) An uncharged conductor is supported by an insulated stand. A positively charged rod is brought near the left end of the conductor, but does not touch it. The right end of the conductor will be:

   A. positive.
   B. negative.
   C. neutral.
   D. a smaller charge than that of the rod.

4) If object X, with a positive charge, is placed in contact with uncharged object Y, what will be the nature of the charge left on object Y?

   A. Positive
   B. Negative
   C. Equal in magnitude to that on X
   D. Negative and less in magnitude than that on X

5) A current in a long, straight horizontal wire produces a magnetic field with magnetic field lines that:

   A. are parallel to the wire.
   B. go out from the wire to infinity.
   C. form circles that go around the wire.
   D. form circles that pass through the wire.

GAMSAT-Prep.com
GOLD STANDARD PHYSICS

GOLD STANDARD GAMSAT-LEVEL PRACTICE QUESTIONS

High-level Importance

6) The diagram below shows three neutral metal spheres, R, S, and T, in contact and on insulating stands.

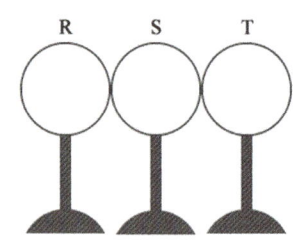

Which of the following diagrams best represents the charge distribution on the spheres when a positively charged insulator rod is brought near the left side of sphere R, but does not touch it?

A.

B.

C.

D.

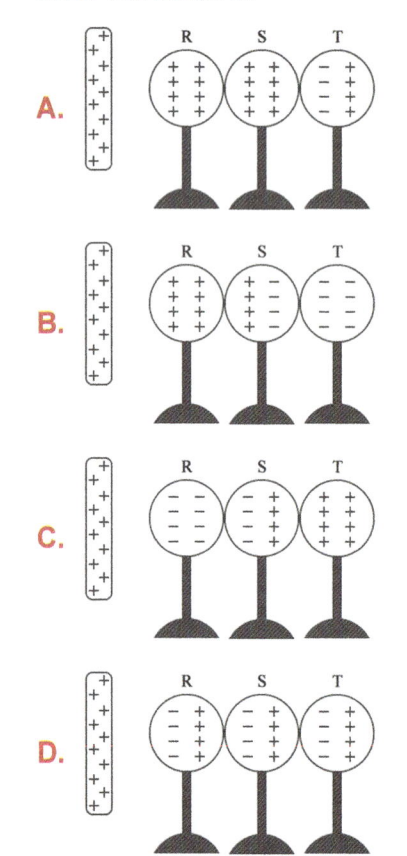

7) The diagram below shows three neutral metal spheres, R, S, and T, which are NOT in contact but are on insulating stands.

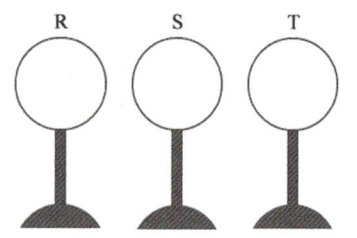

Which of the following diagrams best represents the charge distribution on the spheres when a positively charged insulator rod is brought near the left side of sphere R, but does not touch it?

A.

B.

C.

D.

PHY-128   CHAPTER 9: ELECTROSTATICS AND ELECTROMAGNETISM

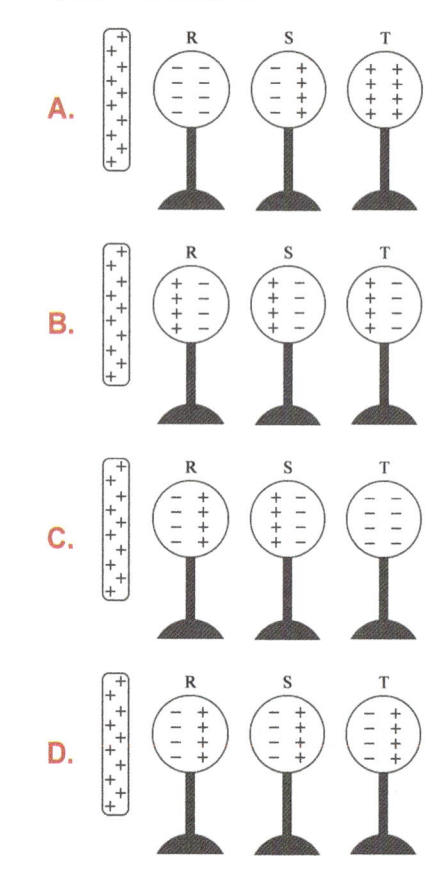

8) Three metal spheres X, Y and Z, are identical in size but carry differing electric charges of −Q, +2Q and −3Q, respectively. The first metal sphere X is brought into contact only with the sphere Y, and then X is brought into contact only with sphere Z. After X contacts spheres Y and Z, in the order described, the charge on sphere X is most consistent with which of the following?

A. −5/4Q
B. −2Q
C. −Q
D. −Q/2

9) If the size of the charge value (magnitude) is tripled for both of two point charges maintained at a constant separation, the mutual force between them will be changed by what factor?

A. 9
B. 1/9
C. 3
D. 1/3

10) The constant k, which appears in the equation for Coulomb's law, is equivalent dimensionally to which of the following? (note: the SI unit of charge is the coulomb, C; if you have forgotten the equation, consider going back to PHY 9.1.2, the highlighted equation, and trying to answer before looking at the worked solution)

A. N/C^2
B. $N·m/C$
C. $N·C^2/m^2$
D. $N·m^2/C^2$

11) Consider 2 charges of magnitude −Q and +4Q as illustrated in the diagram below. At which point will the electric field due to the 2 charges be equal to zero?

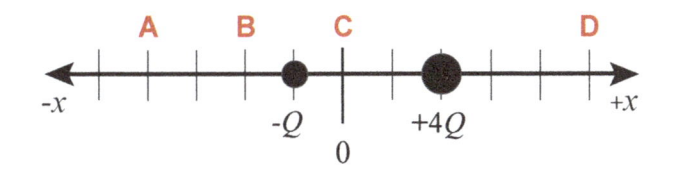

12) Consider the following diagram which reveals a positive test charge that is located between two charged spheres, X and Y. Sphere X has a charge of +3Q and is located 0.6 metres from the test charge. Sphere Y has a charge of −3Q and is located 0.3 metres from the test charge.

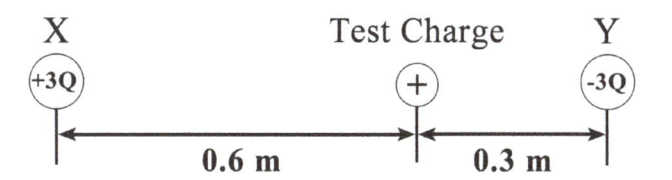

If the magnitude of the force on the test charge due to sphere X is F, what is the magnitude of the force on the test charge due to sphere Y?

A. 4F
B. F/4
C. 2F
D. F/2

13) Two spheres exert a force F on each other. One sphere has a charge of −2Q and it is separated by a distance x from a sphere with a charge of +6Q. If after a change takes place, the force between the two spheres becomes 2F, which of the following could have produced this new result?

A. The charge on both spheres was doubled and the distance between them was halved.
B. The charge on both spheres was doubled.
C. The charge on one of the spheres was increased by a factor of 3.
D. The charge on only one sphere was halved and the distance between them halved.

GAMSAT-Prep.com
GOLD STANDARD PHYSICS

Questions 14–15

The cyclotron is one of the first types of particle accelerators. A magnetic force is applied to a moving charge to bend it into a semicircular path between accelerations by an applied electric field.

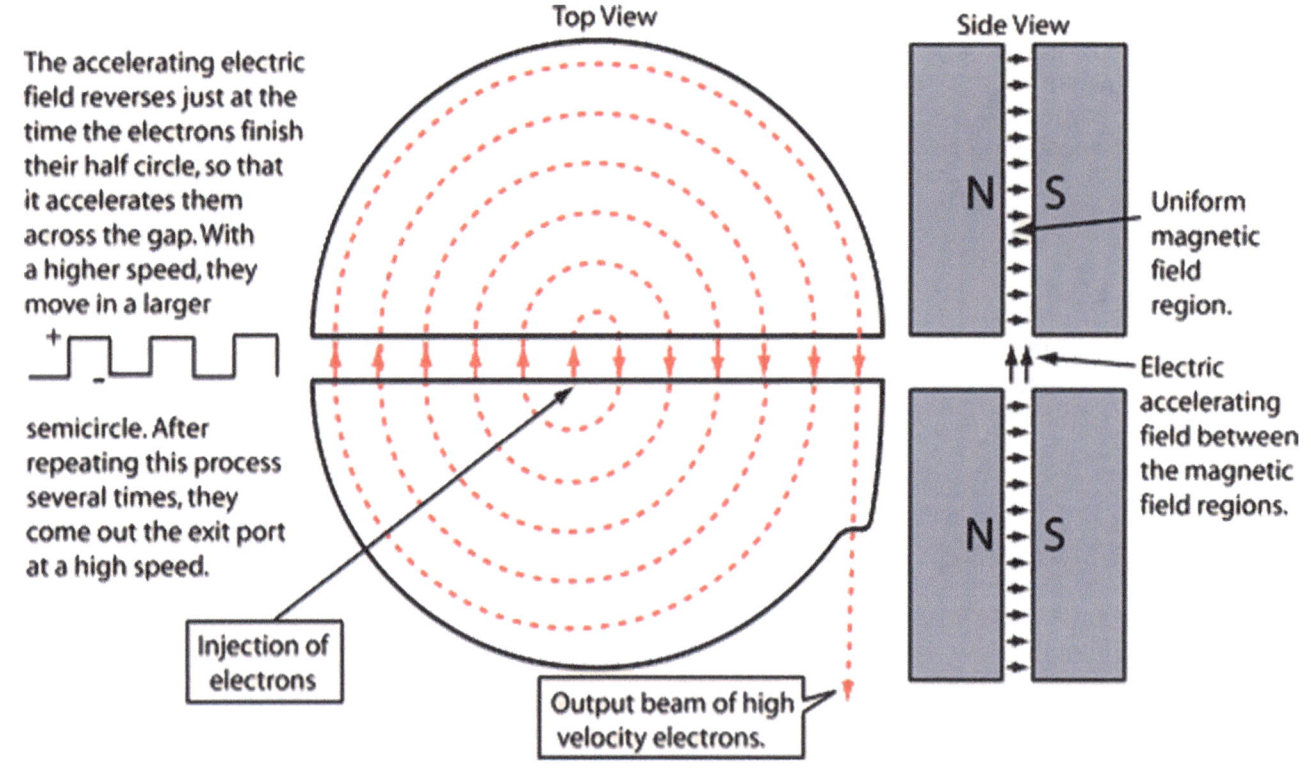

The accelerating electric field reverses just at the time the electrons finish their half circle, so that it accelerates them across the gap. With a higher speed, they move in a larger semicircle. After repeating this process several times, they come out the exit port at a high speed.

Figure 1: Cyclotron: Basic schematic. Note the application of a uniform magnetic field is responsible for the uniform motion in semi-circles; acceleration only occurs across very small gaps identified as parallel, red arrow heads due to an electric field. Large magnets: N – north, S – south.
(ref: Nambikute123; Wikimedia Commons)

With regards to the implicated forces, the following equations may be of value: (1) the electric field force $F = qE$, where q is the charge and E is the electric field; (2) the magnetic force $F = qvB$, where v is the velocity and B is the magnetic field; (3) with regards to the force required to keep the particles in a curved path, the centripetal force $F = mv^2/r$, where r is the radius.

14) Which of the following expressions is most consistent with the velocity of the particle in the cyclotron?

   A. qB/rm
   B. q/Brm
   C. qBr/m
   D. More than one of the above

15) What is the kinetic energy of the particle in the cyclotron?

   A. $(qBr)^2/2m$
   B. $(qBr)^2/2m^2$
   C. $(qBr)/2m$
   D. $(qBr)^2/4m^2$

PHY-130 CHAPTER 9: ELECTROSTATICS AND ELECTROMAGNETISM

GAMSAT MASTERS SERIES

Questions 16–20

One of the fundamental forces of the universe has been used to generate electricity, store information in computers, accurately define abnormalities in the human body, and help to discover the secrets of the universe. This remarkable force is, of course, magnetism.

In 1820 Hans Oersted, a Danish physicist, did the following experiment to confirm the relationship between magnetism and electricity.

Step 1

A wire is placed in the north-south direction with a compass laying besides it. Naturally, the compass needle points in the north-south direction as a result of the Earth's magnetism.

Step 2

The current is switched on and begins to flow in the wire. The compass needle immediately swings 90° to be at a right angle to the wire.

Step 3

The direction of current flow is reversed. The compass needle immediately swings 180° to, again, be at a right angle to the wire.

Note that:

- The Coulomb force F in an electric field E is given by $F = qE$, where q is the charge.
- The centripetal force F with radius r is given by $F = mv^2/r$ where m is the mass and v is the velocity.
- The magnetic force F in a current-carrying wire is perpendicular to both the current and the magnetic field.

16) The acceleration in an electric field is given by:
   A. qE/m.
   B. qEm.
   C. qm/E.
   D. qE.

17) In Step 1 of Oersted's experiment, the wire was placed in the north-south direction. Which of the following is a reasonable explanation for the direction of the wire?
   A. The Earth's magnetic field directs wires in the north-south plane.
   B. The direction was chosen to accelerate the magnetic field.
   C. The direction was chosen to ensure that the compass needle changes direction with the magnetic force.
   D. The east-west direction tends to emit powerful radiation.

GAMSAT-Prep.com
GOLD STANDARD PHYSICS

High-level Importance

Questions 18–20 refer to the following diagram which is based on the experiment in the passage.

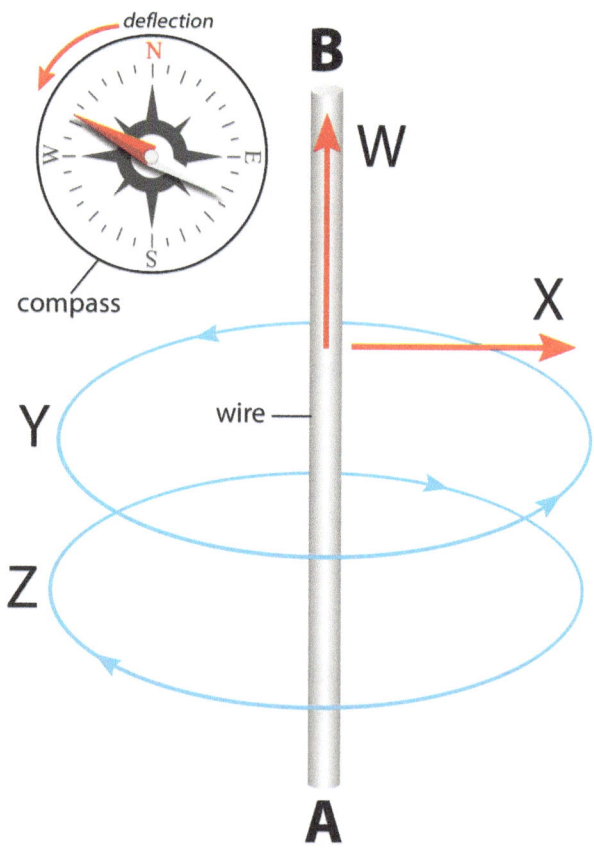

Figure 1: Oersted effect with the needle of the compass in motion. Current flows in the wire from point A to point B.

18) Which vector in Figure 1 represents the magnetic force F?

A. W
B. X
C. Y
D. Z

19) Which vector in Figure 1 represents the magnetic field vector B?

A. W
B. X
C. Y
D. Z

20) Particles were found to simulate the motion of vectors Y and Z which move around the wire at constant velocity. The acceleration associated with such motion is most consistent with which of the following?

(v = velocity, r = radius, m = mass)

A. 0
B. $2\pi r$
C. v^2/r
D. mvr

PHY-132   CHAPTER 9: ELECTROSTATICS AND ELECTROMAGNETISM

GAMSAT MASTERS SERIES

⚠ SPOILER ALERT

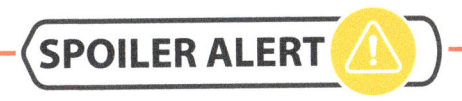

Gold Standard has cross-referenced the content in this chapter to examples from ACER's official GAMSAT practice materials. It is for you to decide when you want to explore these questions since you may want to preserve some of ACER's materials for timed mock-exam practice.

Examples – F = qE meets F = qvB (electromagnetism in a particle accelerator): Q40-43 of 1; charged body in a hollow conductor (electrostatics): Q75-76 of 3; point charges at varying distances (electrostatics): Q109-110 of 3; and finally, a strange one related to knowing the the extreme colours in the visible range of the electromagnetic spectrum (PHY 9.2.4): Q83 of 5. Note that "Q" is followed by the question number, and, for example, "of 1" refers to booklet number 1 which is referenced in the Spoiler Alert table at the end of Chapter 1. The 10 full-length HEAPS GAMSAT practice tests (by Gold Standard and MediRed), exams 1 through 10, contain specific cross-references to this chapter within the worked solutions. Note that the Oersted unit with the application of the right-hand rule is from HEAPS-9.

High-level Importance

Chapter Checklist

- ☐ Access your online account to view answers, worked solutions and discussion boards.
- ☐ Reassess your 'learning objectives' for this chapter: Go back to the first page of this chapter and re-evaluate the top 3 boxes and the Introduction.
    - ☐ Please be sure that you have completed the *Need for Speed* exercises at the beginning of this chapter.
- ☐ Complete a maximum of 1 page of notes using symbols/abbreviations to represent the entire chapter based on your learning objectives. These are your Gold Notes.
- ☐ Consider your multimedia options based on your optimal way of learning:
    - ☐ Download the free Gold Standard GAMSAT app for your Android device or iPhone.
    - ☐ Create your own, tangible study cards or try the free app: Anki.
    - ☐ Record your voice reading your Gold Notes onto your smartphone (MP3s) and listen during exercise, transportation, etc.
    - ☐ Try out the Gold Standard GAMSAT online videos at gamsat-prep.com, or you can try other options on YouTube like Khan Academy or Crash Course Physics.
- ☐ Reassess your schedule for your full-length GAMSAT practice tests: ACER and/or HEAPS exams. Ensure that you have scheduled one full day to complete a practice test and 1-2 days for a thorough assessment of worked solutions while adding to your abbreviated Gold Notes.
- ☐ Reassess your progress in scheduling and/or evaluating stress reduction techniques such as regular exercise (sports), yoga, meditation and/or mindfulness exercises (*see* YouTube for suggestions).

THE PHYSICAL SCIENCES   PHY-133

High-level Importance

GOLD NOTES

ELECTRIC CIRCUITS
Chapter 10

Memorise
* Definition/equation/units: current, resistance
* Ohm's law, resistors in series/parallel
* Capacitance, capacitors in series/parallel
* Kirchoff's laws

Understand
* Battery, emf, voltage, terminal potential
* Internal resistance of the battery, resistivity
* Ohm's law, resistors in series/parallel
* Parallel plate capacitor, series, parallel
* Conductivity, power in circuits, Kirchoff's laws
* Capacitor discharge curve: a quite 'famous' example of exponential decay

Importance
Medium level: 7% of GAMSAT Physics questions released by ACER are related to content in this chapter (in our estimation).
* Note that approximately **75%** of the questions in GAMSAT Physics are related to just 6 chapters: 1, 4, 6, 9, 11 and 12.

GAMSAT-Prep.com

Introduction

Electric circuits are closed paths which includes electronic components (i.e. resistors, capacitors, power supplies) through which a current can flow. There are 3 basic laws that govern the flow of current in an electrical circuit: Ohm's law and Kirchoff's first and second laws.

Multimedia Resources at GAMSAT-Prep.com

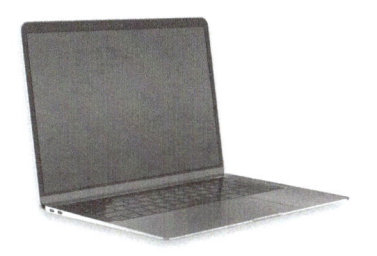

Open Discussion Boards 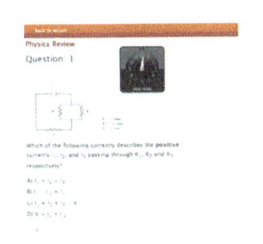   Foundational Videos   Flashcards 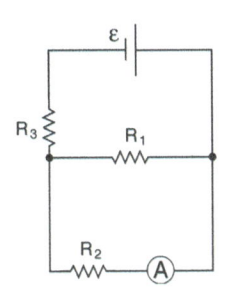   Special Guest

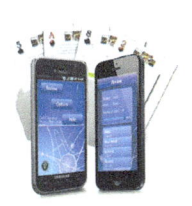

THE PHYSICAL SCIENCES   PHY-135

* The real GAMSAT may have advanced-level information presented (i.e. in a passage) but previous knowledge of said information is not required to answer the questions that would follow. Practice questions at the end of this chapter, as well as ACER and GS (HEAPS) practice GAMSATs can help you clarify this point.

GAMSAT-Prep.com
GOLD STANDARD PHYSICS

10.0 GAMSAT has a *Need for Speed*!

Section Number	GAMSAT Physics *Need for Speed* Exercises
10.1	How does electrical current relate to charge? What are all of the SI units involved in that relationship?
	What is Ohm's law?
10.2	What are the SI units for resistance? Provide an example of equivalent units based on Ohm's Law.
	What are the SI units for power? Also, provide an equivalent set of SI units for power.
	How does power relate to current?
	How can you calculate the equivalent resistance across 3 resistors in series?
	How can you calculate the equivalent resistance across 3 resistors in parallel?
10.3.1	In the diagram below, label the charges on the battery and show the direction of the current going through each resistor. What is the relationship between the current coming from the battery and the currents going through R_1 and R_2?
10.4	How is capacitance related to charge?
	How can you calculate the equivalent capacitance across 3 capacitors in series?
	How can you calculate the equivalent capacitance across 3 capacitors in parallel?

Medium-level Importance

PHY-136 CHAPTER 10: ELECTRIC CIRCUITS

10.1 Current

Before discussing current in terms of electricity, let's explore your understanding of current in terms of water (e.g. a stream or river). If forced to define current, some students might say: It is the amount of water passing a point over time. You might use some Physics language (PHY 6.1.3) and proclaim: It is the volume of water passing a point divided (over!) time. And so it is with electricity, but instead of considering water, we must consider charge.

Thus the current (*I*) is the amount of charge (*Q*) that flows past a point in a given amount of time (*t*),

$$I = Q/t = \text{amperes} = \text{coulombs/sec.}$$

Current is caused by the movement of electrons between two points of significant potential difference of an electric circuit. Free electrons will accelerate towards the positive connection. As they move they will collide with atoms in the substance, losing energy which we observe as heat. The net effect is a drift of electrons at a roughly constant speed towards the positive connection. The motion of electrons is an *electric current*.

As electrons are removed by the electric potential source at the positive connection, electrons are being injected at the negative connection. The potential can be considered as a form of *electron pump*.

This model explains many observed effects.

If the magnitude of the electric potential is increased, the electrons will accelerate faster and their mean velocity will be higher, i.e., the current is increased. The collisions between electrons and atoms transfer energy to the atoms. The collisions manifest themselves as heat. This effect is known as *Joule heating*. Materials such as these are termed ohmic conductors, since they obey the well-known Ohm's law:

$$V = IR$$

where *V* is the voltage, *I* is the current, and *R* is the resistance.

The potential difference is maintained by a voltage source (emf). The direction of current is taken as the direction of positive charge movement, by convention. It is

Figure III.B.10.0: Water flowing in a closed circuit of pipes vs current flowing in a closed electric circuit. Note that the battery is the electrical pump being the source of electric potential (voltage, *emf*; PHY 10.3) driving the current past the resistance (PHY 10.2) in the electric circuit.

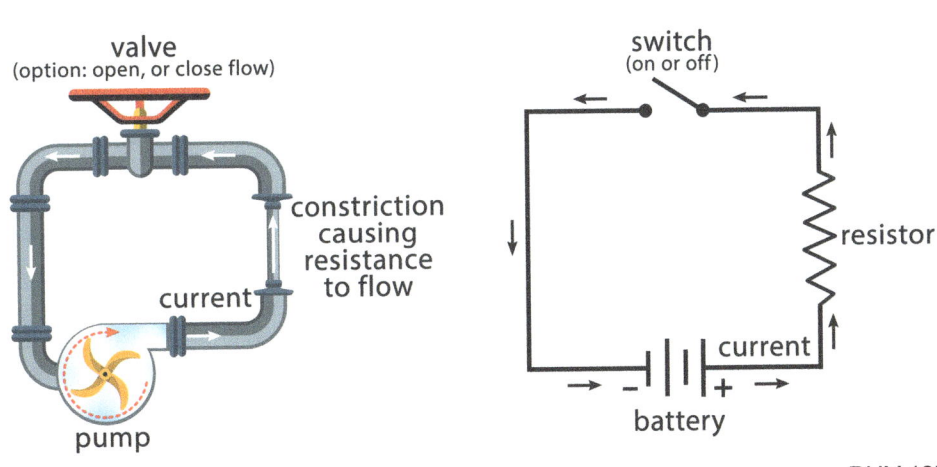

represented on a circuit diagram by arrows. Ammeters are used to measure the flow of current and are symbolised as in Figure III.B.10.1.

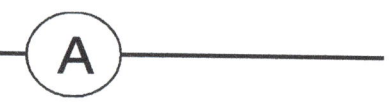

Figure III.B.10.1: Symbol of an ammeter.

10.2 Resistance, Resistivity, Series and Parallel Circuits

Resistance (R) is the measure of opposition to the flow of electrons in a substance. Resistivity (ρ) is an inherent property of a substance. It varies with temperature. For example, the resistivity of metals increases with increasing temperature.

Resistance is directly proportional to resistivity and length l (e.g. the length of a wire) but inversely proportional to the cross-sectional area A.

$$R = \rho l/A$$

Resistance increases with temperature because the thermal motion of molecules increases with temperature and results in more collisions between electrons which impede their flow.

The units of resistance are ohms, symbolised by Ω (omega). From Ohm's law, 1 ohm = 1 volt/ampere.

When a positive current flows across a resistor, there is a voltage decrease and an energy loss:

energy loss = Vq = VIt = joules

power loss (P) = VIt/t = VI = watts

watts = volts × amperes = joules/sec.

The energy loss may be used to perform work. These relations hold for power (P),

$$P = VI = (IR)(I) = I^2R = V(V/R) = V^2/R.$$

constant (normal) resistance
"classic" image of resistor

"modern" image of resistor

variable resistance (rheostat)

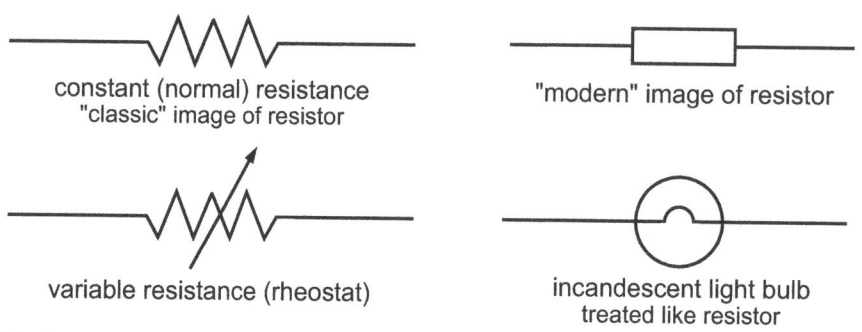

incandescent light bulb treated like resistor

Figure III.B.10.2: Representations of resistors. Note that the filament inside of a light bulb (= *incandescent lamp* or *globe*) is a resistor. Because it resists the flow of current, it becomes hot and glows providing light. This is why a light bulb in a circuit is treated exactly like a resistor. The brightness of a light bulb depends on how much power it loses (= *dissipates*; $P = VI$). Consequently, when you are shopping to compare the brightness among similar types of light bulbs, the higher the number of watts, the brighter the bulb will be. Consider briefly revising SI units: GM 2.1.3.

GAMSAT MASTERS SERIES

Circuit elements are either in series or in parallel. Two components are in series when they have only one point in common; that is, the current travelling from one of them back to the emf source must pass through the other. In a complete series circuit, or for individual series loops of a larger mixed circuit, the current (I) is the same over each component and the total voltage drop in the circuit elements (resistors, capacitors, inductors, internal resistance of emf sources, etc.) is equal to the sum V_t of all the emf sources. The value of the equivalent resistance R_{eq} in a series circuit is:

$$R_{eq} = R_1 + R_2 + R_3 + \ldots$$

Figure III.B.10.2a: Resistors connected in series.

Two components are in parallel when they are connected to two common points in the circuit; that is, the current travelling from one such element back to the emf source need not pass through the second element because there is an alternate path.

In a parallel circuit, the total current is the sum of currents for each path and the voltage is the same for all paths in parallel. The equivalent resistance in a parallel circuit is:

$$1/R_{eq} = 1/R_1 + 1/R_2 + 1/R_3 + \ldots$$

Figure III.B.10.2b: Resistors connected in parallel.

10.2.1 Resistance Problem in Series and Parallel

Determine the equivalent resistance between points A and B in Figure III.B.10.3.

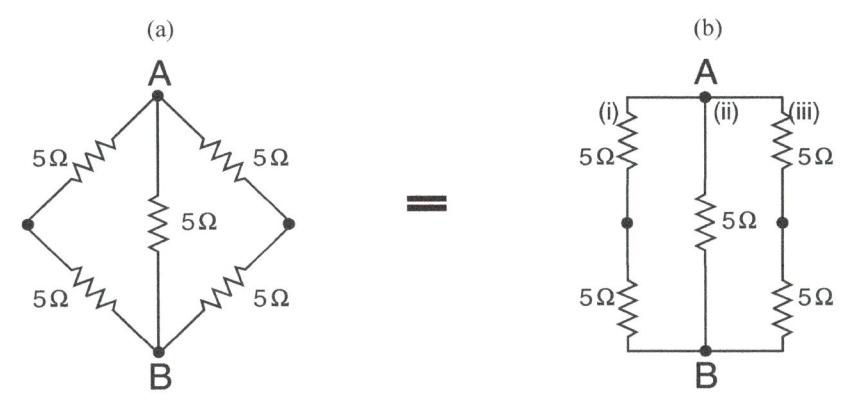

Figure III.B.10.3: Equivalent resistance.
(a) The problem as it could be presented; (b) the way you should interpret the problem.

THE PHYSICAL SCIENCES PHY-139

- Wire (i) has two resistors in a row (*in series*): $R_{(i)} = 5 + 5 = 10\ \Omega$

- Wire (ii) has only one resistor: $R_{(ii)} = 5\ \Omega$

- Wire (iii) has two resistors in series: $R_{(iii)} = 5 + 5 = 10\ \Omega$

Between A and B we have three resistor systems in parallel: (i), (ii) and (iii), thus

$$1/R_{eq} = 1/R_{(i)} + 1/R_{(ii)} + 1/R_{(iii)}$$
$$= 1/10 + 1/5 + 1/10 = 4/10$$

multiply through by $10R_{eq}$ to get: $10 = 4R_{eq}$

thus $R_{eq} = 10/4 = 2.5\ \Omega$.

10.3 Batteries, Electromotive Force, Voltage, Internal Resistance

An *electromotive force* (*emf*, symbol ℰ and measured in volts), is the electrical action produced by a non-electrical source. Sources of emf are batteries (conversion of chemical energy to electrical energy) and generators (conversion of mechanical energy to electrical energy). A transducer is a device that converts energy from one form to another.

The source of emf, the transducer, does work on each charge to raise it from a lower potential to a higher potential (i.e. the 'pump' analogy from PHY 10.1).

Then as the charge flows around the circuit (naturally from higher to lower potential) it loses energy which is replaced by the emf source again.

energy supplied = energy lost

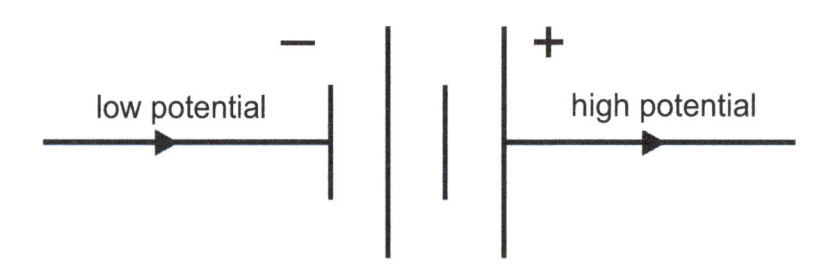

Figure III.B.10.4: Symbol of an emf source. Arrows show the normal direction of current. An electromotive force (emf) source maintains between its terminal points, a constant potential difference. The emf source replaces energy lost by moving electrons.

Energy is lost whenever a charge (as current) passes through a resistor. The units of emf are volts. The actual voltage delivered to a circuit is not equal to the value of the source. This is reduced by an internal voltage lost which represents the voltage loss by the *internal resistance (r)* of the source itself. The net voltage is called the terminal voltage or *terminal potential* V_t.

Figure III.B.10.5:
Simplified symbol of an emf source.

$V_t = V - Ir = IR_t$

I, R_t = totals for the circuit; V = maximal voltage output of the emf source.

When two emf sources are connected in opposition, (positive pole to positive pole) the charge loses energy when passing in the second emf source.

Therefore, if there is more than one emf source in a circuit, the total emf is the sum of the individual emf sources not in opposition reduced by the sum of individual sources in opposition in a given direction.

10.3.1 Kirchoff's Laws and a Multiloop Circuit Problem

Given that the emf of the battery $\varepsilon = 12$ volts and the resistors $R_1 = 12\ \Omega$, $R_2 = 4.0\ \Omega$, and $R_3 = 6.0\ \Omega$, determine the reading in the ammeter (*see* Figure III.B.10.6).

Ignore the internal resistance of the battery.

{*The ammeter will read the current which flows through it which is i_2*}

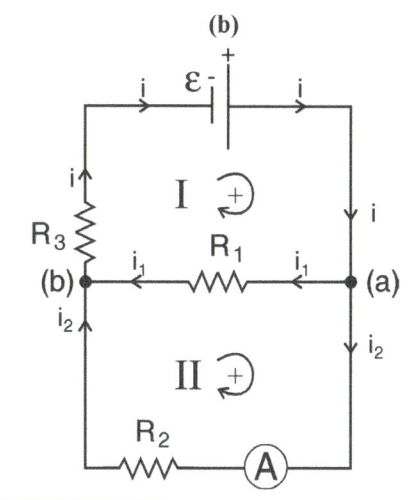

Figure III.B.10.6: A multiloop circuit.
(**a**) The problem as it could be presented; (**b**) the way you should label the diagram. Note that the current emanates from the positive terminal and is the same current i which returns to the emf source.

GAMSAT-Prep.com
GOLD STANDARD PHYSICS

Kirchoff's Law I (*the junctional theorem*): when different currents arrive at a point (= *junction*, as in points (*a*) and (*b*) in the labelled diagram) the sum of current equals zero.

We can arbitrarily define all current *arriving* at the junction as <u>positive</u> and all current *leaving* as <u>negative</u>.

Kirchoff's Law I	$\Sigma i = 0$ at a junction

Thus at junction (a) $i - i_1 - i_2 = 0$

And for junction (b) $i_1 + i_2 - i = 0$

Both (a) and (b) reduce to equation (c):

$$i = i_1 + i_2$$

Kirchoff's Law II (*the loop theorem*): the sum of voltage changes in one continuous loop of a circuit is zero. A single loop circuit is simple since the current is the same in all parts of the loop hence the loop theorem is applied only once.

In a multiloop circuit (loops *I* and *II* in the labelled diagram), there is more than one loop thus the current in general will not be the same in all parts of any given loop. We can arbitrarily define all voltage changes around the loop in the *clockwise* direction as <u>positive</u> and in the *counterclockwise* direction as <u>negative</u>.

Thus if by moving in the clockwise direction we can move from the battery's negative terminal (*low potential*) to its positive terminal (*high potential*), the value of the emf ε is negative.

Kirchoff's Law II	$\Sigma \Delta V = 0$ in a loop

Thus in loop *I* (recall: $V = IR$)

$$i_1 R_1 + i R_3 - \varepsilon = 0$$

And in loop *II*

$$i_2 R_2 - i_1 R_1 = 0$$

We now have simultaneous equations. There are three unknowns (i, i_1, i_2) and three equations (c, loop *I*, and loop *II*). We need only solve for the current i_2 which runs through the ammeter.

Substitute (c) into loop I

$$i_1 R_1 + (i_1 + i_2) R_3 - \varepsilon = 0$$

Thus

$$i_1 R_1 + i_1 R_3 + i_2 R_3 - \varepsilon = 0$$

Substitute i_1 from loop *II* where $i_1 = i_2 R_2 / R_1$, hence

$$i_2 R_2 + i_2 R_2 R_3 / R_1 + i_2 R_3 = \varepsilon$$

Begin isolating i_2

$$i_2 (R_2 + R_2 R_3 / R_1 + R_3) = \varepsilon$$

Isolate i_2

$$i_2 = \varepsilon (R_2 + R_2 R_3 / R_1 + R_3)^{-1}$$

Substitute

$$i_2 = 12[4 + (4)(6)/(12) + 6]^{-1} = 12/12 = 1.0 \text{ ampere.}$$

10.4 Capacitors and Dielectrics

A camera flash requires a lot of energy quickly in order to produce a very bright flash. A battery does not typically have sufficient power to do the job. An array of *capacitors* can store enough energy and release it very quickly across the bulb filament.

Capacitors store and separate charge. Capacitors can be filled with dielectrics which are materials which can increase capacitance. The capacitance (C) is an inherent property of a conductor and is formulated as:

C = charge/electric potential = Q/V = farad = coulomb/volt

By examining the preceding units, you can conclude that the capacitance is the number of coulombs that must be transferred to a conductor to raise its potential by one volt.

The amount of charge that can be stored depends on the shape, size, surroundings and type of the conductor.

The higher the dielectric strength (i.e., the electric field strength at which a substance ceases to be an insulator and becomes a conductor) of the medium, the greater the capacitance of the conductor.

A capacitor is made of two or more conductors with opposite but equal charges placed near each other.

A common example is the parallel plate capacitor. The important formulas for capacitors are:

1) $C = Q/V$ where V = the potential between the plates

2) $V = Ed$ where E = electric field strength, and d = distance between the plates

3) C is directly proportional to the surface area A of the plates and inversely pro-

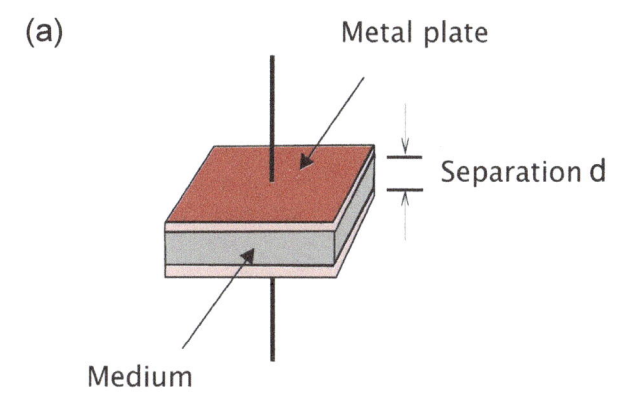

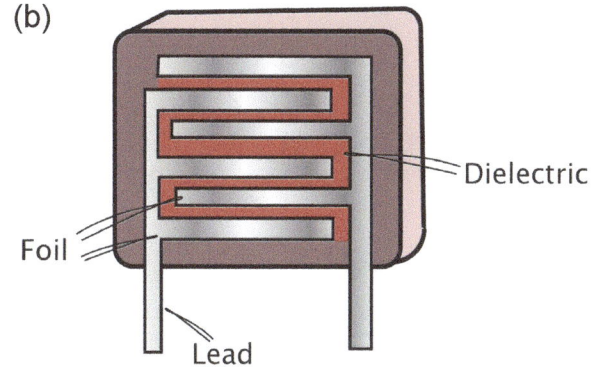

Figure III.B.10.7: (a) Parallel plate capacitor; (b) Ceramic capacitor.

portional to the distance between the plates

$$C = \varepsilon_o A/d$$

for air as a medium between the plates. If the capacitor contains a dielectric, the above equation would be multiplied by the factor κ (= *dielectric constant*) whose value depends on the dielectric being used.

4) The equivalent capacitance C_{eq} for capacitors arranged in series and in parallel is:

Series: $1/C_{eq} = 1/C_1 + 1/C_2 + 1/C_3 \ldots$

Parallel: $C_{eq} = C_1 + C_2 + C_3 \ldots$

The dielectric substances set up an opposing electric field to that of the capacitor which decreases the net electric field and allows the capacitance of the capacitor to increase ($C = Q/Ed$). The molecules of the dielectric are dipoles which line up in the electric field.

{cf. Figure III.B.9.5 from PHY 9.1.5, and Figure III.B.10.8 in this section}

The energy associated with each charged capacitor is:

Potential Energy (PE) = W = $(1/2V)(Q)$ = $1/2QV$

also

$$W = 1/2(CV)(V) = 1/2CV^2$$

and

$$W = 1/2Q(Q/C) = 1/2Q^2/C.$$

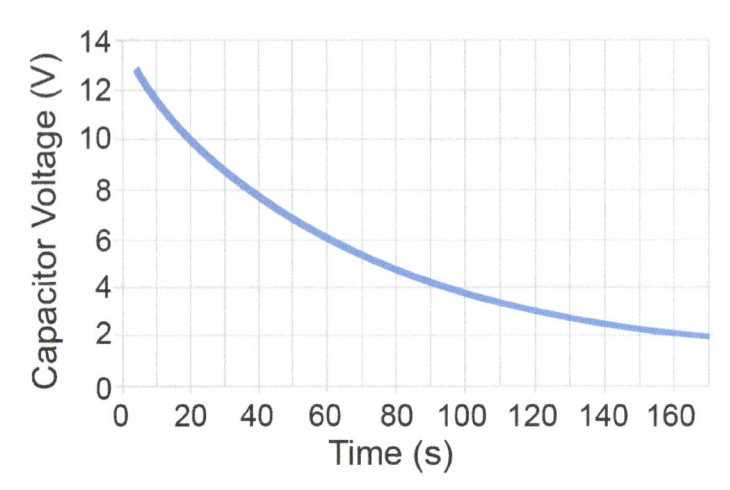

Medium-level Importance

Figure III.B.10.7.1: Capacitor discharge curve. A capacitor is first charged by connecting it to a power supply. In this example, the capacitor is charged up to 14 volts. When the capacitor discharges through a resistor, the charge drains rapidly at first then decreases gradually. This pattern of decrease can be described as *exponential decay* and can be found in many areas of science (other examples: first and second order reactions in General Chemistry, CHM 9.2; radioactive decay in Physics, PHY 12.4).

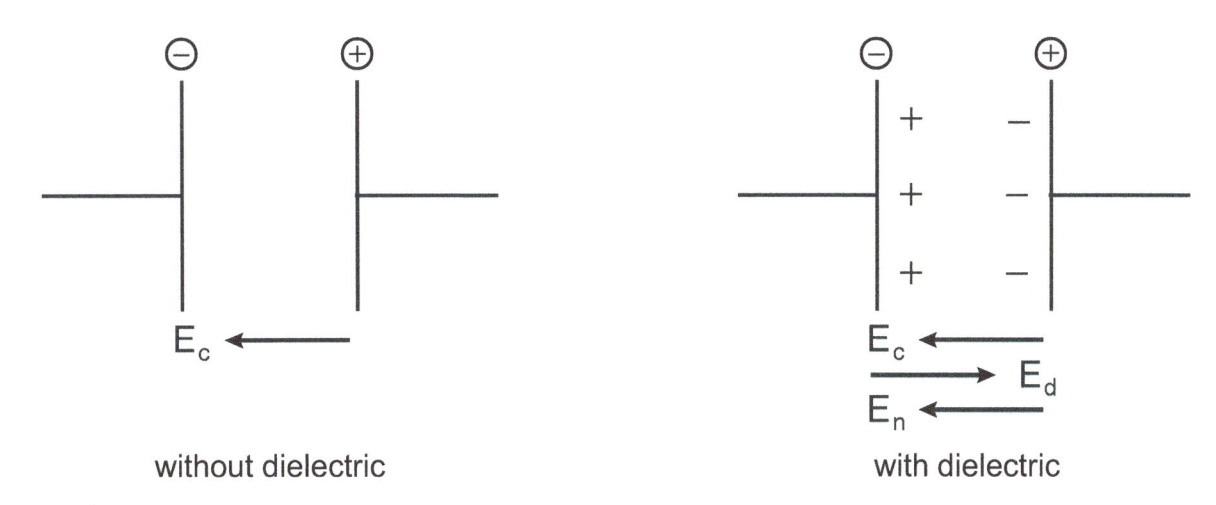

Figure III.B.10.8: Capacitors and dielectrics.
Note that the capacitor is symbolised by two parallel lines of equal length. The electric fields: E_c generated by the capacitor, E_d generated by the dielectric, and E_n is the resultant electric field.

10.5 Root-Mean-Square Current and Voltage

DC (*direct current*) circuits contain a continuous current. Thus calculating power output is quite simple using $P = I^2R = IV$. However, AC (*alternating current*) circuits pulsate; consequently, we must discuss the average power output P_{av} where

$$P_{av} = (I_{rms})^2 R = (I_{rms})(V_{rms})$$

which is true for a purely resistive load (i.e. all circuit power is dissipated - lost - by the resistor/s) where the root-mean-square (*rms*) values are determined from their maximal (*max*) values:

$$I_{rms} = I_{max}/\sqrt{2} \quad \text{and} \quad V_{rms} = V_{max}/\sqrt{2}.$$

Thus by introducing the *rms* quantities the equations for DC and AC circuits have the same forms. AC circuit voltmeters and ammeters have their scales adjusted to read the *rms* values.

GAMSAT-Prep.com
GOLD STANDARD PHYSICS

CHAPTER 10: Electric Circuits

GOLD STANDARD FOUNDATIONAL GAMSAT PRACTICE QUESTIONS

1) The SI unit of electric current, the ampere, is equivalent to which of the following?

   A. ohm/volt
   B. volts/ohm
   C. second/coulomb
   D. volts/second

2) All of the following are different representations of the same unit EXCEPT one. Which one is the EXCEPTION?

   A. (volt)/(second)
   B. (joule)/(second)
   C. watt
   D. (volt)(ampere)

3) A current of 2.0 A is passed through a wire for 1.5 minutes. How many electrons passed through the wire?

   Note that the charge on an electron is 1.6×10^{-19} C. If you need a hint, it is upside down at the bottom of this page.

   A. 1.1×10^{21}
   B. 2.5×10^{19}
   C. 1.1×10^{17}
   D. 2.5×10^{15}

4) In a flashlight, a battery provides a total of 3.0 volts to a bulb. If the flashlight bulb has an operating resistance of 3.0 ohms, the current through the bulb is which of the following?

   A. 0.33 A
   B. 0.50 A
   C. 1.0 A
   D. 9.0 A

5) If the potential difference applied to a fixed resistance is doubled, the power dissipated by that resistance:

   A. quarters.
   B. halves.
   C. doubles.
   D. quadruples.

6) The unit of capacitance, the farad, is dimensionally equivalent to which of the following?

   A. V/C
   B. C/V
   C. V•C
   D. V/J

7) Consider two parallel metal plates carrying opposite electrical charges each with a magnitude of Q. The plates are separated by a distance d and each plate has an area A. Consider the following situations:

   I. Increasing d
   II. Increasing A
   III. Increasing Q

   Which of the following would have the effect of reducing the potential difference between the plates?

   A. I only
   B. II only
   C. III only
   D. I, II and III

Hint for Question 3: First, define current because that will link to time; the rest is dimensional analysis (PHY 2.2).

PHY-146 CHAPTER 10: ELECTRIC CIRCUITS

8) A 0.50-microfarad capacitor is connected to an 800 V battery. Determine the charge on the capacitor.

   A. 4.0×10^{-1} mC
   B. 6.3×10^{-2} μC
   C. 0.020 mC
   D. 0.040 μC

9) If three 3.0-F capacitors are connected in parallel, what is the combined capacitance?

   A. 9.0 F
   B. 3.0 F
   C. 1.0 F
   D. 0.33 F

10) Given the directions and magnitudes in amperes of the current in the copper wires below, what is the magnitude of current in wire R?

    Q = 7 A, T = 8 A, S = 4 A, U = 11 A

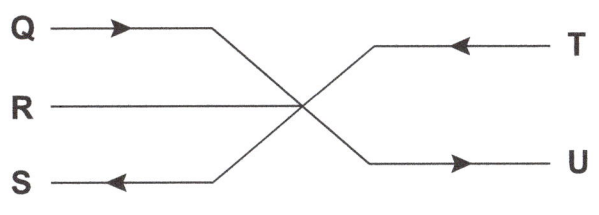

    A. 0 A
    B. 7 A
    C. 15 A
    D. 18 A

High-level Importance

GOLD STANDARD GAMSAT-LEVEL PRACTICE QUESTIONS

11) Which of the following graphs is most consistent with the relationship between electrical power and current in a resistor that obeys Ohm's law?

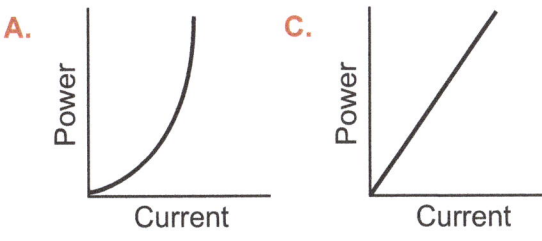

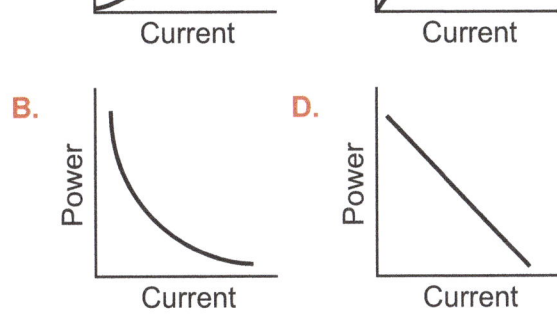

    A. (Power vs Current, increasing exponential-like curve)
    B. (Power vs Current, decreasing curve)
    C. (Power vs Current, linear increasing)
    D. (Power vs Current, linear decreasing)

12) A 12-volt battery is connected to a 6.0-ohm resistor and a 3.0-ohm resistor as shown in the following diagram.

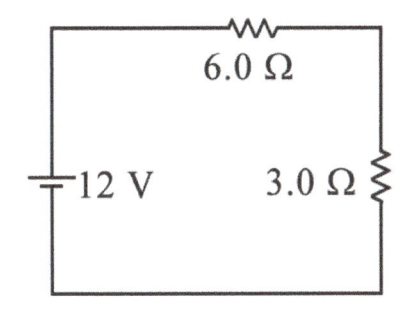

    What is the current in the 3.0-ohm resistor?

    A. 0.5 A
    B. 1.0 A
    C. 1.3 A
    D. 2.0 A

THE PHYSICAL SCIENCES   PHY-147

13) Consider the following circuit where all 3 resistors have equal resistances.

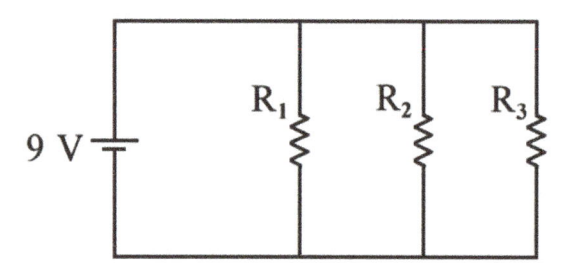

All of the following is correct EXCEPT one. Which of the following is the EXCEPTION?

A. The largest current will pass through R_1.
B. The net resistance of the circuit is less than R_2.
C. The voltage across R_3 is 9 volts.
D. The power dissipated in R_3 could be 18 watts.

Questions 14–16

A defibrillator delivers a dose of electric current (often called a countershock) to the heart. A defibrillator works by using a moderately high voltage (e.g., hypothetical Brand Q uses between 200 and 1000 volts) to pass an electric current through the heart so it's shocked into working normally again.

Depending on the settings of the defibrillator and the resistance across the chest, the patient's heart could receive roughly 300 joules of electrical energy (about as much as a 100-watt incandescent lamp uses in three seconds).

14) If the maximum voltage was applied and a current of 50 amps was used, which of the following would be most consistent with the power of a Brand Q defibrillator?

A. 50 mW
B. 20 MW
C. 50 kW
D. 20 kW

15) Based on the information provided, determine the resistance across the person's chest given the same defibrillator.

A. 0.2 ohms
B. 2 ohms
C. 20 ohms
D. 200 ohms

16) Based on the information provided, what is the energy delivered to the patient in 8 ms?

A. 0.4 kJ   C. 40 kJ
B. 4 kJ   D. 400 kJ

17) Consider the following circuits where all of the cells and globes are identical, and the internal resistances of the cells are negligible. Which circuit would have the brightest globe?

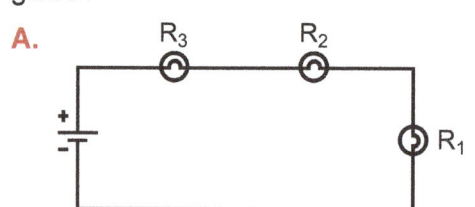

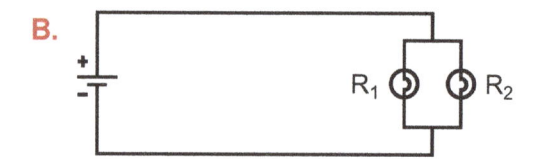

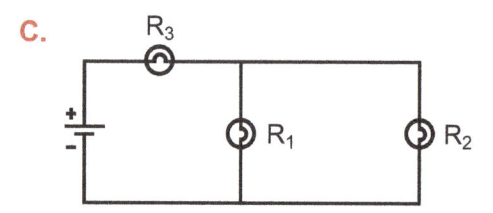

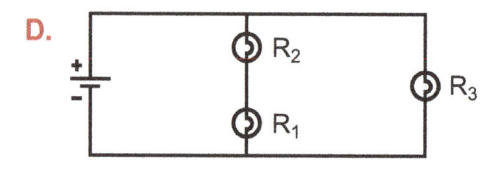

A.
B.
C.
D.

PHY-148   CHAPTER 10: ELECTRIC CIRCUITS

18) Consider Figure 1.

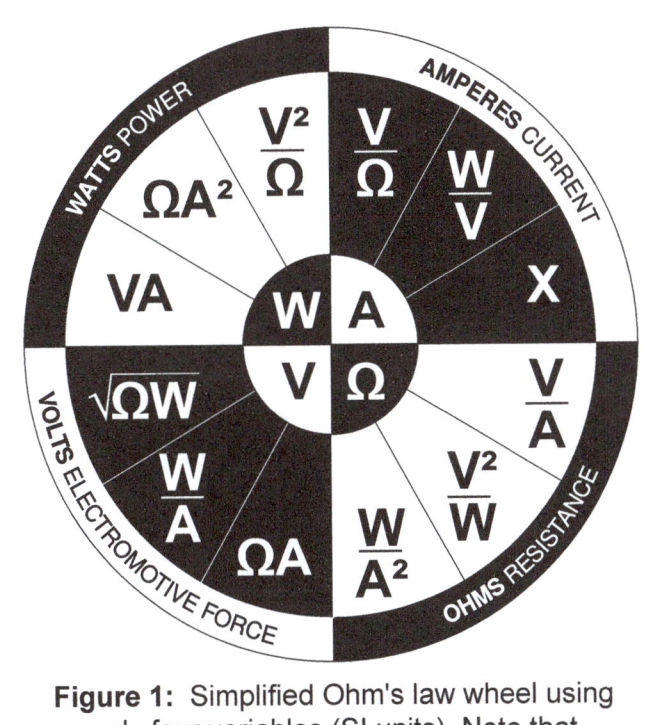

Figure 1: Simplified Ohm's law wheel using only four variables (SI units). Note that one expression is missing and has been replaced by the letter X.
(Edited from Per Mejdal Rasmussen; Wikimedia Commons)

Which of the following expressions is most likely to represent X?

A. $\sqrt{W/\Omega}$
B. $\sqrt{W/\Omega}$
C. $W\Omega^2$
D. WA^2

19) The circuit below shows four identical globes connected to an ideal battery with negligible internal resistance. Rank the globes in order from brightest to dimmest.

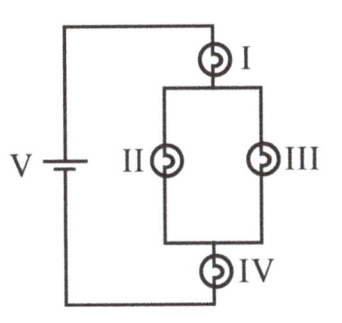

A. I > II = III > IV
B. II = III > I = IV
C. I = IV > II = III
D. I = II = III = IV

20) Consider the following diagram where all capacitors are 1.0 microfarads.

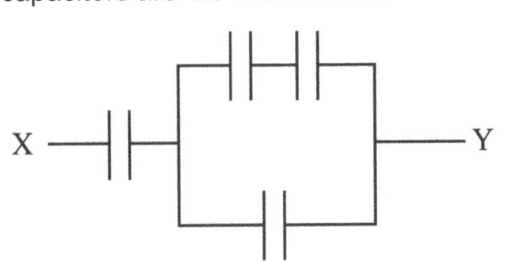

What is the equivalent capacitance between points X and Y?

A. 0.4 microfarads
B. 0.6 microfarads
C. 1.0 microfarads
D. 1.4 microfarads

GAMSAT-Prep.com
GOLD STANDARD PHYSICS

High-level Importance

> ### ⚠ SPOILER ALERT
>
> Gold Standard has cross-referenced the content in this chapter to examples from ACER's official GAMSAT practice materials. It is for you to decide when you want to explore these questions since you may want to preserve some of ACER's materials for timed mock-exam practice.
>
> **Examples** – Globes in series and parallel: Q27 of 2; capacitors: Q60-61 of 3; simple circuit analysis, emf, current: Q10-11 of 4. Note that "Q" is followed by the question number, and, for example, "of 1" refers to booklet number 1 which is referenced in the Spoiler Alert table at the end of Chapter 1. The 10 full-length HEAPS GAMSAT practice tests (by Gold Standard and MediRed), exams 1 through 10, contain specific cross-references to this chapter within the worked solutions. Note that the defibrillation unit with dimensional analysis is from HEAPS-7.

Chapter Checklist

- ☐ Access your online account to view answers, worked solutions and discussion boards.

- ☐ Reassess your 'learning objectives' for this chapter: Go back to the first page of this chapter and re-evaluate the top 3 boxes and the Introduction.

    - ☐ Please be sure that you have completed the *Need for Speed* exercises at the beginning of this chapter.

- ☐ Complete a maximum of 1 page of notes using symbols/abbreviations to represent the entire chapter based on your learning objectives. These are your Gold Notes.

- ☐ Consider your multimedia options based on your optimal way of learning:

    - ☐ Download the free Gold Standard GAMSAT app for your Android device or iPhone.
    - ☐ Create your own, tangible study cards or try the free app: Anki.
    - ☐ Record your voice reading your Gold Notes onto your smartphone (MP3s) and listen during exercise, transportation, etc.
    - ☐ Try out the Gold Standard GAMSAT online videos at gamsat-prep.com, or you can try other options on YouTube like Khan Academy or Crash Course Physics.

- ☐ Reassess your schedule for your full-length GAMSAT practice tests: ACER and/or HEAPS exams. Ensure that you have scheduled one full day to complete a practice test and 1-2 days for a thorough assessment of worked solutions while adding to your abbreviated Gold Notes.

- ☐ Reassess your progress in scheduling and/or evaluating stress reduction techniques such as regular exercise (sports), yoga, meditation and/or mindfulness exercises (*see* YouTube for suggestions).

LIGHT AND GEOMETRICAL OPTICS
Chapter 11

Memorise
* Equations: PHY 11.3, 11.4, 11.5
* Rules for drawing ray diagrams

Understand
* Rules/equations: reflection, refraction, Snell's law
* Dispersion, total internal reflection
* Mirrors, lenses, real/virtual images
* Ray diagrams
* Lens strength, aberration

Importance
High level: 14% of GAMSAT Physics questions released by ACER are related to content in this chapter (in our estimation).
* Note that approximately **75%** of the questions in GAMSAT Physics are related to just 6 chapters: 1, 4, 6, 9, 11 and 12.

GAMSAT-Prep.com

Introduction

Geometrical optics describes the propagation of light in terms of "rays." Rays are then bent at the interface of 2 rather different substances (i.e. air and glass) thus the ray may change direction. A basic understanding of the equations and the geometry of light rays is necessary for solving problems in geometrical optics. Discrete questions regarding total internal reflection are frequent. Usually for the real GAMSAT, they will provide you with the optics equations to solve problems when needed. However, sometimes knowing the equation will give you an edge for "theoretical" questions and this is why we recommend that many optics equations be memorised.

Multimedia Resources at GAMSAT-Prep.com

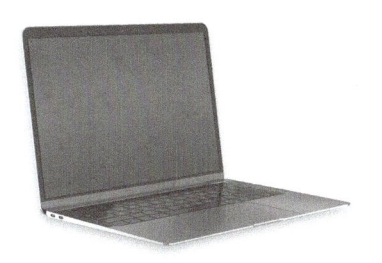

Open Discussion Boards   Foundational Videos   Flashcards   Special Guest

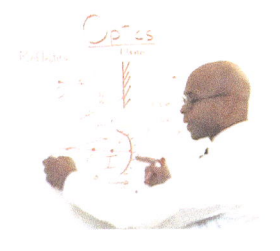

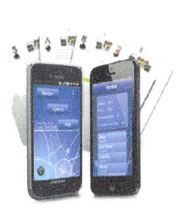

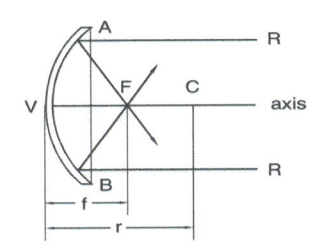

* The real GAMSAT may have advanced-level information presented (i.e. in a passage) but previous knowledge of said information is not required to answer the questions that would follow. Practice questions at the end of this chapter, as well as ACER and GS (HEAPS) practice GAMSATs can help you clarify this point.

GAMSAT-Prep.com
GOLD STANDARD PHYSICS

11.0 GAMSAT has a *Need for Speed*!

High-level Importance

Section Number	GAMSAT Physics *Need for Speed* Exercises
11.1	When light moves within a transparent medium with a uniform composition (*homogeneous*; e.g. either in air, or glass, or water), does it move in a curved path or in a straight-line path?
11.3	Consider the image below. What is the relationship between θ_i and θ_r?
	What is the difference between a real image and a virtual image?
	For a plane mirror (i.e. a flat mirror, the type that you might look at daily!): ▶ Is the image real or virtual? ▶ Is the image erect (right side up) or inverted (upside down)? ▶ Is the image identical to the object or left-right (*laterally*) reversed? ▶ Does the image appear to be just as far behind the mirror as the object is in front of the mirror, or is the distance more or less than that?
	Give one example of a concave mirror. Give one example of a convex mirror.
	Four light rays labelled "R" strike the mirrors below (i.e. are *incident* to the mirrors). Draw 4 arrows to show the general direction of the light rays after bouncing off the mirrors (i.e. the *reflected* rays). Concave mirror Convex mirror

PHY-152   CHAPTER 11: LIGHT AND GEOMETRICAL OPTICS

11.4	Define refraction.	
	The incident ray I strikes the surface S of a medium with a lower index of refraction. N is the normal line. Draw the general direction of the refracted ray.	
	Consider light moving through a medium and then encounters a second medium that has a smaller index of refraction. If the angle of incidence is greater than the critical angle, what happens to the light after it reaches the surface boundary (*interface*)?	
	A. Totally absorbed	
	B. Totally reflected	
	C. Totally transmitted	
	D. Partly transmitted and partly absorbed	
11.5	Light strikes 2 lenses as shown. Draw the direction of the refracted light rays.	
	Convex lens	Concave lens

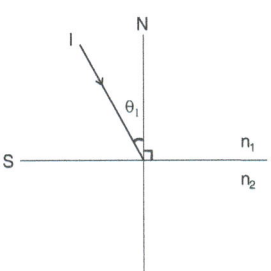

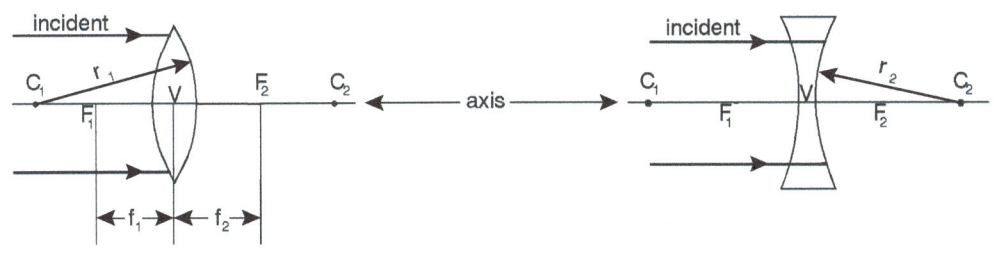

11.6

Property	Light	Sound
Travel through a vacuum?	Yes/No	Yes/No
Can they be reflected?	Yes/No	Yes/No
Can they be refracted?	Yes/No	Yes/No
Can they be diffracted?	Yes/No	Yes/No
Can they interfere? (if so, provide examples)	Yes/No	Yes/No
Variation in frequency from low to high (*What is the range of colours for light? What is the range of pitch for sound?*)		

11.1 Generalities

Geometrical optics describes the movement of light in terms of rays. It is often a very useful approximation of the propagation of light, which itself has a dual nature:

- *particulate*: referring to a packet of energy called a photon when one wants, for example, to explain the photoelectric effect (= an experiment whereby light is shone onto a material resulting in the emission of electrons; General Chemistry, Chapter 2, GAMSAT-level MCQs).

- *wavy*: when one wants to explain, for example, light interference and diffraction (PHY 7.1.3, Fig. III.B.7.5.1).

The simplifying assumptions of geometrical optics include that light rays:

1) propagate in straight-line paths as they travel in a homogeneous medium (e.g. either in air, or glass, or water);

2) bend, and sometimes split in two, at the interface (i.e. boundary) between two dissimilar media (e.g. light hits the surface of water, some light is reflected on the surface, some light is bent – *refracted* - as it enters the water);

3) follow curved paths in a medium with a different ability to bend light (*refractive index*);

4) may be absorbed or reflected.

11.2 Polarisation

Another special feature of light is related to its wave-like characteristic: Polarisation. Natural light generally has random polarisation and can be deemed unpolarised. Polarised waves are light waves in which the vibrations occur in a single plane. Plane-polarised light consists of waves in which the direction of vibration is the same for all waves (in Physics, a *plane* is simply a flat, 2-dimensional surface; cf. PHY 3.2). The process of transforming unpolarised light into polarised light is known as *polarisation*.

An electromagnetic field is described as having at every point of the field two perpendicular vectors: *the electric field vector E* and *the magnetic induction field vector B*.

The electromagnetic wave front is polarised in a straight line when E and B are fixed at all times. Thus, the most common scenario, linearly polarised light, is light that has waves in only one plane.

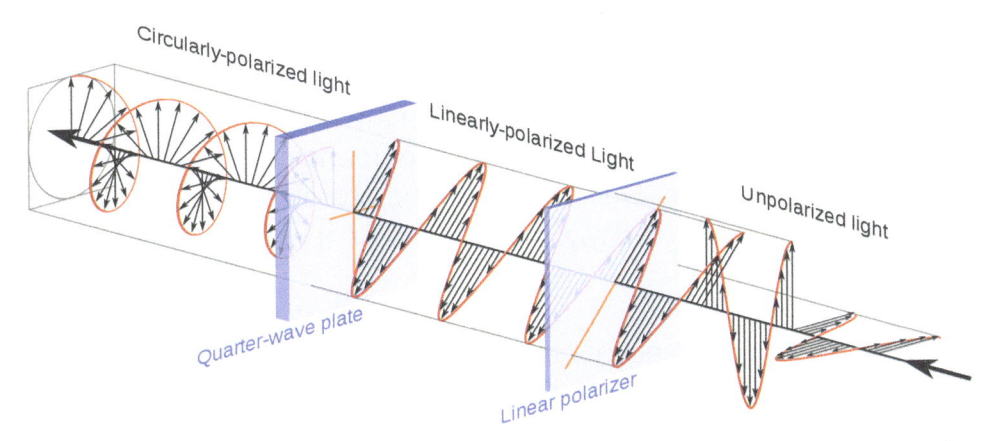

Figure III.B.11.0: Polarisation. On the right side of the diagram, we see light waves in 3 different planes (*such a tiny number is a gross simplification for normal light*). The linear polariser, represented with an orange line at a positive 45° angle, filters out one plane which is now consistent with linearly-polarised, plane-polarised light. The design of the quarter-wave plate, also represented in orange, is such that it can filter light in a way as to generate circularly-polarised light.

11.3 Reflection, Mirrors

Reflection occurs when light hits a surface and bounces off. An uneven surface reflects light diffusely, scattering it, but an even surface like a mirror reflects light in a very precise way. This is one of the reasons why you can see your image in a mirror but not in, say, a brick wall with reflective paint.

Law of Reflection: This law says that the angle of incidence is always equal to the angle of reflection.

If you draw a line perpendicular to the mirror at the point where the light hits (= the "normal" line), the **angle of incidence** (θ_i) is the angle formed by that line and the incoming light ray. Similarly, the **angle of reflection** (θ_r) is the angle formed by the perpendicular and the reflected light ray.

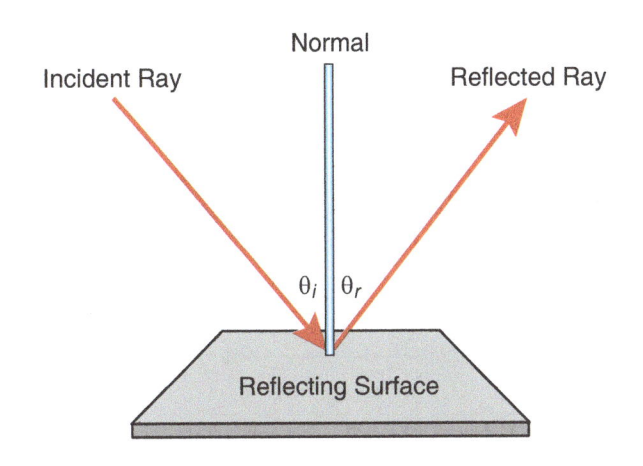

Using the law of reflection, this must always be true: $\theta_i = \theta_r$. Thus, any plane-mirror problem turns into a simple geometry and/or trigonometry problem involving lines and angles (GM 4, 5).

And so, from a technical standpoint, reflection is the process by which light rays

GAMSAT-Prep.com
GOLD STANDARD PHYSICS

(= *imaginary lines drawn perpendicular to the advancing wave fronts*) bounce back into a medium from a surface with another medium (*versus being refracted or absorbed*). The ray that arrives is the *incident* ray while the ray that bounces back is the *reflected* ray. To summarise:

1) the angle of incidence (θ_i) equals the angle of reflection (θ_r) at the normal (*N*, the line perpendicular to the surface)

2) θ_i, θ_r and N all lie in the same plane.

After a ray strikes a mirror or a lens it forms an image. A <u>virtual image</u> has no light rays passing through it and cannot be projected upon a screen.

A <u>real image</u> has light rays passing through it and can be projected upon a screen.

Mirrors have a plane (2D, flat) surface, like an ordinary household mirror, or a non-plane surface. For a plane mirror, all incident light is reflected in parallel off the mirror and therefore all images seen are virtual, erect, left-right reversed and appear to be just as far (perpendicular distance) behind the mirror as the object is in front of the mirror (you can experiment with these assertions yourself!).

In other words, the object (*o*) and the image (*i*) distances have the same magnitudes but have opposite directions ($i = -o$).

Spherical mirrors are non-plane mirrors which may have the reflecting surface convex (*diverges light*) or concave (*converges light*). We will see that the images formed by a converging mirror (concave) are like those for a converging lens (convex); and diverging mirrors (convex) and a diverging lens (concave) also form similar images.

Examples:
- concave mirror: headlights of a car, make-up mirror, the inside of a shiny spoon;
- convex mirror: car's side-view mirror, security mirrors, the outside of a shiny spoon.

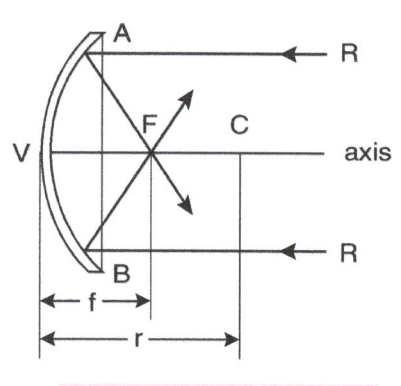

Concave (converging) 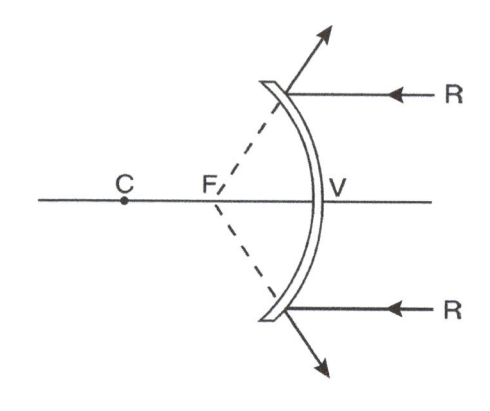 Convex (diverging)

Figure III.B.11.1: Reflection by spherical mirrors. R = the light rays.

CHAPTER 11: LIGHT AND GEOMETRICAL OPTICS

The terminology for spherical mirrors is (*see* Figure III.B.11.1):

r = radius of curvature (distance from C to V)
C = centre of curvature
F = focal point (AKA 'principal' focus)
V = vertex (centre of the mirror itself)
axis = 'central' or 'optical' axis = line through C and V
f = focal length (distance from F to V)
i = image distance (distance from V to image along the axis)
o = object distance (distance from V to object along the axis)
AB = linear aperture (cord connecting the ends of the mirror; the larger the aperture, the better the resolution).

As a rule, capital letters refer to a point (*or position*) and small case letters refer to a distance.

With concave (spherical) mirrors the incident light is converged toward the axis. The path of light rays is as follows:

1)
if o < f, then the image is virtual and erect;
if o > f, then the image is real and inverted;
if o = f, then no image is formed;
2)
if o < r, then the image is enlarged in size;
if o > r, then the image is reduced in size;
if o = r, then the image is the same.

The relations are similar to those for a converging lens (convex). With convex (spherical) mirrors, the incident light is diverged from the axis after reflection. It is the backward extension (dotted lines in the diagram) that may pass through the focal point F. The path of light rays are as follows:

1) Incident rays parallel to the axis have backward extension of their reflections through F (*see* Figure III.B.11.1);
2) incident rays along a radius (that would pass C if extended) reflect back along themselves;
3) incident rays that pass through F (if extended) reflect parallel to the axis.

The image formed for a convex mirror is always virtual, erect and smaller than the object {Convex mirror = REV: Reduced, Erect, Virtual}. The mirror equation and the derivations from it allow the above relations between object and image to be calculated instead of memorised. The equation is valid for convex and concave mirrors:

$$1/i + 1/o = 1/f$$

$$f = r/2$$

$$M = magnification = -i/o.$$

Convention for concave and convex mirrors:
- for i and o, *positive* values mean real, negative values mean virtual;
- for r and f, *positive* values mean converging, negative values mean diverging;
- for M, a *positive* value means erect, negative is inverted;
- for M > 1 the image is enlarged, M < 1 the image is diminished.

11.4 Refraction, Dispersion, Refractive Index, Snell's Law

Refraction is the bending of light as it passes from one transparent medium to another and is caused by the different speeds of light in the two media.

If θ_1 is taken as the angle (to the normal) of the incident light and θ_2 is the angle (to the normal) of the refracted light, where 1 and 2 represent the two different media, the following relations hold (Snell's Law):

where v = velocity and λ = wavelength.

$$\frac{\sin \theta_1}{\sin \theta_2} = \frac{v_1}{v_2} = \frac{n_2}{n_1} = \frac{\lambda_1}{\lambda_2}$$

$$n = \frac{\text{speed of light in vacuum}}{\text{speed of light in medium}} = \frac{c}{v}$$

$c = 3 \times 10^8$ m/sec or 181,000 mi/sec
$n = 1.0$ for air, $n = 1.33$ for H_2O
$n = 1.5$ for glass (at $\lambda = 589$ nm)
n = the refractive index which is a property of the medium
n_1 = refractive index of medium 1
n_2 = refractive index of medium 2
N = normal line to the surface
S = surface line, represents the separation between the two media = interface = boundary)
I = incident light = ray = beam
R = refracted light (= ray = beam)

The speed at which light propagates through transparent materials, such as glass, water or air, is less than c, as you can tell from index of refractions above.

The angle θ is smaller (closer to the normal, e.g. θ_1) in the more optically dense (higher n) medium.

Also the smaller wavelength of the incident light (i.e. toward the violet end), the closer θ_2 is to the normal (i.e. it is smaller than θ_1).

This means longer wavelengths travel faster in a medium than shorter wavelengths (i.e. shorter wavelengths are more subject to refraction).

This leads to *dispersion* which is the separation of white light (= *all colours together*) into individual colours by this differential refraction. For example, a prism disperses white light (*see* PHY 9.2.4).

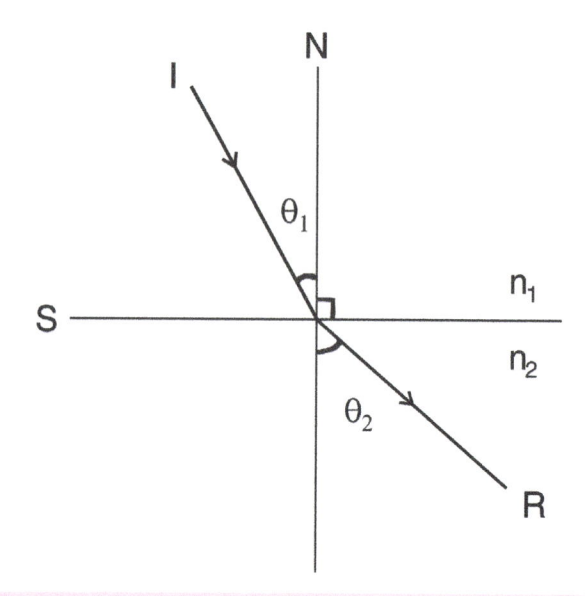

Figure III.B.11.2: Refraction. Note that in this case, the incident ray I bends (*refraction*) further from the normal line N than its original heading. This indicates that it has entered a 'faster' medium, less optically dense, thus $n_2 < n_1$.

The laws of refraction are:

1) The incident ray, the refracted ray and the normal ray all lie in the same plane.
2) The path of the ray (incident and refracted parts) is reversible.

When light passes from a more optically dense (higher n) medium into a less optically dense medium (lower n), there exists an angle of incidence such that the angle of refraction θ_2 is 90°. This special angle of incidence is called the critical angle θ_c.

This is because when the angle of incidence is less then θ_c refraction occurs. If the angle of incidence is equal to θ_c, then neither refraction nor reflection occur.

And if $\theta_1 > \theta_c$, then total internal reflection (ray is reflected back into the more optically dense medium) occurs. The θ_c is found from Snell's Law (*Need for Speed* answer B):

$$n_1 \sin\theta_c = n_2 \sin\theta_2$$

and $\theta_2 = 90° \Rightarrow \sin\theta_2 = 1$

giving $n_1 \sin\theta_c = n_2 \times 1$

finally $\sin\theta_c = n_2/n_1$

where $n_2 < n_1$.

When looking at an object under water from above the surface, the object appears closer than it actually is. This is due to refraction. In general:

apparent depth/actual depth $= n_2/n_1$

where n_2 = the medium of the observer, and n_1 = the medium of the object.

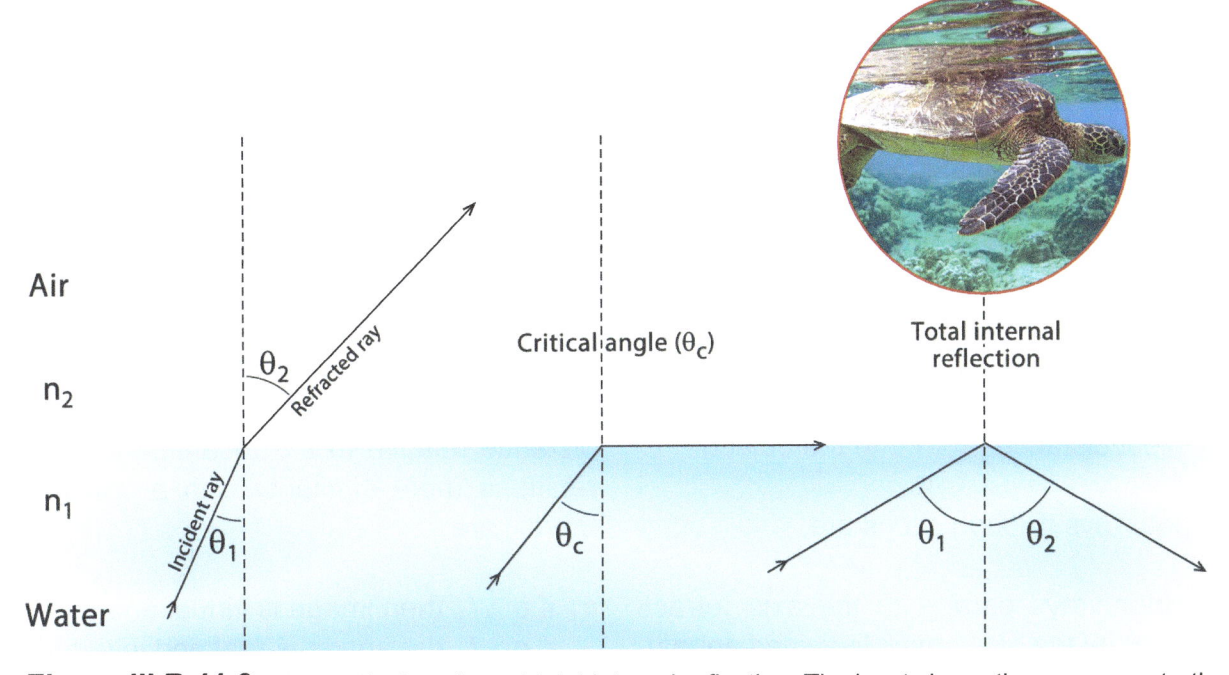

High-level Importance

Figure III.B.11.3: The critical angle and total internal reflection. The inset shows the green sea turtle, *Chelonia mydas*, and its reflection seen at the interface (boundary) where air and water meet.
(Inset photo: TheBrockenInaGlory 2008, Wikimedia Commons.)

THE PHYSICAL SCIENCES   PHY-159

11.5 Thin Lens, Diopters

A lens is a transparent material which refracts light. **Converging lenses refract toward the axis, and diverging lenses refract the light away from the axis.**

A converging lens is wider at the middle than at the ends, and the diverging lens is thinner at the middle than at the ends.

Convex lens

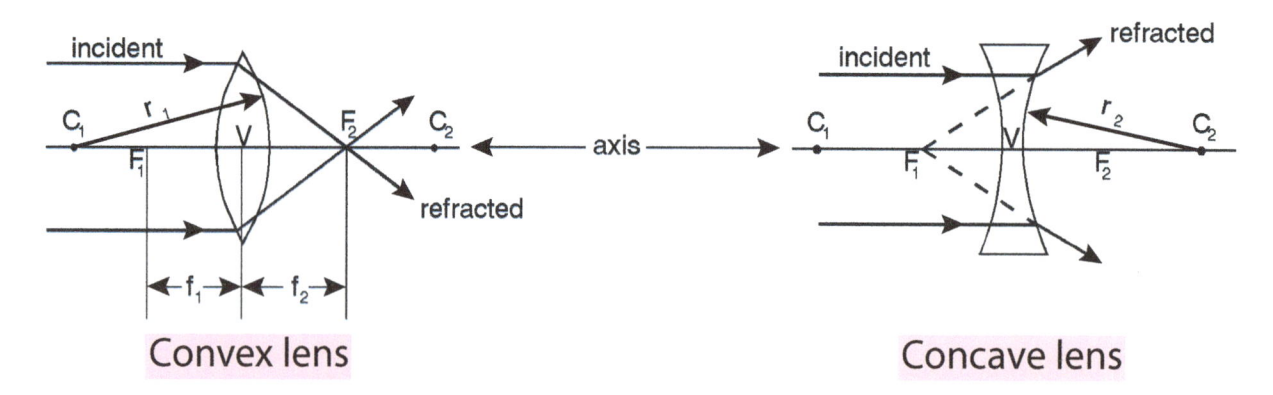

Concave lens

Figure III.B.11.4: Refraction by spherical lenses; r = the radius of curvature.

If the surface is convex, r is positive (e.g., r_1). If the surface is concave, r is negative (e.g., r_2). Subscript 1 refers to the incident side, 2 refers to the refracted side.

C = centre of curvature, F = focal point
V = the optical centre of the lens or vertex
axis = line through C and V

f = focal length is the distance between V and F
i = image distance (from V to the image)
o = object distance (from V to the object).

The path rays through a lens are:

1) incident rays parallel to the axis refract through F_2 of the converging lens, and appear to come from F_1 of a diverging lens (backward extensions of the refracted ray, see dotted line on diverging diagram);

2) an incident ray through F_1 of a converging lens or through F_2 of a diverging lens (if extended) are refracted parallel to the axis;

3) incident rays through V are not deviated (refracted).

For a converging lens (e.g., convex) the image formed depends on the object distance relative to the focal length (f). The relations (note similarity with a converging mirror) are:

1) if $o < f_1$, then image is virtual and erect;
if $o > f_1$, the image is real and inverted;
if $o = f_1$, then no image is formed;

2) if $o < 2f_1$, then the image is enlarged in size;
if $o > 2f_1$, then the image is reduced in size;
if $o = 2f_1$, then the image is the same;
remember $2f_1 = r$.

For a diverging lens (e.g., concave), the image is always virtual, erect and reduced in size as for a diverging mirror (REV, cf. PHY 11.4).

The above relations can be calculated rather than memorised by use of the lens equation and derivations from it,

1) $1/o + 1/i = 1/f$ (lens equation, same as the mirror equation)

2) $D = 1/f = (n-1)(1/r_1 - 1/r_2)$, (lens maker's equation, n = index of refraction)

A <u>magnifying glass</u> (or "hand lens") is a convex lens that is used to produce a magnified image of an object. The lens is usually mounted in a frame with a handle. You can determine from the preceding rules that, in order to have an image that is erect (upright) and magnified for easier viewing, the object distance must be less than the focal length of the convex lens.

3) diopters $(D) = 1/f$ where f is in metres, measures the refractive *power* of the lens; the larger the diopters, the stronger the lens. The diopters has a positive value for a converging lens and a negative value for a diverging lens.

To get the refractive power (D) of lenses in series just add the diopters which can then be converted into focal length:

$$D_T = D_1 + D_2 = 1/f_T \text{ (T = total)}.$$

4) Note that you can add only inverses of focal lengths:

$$1/f_T = 1/f_1 + 1/f_2 \ldots$$

5) M = Magnification = $-i/o = M_1 M_2$ for lenses in series.

Convention for both concave and convex lenses *and* mirrors (PHY 11.3):
- for i and o, positive values mean real, negative values mean virtual;
- for r and f, positive values mean converging, negative values mean diverging;
- for M, a positive value means erect, negative is inverted.
- for $M > 1$ the image is enlarged, $M < 1$ the image is diminished.

The lens equation holds only for thin lenses (the thickness is small relative to other dimensions). For combination of lenses not in contact with each other, the image is found for the first lens (nearer the object) and then this image is used as the object of the second lens to find the image formed by it.

It should be noted that since concave lenses are concave on both sides they are sometimes called *biconcave*. Likewise, convex lenses may be called *biconvex*.

11.5.1 Lens Aberrations

High-level Importance

In practice, the images formed by various refracting surfaces, as described in the previous section, fall short of theoretical perfection. Imperfections of image formation are due to several mechanisms or *aberrations*.

For example a nick or cut in a convex lens might create a microscopic area of concavity. Thus the light ray which strikes the aberration diverges instead of converging. Therefore the image will be less sharp or clear as the number or sizes of the aberrations increase.

11.6 Light vs. Sound

Property	Light	Sound
Travel through a vacuum?	Yes	No, can only pass through a solid, liquid or gas.
Can they be reflected?	Yes	Yes
Can they be refracted?	Yes	Yes
Can they be diffracted?	Yes	Yes
Can they interfere?	Yes, e.g. bright vs dark	Yes, e.g. loud vs quiet
Variation in frequency from low to high	Red light to violet light	Low pitch (note) to high pitch

Table III.B.11.1: Comparing light and sound waves, GAMSAT Physics Chapters 7, 8 and 11. What about water waves like those you can see at the beach (after finishing your GAMSAT studies!)? Water waves are quite similar to sound waves (transverse, can be reflected, refracted and diffracted) but, of course, the velocity is not standard. Maximal destructive interference would create calm waters (for sound, similar to quiet), whereas maximal constructive interference could be caused by an earthquake (or other disturbance) and produce a tsunami (for sound, extremely loud similar to a volcanic eruption or standing right beside the speakers at a concert in a football stadium!).

CHAPTER 11: Light and Geometrical Optics

GOLD STANDARD FOUNDATIONAL GAMSAT PRACTICE QUESTIONS

1) All of the following are true concerning an image that is formed by reflection from a plane surface EXCEPT one. Which one is the EXCEPTION?

   A. The image is real.
   B. The image is upright.
   C. The image appears laterally inverted.
   D. It is as far behind the surface as the object is in front of it.

2) A light ray is directed downward passing through point B and hitting a flat mirror angled to the horizontal as illustrated below. Which point labelled in the diagram is most consistent with the point through which the reflected ray from the mirror will pass?

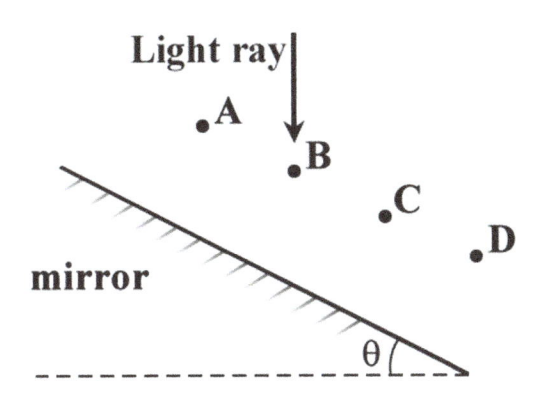

3) Consider a person standing 0.6 m from a plane mirror. How far is the image from that person?

   A. 0 m
   B. 0.6 m
   C. 1.2 m
   D. 1.8 m

4) A concave mirror forms a real image at 10 cm from the surface along the principal axis to the mirror. If the corresponding object is at a 5.0 cm distance to the mirror, what is the mirror's focal length?

   Note: The mirror equation (o = object distance; i = image distance; f = focal length), $1/o + 1/i = 1/f$

   A. 3.3 cm
   B. 5.0 cm
   C. 7.5 cm
   D. 10 cm

5) Consider the following diagram of an object at position X, an image at position Y (somewhere to the right of F but may be on either side of the mirror) and the focal length of the convex mirror at position F.

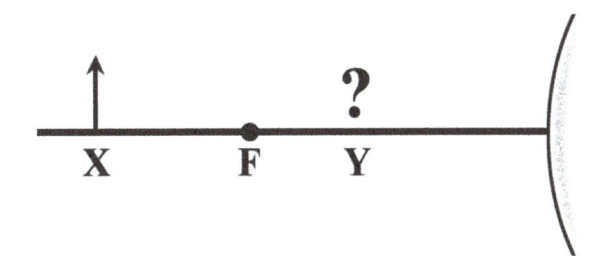

   The image at position Y would be expected to be:

   A. virtual, reduced and upright.
   B. real, reduced and upright.
   C. virtual, reduced and inverted.
   D. virtual, enlarged and upright.

GAMSAT-Prep.com
GOLD STANDARD PHYSICS

High-level Importance

6) Consider the following ray diagram of light reflected from a concave mirror where the focal point f (i.e. the principal focus) is as indicated. Where along the principal axis is the image located?

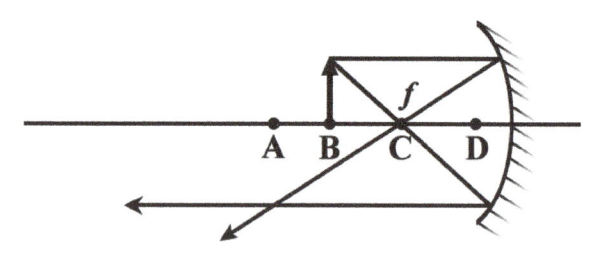

7) Consider the following diagram with an object at position O which is at a distance r in front of (to the left in the diagram) a convex, spherical mirror. The mirror has a centre of curvature at position C and the radius of curvature is distance r.

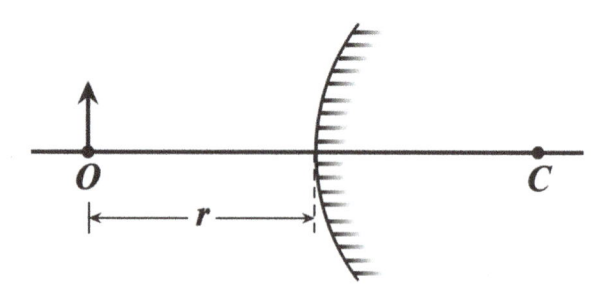

Which of the following is most consistent with the position of the image?

A. Distance r to the right of the mirror
B. Distance r to the left of the mirror
C. Distance r/3 to the right of the mirror
D. Distance r/3 to the left of the mirror

8) If light rays from the sun strike the surface of water at an angle, which of the following is most consistent with the properties of the light once it enters the water?

A. The light's speed, frequency and wavelength change.
B. The light's wavelength and speed change, but the frequency stays the same.
C. The light's speed and frequency change, but the wavelength stays the same.
D. The light's wavelength and frequency change, but the light's speed stays the same.

9) An object O is located at 0.60 m to the left of a convex lens with a focal length of 1.0 m, where is the image of the object located? (if you think that it is applicable, you can use the mirror/lens equation referenced in Question 4)

A. At infinity
B. 1.5 m to the left of the lens
C. 0.15 m to the right of the lens
D. 1.5 m to the right of the lens

10) Which of the following is true of an image created from an object located at any point in front of a convex mirror?

A. It is magnified.
B. It is real.
C. It is erect.
D. None of the above

PHY-164   CHAPTER 11: LIGHT AND GEOMETRICAL OPTICS

GAMSAT MASTERS SERIES

GOLD STANDARD GAMSAT-LEVEL PRACTICE QUESTIONS

11) A 10-year old boy is 1.4 metres tall and preparing for a play in which he wears a top hat that extends the boy's height by 10 cm. What is the size of the smallest mirror that would permit the boy to see his shoes and the top of his hat while standing?

   A. 0.75 m
   B. 1.4 m
   C. 1.5 m
   D. Cannot be determined without knowing how far he is standing from the mirror.

12) Consider the following diagram in which a laser directs a ray of light at the surface of water.

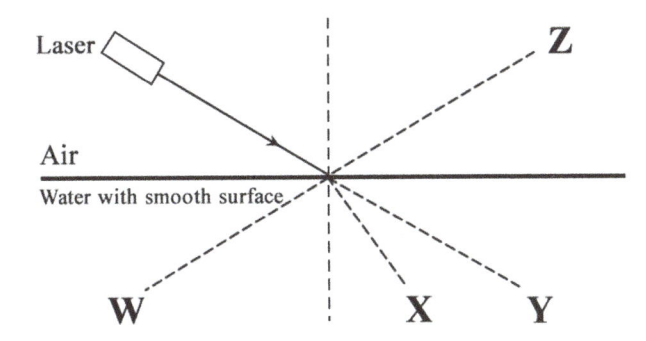

   Which regions are most likely to be illuminated by the laser?

   A. W and Y
   B. Y and Z
   C. X and Z
   D. X and W

13) A biologist in a boat is trying to shoot a shark swimming in the water with a laser tag. Once she sees the shark in the barrel of her scope, she should aim in which of the following directions?

   A. Above
   B. Below
   C. In front
   D. Behind

14) A rectangular block of glass is pushed upwards directly into the path of light rays emerging from a convex lens as shown in the ray diagram. As a result, the point *i* where the light rays cross will move in which direction?

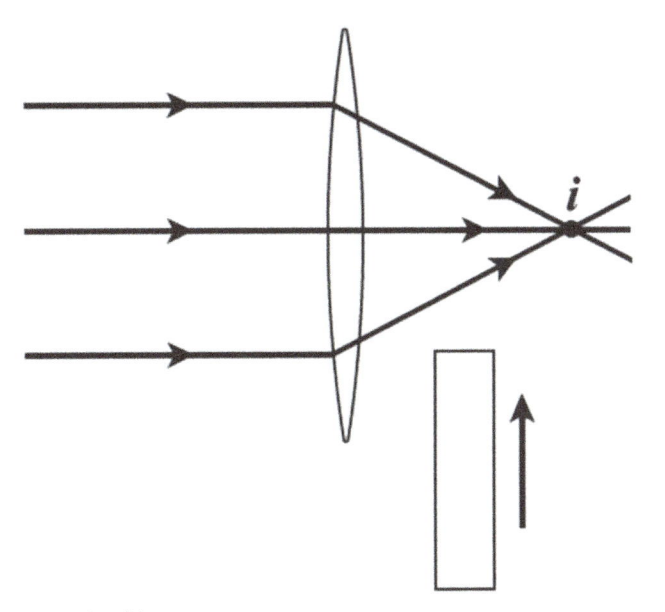

   A. Up
   B. Down
   C. Right
   D. Left

High-level Importance

THE PHYSICAL SCIENCES   PHY-165

GAMSAT-Prep.com
GOLD STANDARD PHYSICS

Questions 15–18

Flexible endoscopes have revolutionised many areas of diagnostic medicine by helping to visualise internal structures such as the respiratory tract, stomach, and colon. Unlike a rigid endoscope, a flexible endoscope can bend and thus go around "corners." The consequence is less discomfort for the patient and the endoscope can be advanced farther into the cavity under examination.

A typical endoscope has various channels, such as for irrigation, suction, surgical manipulation, illumination, and imaging. The image from the patient is transmitted along bundles of optical fibers containing separate layers of glass, or more specifically, silica. Each optical fiber consists of a cylindrical *core* surrounded by a *cladding*. Light enters one end of a fiber and is total internally reflected repeatedly until it exits the fiber at the opposite end. Because of the difference in the index of refraction of the two layers, total internal reflection confines the light waves within the core of the fiber.

A model for a segment of an optical fiber in longitudinal section is shown in Figure 1. A beam of light enters one end of the fiber at an angle with respect to the axis of the fiber. Assume that the interface between the air and the optical fiber is a flat plane.

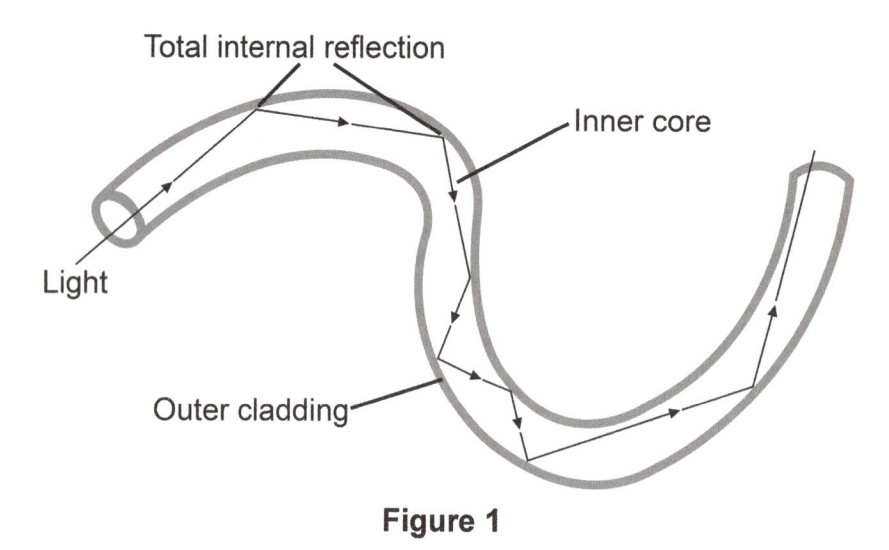

Figure 1

The optical density of a material is given by the index of refraction n. Snell's law states that the ratio of the sines of the angles of incidence and refraction is equivalent to the reciprocal of the ratio of the indices of refraction.

15) For the best image quality, which of the following conditions should be met?

   I. The cladding must have a higher optical density than the core.
   II. Light rays must be incident to the core-cladding interface at angles of incidence greater than the critical angle.
   III. The core must not absorb a significant amount of light.

   A. II only
   B. I and II only
   C. II and III only
   D. I, II and III

16) The critical angle of the core-cladding interface is given by:

   A. critical angle = $\sin^{-1}(n_{cladding}/n_{core})$
   B. critical angle = $\sin^{-1}(n_{core}/n_{cladding})$
   C. critical angle = $\sin^{-1}(1/n_{core})$
   D. critical angle = $\sin^{-1}(1/n_{cladding})$

17) Consider the following graphs of the sine of the angle of refraction (y-axis) vs. the sine of the angle of incidence (x-axis). Which of the following is consistent with Snell's law?

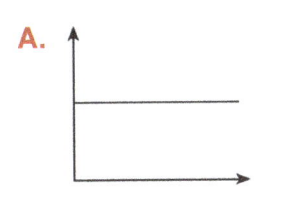

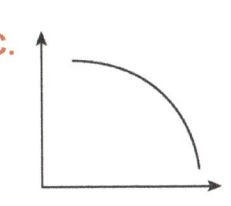

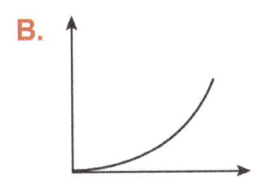

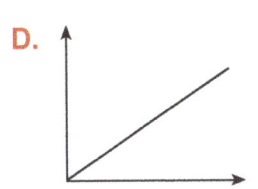

   A.
   B.
   C.
   D.

18) A spherical air bubble is rising in a small pool of clear gastrointestinal fluid and is illuminated from one side by an endoscope. What happens to a ray of light incident on the air bubble at A?

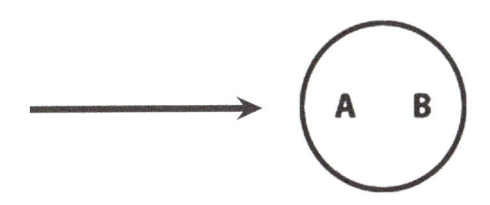

   A. Reflection at both surfaces
   B. Reflection at A; no reflection at B
   C. Reflection at B; no reflection at A
   D. No reflection at either surface

19) Consider the following ray diagrams, where the object point O, the image point I and the focal points F_1 and F_2 of a concave lens are indicated. Which diagram is accurate?

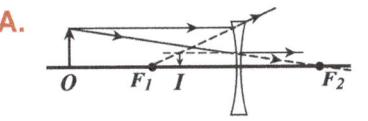

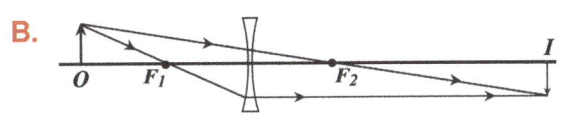

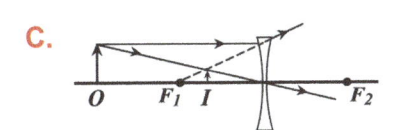

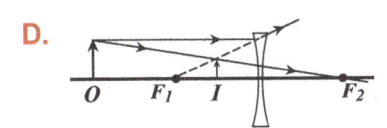

   A.
   B.
   C.
   D.

GAMSAT-Prep.com
GOLD STANDARD PHYSICS

Questions 20–24

Consider the diagram of the human eye.

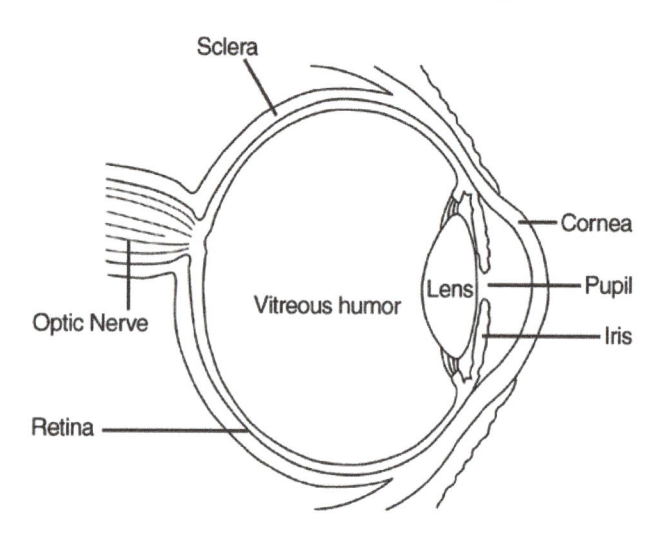

Figure 1: Basic anatomy of the human eye

Like any wave, the speed of a light wave is dependent upon the properties of the medium. In the case of an electromagnetic wave, the speed of the wave depends upon the optical density of that material. One indicator of the optical density of a material is the index of refraction value of the material. Index of refraction values (represented by the symbol n) are numerical index values that are expressed relative to the speed of light in a vacuum.

Component	Index of Refraction
Air	1
Cornea	1.38
Vitreous humour	1.34
Lens	1.40

Myopia (also known as near-sightedness or short-sightedness) and *hyperopia* (also known as far-sightedness or long-sightedness) are among the most common anomalies of vision. Someone with myopia can see near objects clearly, but cannot focus properly on distant objects. This is caused by the eyeball being elongated, so that the distance between the lens and the retina is too great.

Someone with hyperopia can see distant objects clearly, but cannot focus properly on near objects. This is because the lens focuses the sharpest image behind the retina, instead of on it.

Artificial (glass or plastic) lenses are sometimes used to correct visual anomalies. The thin lens equation relates the object distance to the lens o, the image distance to the lens i, and the focal length f of a lens as follows:

$$1/o + 1/i = 1/f$$

20) To focus an image on the retina, the components of the eye which are primarily implicated are which of the following?

A. Pupil and vitreous humour
B. Iris and cornea
C. Cornea and lens
D. Lens and iris

21) The greatest deviation (*refraction*) of light would be expected at which of the following boundaries?

A. Lens – vitreous humour
B. Cornea – air
C. Pupil – lens
D. Cornea – lens

PHY-168 CHAPTER 11: LIGHT AND GEOMETRICAL OPTICS

22) Which of the following lenses would most reasonably be used to correct myopia and hyperopia, respectively?

A. Convex, convex
B. Convex, concave
C. Concave, convex
D. Concave, concave

23) The power of a lens is its ability to bend light: the greater the power, the greater the refraction of light. The power of a lens is measured in dioptres (D) which is equal to the inverse of the focal length calculated in metres. What is the refractive power of a thin convex lens with a focal length of 0.50 cm?

A. 0.2 D
B. 2.0 D
C. 20 D
D. 200 D

24) An intern in dermatology is using a magnifying glass with a convex lens to examine moles on her patient's skin in order to rule out characteristics of melanoma. She is holding the magnifying glass near her eye, within the focal length of the lens. Which of the following is most accurate?

A. The image will be inverted and real.
B. If the mole's distance to the magnifying glass is within the focal distance, then the image will be upright, virtual and enlarged.
C. If the mole is exactly at the focal length of the magnifying glass, she will be able to see the image most clearly.
D. Neither **A**, nor **B**, nor **C** is correct.

25) Consider the following diagram of an object at position O located to the left of a converging lens and the focal points F_1 and F_2 of the lens.

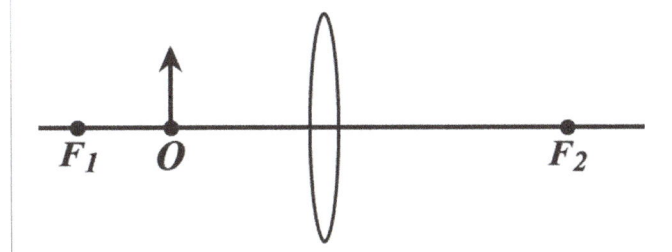

Which of the following best describes the image that would be formed?

A. Real, upright, and larger than the object
B. Real, inverted, and smaller than the object
C. Virtual, upright, and larger than the object
D. Virtual, upright, and smaller than the object

GAMSAT-Prep.com
GOLD STANDARD PHYSICS

High-level Importance

⚠ SPOILER ALERT

Gold Standard has cross-referenced the content in this chapter to examples from ACER's official GAMSAT practice materials. It is for you to decide when you want to explore these questions since you may want to preserve some of ACER's materials for timed mock-exam practice.

Examples – Very easy lens-equation questions with the equations provided: Q22-23 of 1; do you really understand what inversion of an image means? OK: Q22 of 2; does frequency change when light enters a medium with a different index of refraction and what about wavelength? PHY 11.4, a rare example of pure knowledge required: Q39 of 2; convex and concave lenses using the lens and magnification equations, a classic unit: Q40-43 of 4; although it seems to be about lenses, it is pure GAMSAT Maths: Q37-39 of 5. Note that "Q" is followed by the question number, and, for example, "of 1" refers to booklet number 1 which is referenced in the Spoiler Alert table at the end of Chapter 1. The 10 full-length HEAPS GAMSAT practice tests (by Gold Standard and MediRed), exams 1 through 10, contain specific cross-references to this chapter within the worked solutions. Note that the eye unit is a rare visitor from HEAPS-1 but we completely changed 2 of the questions in that unit for this book; the endoscopy unit with total internal reflection is from HEAPS-5; the diverging-lens, ray-diagram question is from HEAPS-8.

Chapter Checklist

- ☐ Access your online account to view answers, worked solutions and discussion boards.
- ☐ Reassess your 'learning objectives' for this chapter: Go back to the first page of this chapter and re-evaluate the top 3 boxes and the Introduction.
    - ☐ Please be sure that you have completed the *Need for Speed* exercises at the beginning of this chapter.
- ☐ Complete a maximum of 1 page of notes using symbols/abbreviations to represent the entire chapter based on your learning objectives. These are your Gold Notes.
- ☐ Consider your multimedia options based on your optimal way of learning:
    - ☐ Download the free Gold Standard GAMSAT app for your Android device or iPhone.
    - ☐ Create your own, tangible study cards or try the free app: Anki.
    - ☐ Record your voice reading your Gold Notes onto your smartphone (MP3s) and listen during exercise, transportation, etc.
    - ☐ Try out the Gold Standard GAMSAT online videos at gamsat-prep.com, or you can try other options on YouTube like Khan Academy or Crash Course Physics.
- ☐ Reassess your schedule for your full-length GAMSAT practice tests: ACER and/or HEAPS exams. Ensure that you have scheduled one full day to complete a practice test and 1-2 days for a thorough assessment of worked solutions while adding to your abbreviated Gold Notes.
- ☐ Reassess your progress in scheduling and/or evaluating stress reduction techniques such as regular exercise (sports), yoga, meditation and/or mindfulness exercises (*see* YouTube for suggestions).

ATOMIC AND NUCLEAR STRUCTURE
Chapter 12

Memorise
* Basic atomic and nuclear structure
* Define 'isotopes'
* Equation for half-life

Understand
* Basic atomic structure, amu
* Fission, fusion; the Bohr model of the atom
* Isotopes and the calculation for weighted average
* Problem-solving for half-life
* Quantised energy levels for electrons
* Fluorescence

Importance
High level: 15% of GAMSAT Physics questions released by ACER are related to content in this chapter (in our estimation).
* Note that approximately **75%** of the questions in GAMSAT Physics are related to just 6 chapters: 1, 4, 6, 9, 11 and 12.

GAMSAT-Prep.com

Introduction

Atomic structure can be summarised as a nucleus orbited by electrons in different energy levels. Transition of electrons between energy levels and nuclear structure (i.e. protons, neutrons) are important characteristics of the atom.

Multimedia Resources at GAMSAT-Prep.com

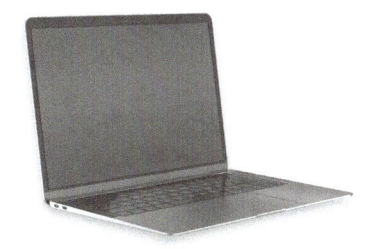

Open Discussion Boards   Foundational Videos   Flashcards   Special Guest

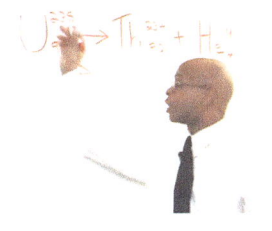

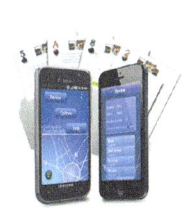

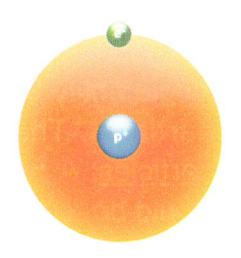

THE PHYSICAL SCIENCES   PHY-171

* The real GAMSAT may have advanced-level information presented (i.e. in a passage) but previous knowledge of said information is not required to answer the questions that would follow. Practice questions at the end of this chapter, as well as ACER and GS (HEAPS) practice GAMSATs can help you clarify this point.

GAMSAT-Prep.com
GOLD STANDARD PHYSICS

12.0 GAMSAT has a *Need for Speed*!

Section Number	GAMSAT Physics *Need for Speed* Exercises
12.1	The hydrogen atom is composed of how many protons, electrons and neutrons?
12.2	How do the 3 carbon isotopes differ?
	How are different elements distinguished?
	How many protons and neutrons are in $^{13}_{6}C$?
12.3	What is the mass and charge of a gamma (γ) ray?
12.4	What number must **X** be? (*note: no periodic table is required*) $$^{238}_{92}U \rightarrow {}^{X}_{90}Th + {}^{4}_{2}He^{2+}$$
	What is the equation for the calculation of half-life?
	If a radioactive substance has a half-life of 9 years, what fraction would remain radioactive after 27 years?

High-level Importance

12.1 Protons, Neutrons, Electrons

Only recently, with high-resolution electron microscopes, have large atoms been visualised. However, for years their existence and properties have been inferred by experiments. Experimental work on gas discharge effects suggested that an atom is not a single entity but is itself composed of smaller particles. These were termed <u>elementary particles</u>. A more encompassing expression would be "subatomic" particles.

The atom appears as a small solar system with a heavy nucleus composed of positive particles and neutral particles: *protons and neutrons*. Around this nucleus, there are clouds of negatively charged particles, called *electrons*. The mass of a neutron is slightly more than that of a proton (both ≈ 1.7×10^{-24} g); the mass of the electron is considerably less (9.1×10^{-28} g).

Since an atom is electrically neutral, the negative charge carried by the electrons must be equal in magnitude (but opposite in sign) to the positive charge carried by the protons.

Experiments with electrostatic charges have shown that ==opposite charges attract==

(and like charges repel), so it can be considered that electrostatic forces (PHY 9.1) hold an atom together. The difference between various atoms is therefore determined by their *composition*.

A hydrogen atom consists of one proton and one electron (no neutron); a helium atom of two protons, two neutrons and two electrons. They are shown in diagram form in Figure III.B.12.1a.

(a) (b)

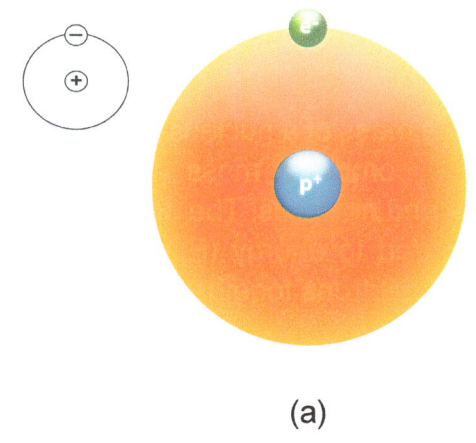

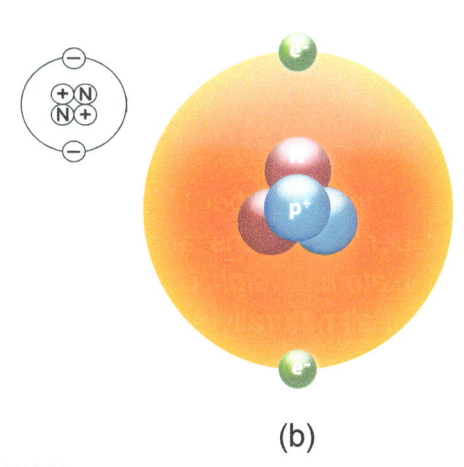

Figure III.B.12.1a: Atomic structure simplified: (a) hydrogen atom; (b) helium atom. The images above are a summary of key features of the 2 simplest atoms. The insets (black and white) are basic sketches, while in colour is essentially a cartoon for several reasons including: 1) the actual proportions cannot be drawn to scale because the space between the nucleus and electrons is too great and the electron itself is far smaller; 2) the actual position of an electron cannot be known (CHM 2.1; though the orange cloud is supposed to be a reminder); 3) subatomic particles do not have colour in any traditional sense.

12.2 Isotopes, Atomic Number, Atomic Weight

A proton has a mass of 1 a.m.u. (*atomic mass unit*) and a charge of +1, whereas, a neutron has a mass of 1 a.m.u. and no charge. The *atomic number* (AN) of an atom is the number of protons in the nucleus. In an atom of neutral charge, the atomic number (AN) is also equal to the number of electrons.

The atomic number is conventionally represented by the letter "Z". Each of the chemical elements has a unique number of protons which is identified by its own atomic number "Z". As an example, for the hydrogen H element, Z = 1 and for Na, Z = 11.

An *element* is a group of atoms with the same AN. *Isotopes* are elements which have the same atomic number (Z) but different number of neutrons and hence a different mass number (MN). As an example, the three carbon isotopes differ only in the number of neutrons and therefore have the same

GAMSAT-Prep.com
GOLD STANDARD PHYSICS

High-level Importance

number of protons and electrons but differ in mass and are usually represented as follows: C-12, C-13 and C-14 or more specifically as follows: $^{12}_{6}C$, $^{13}_{6}C$ and $^{14}_{6}C$ (*see* Fig. III.B.12.1b). It is therefore the number of protons that distinguishes elements from each other. The *weighted average* follows the natural abundance of the various isotopic compositions of an element.

The *mass number* (*MN*) of an atom is the number of protons and neutrons in an atom. The *atomic weight* (*AW*) is the weighted average of all naturally occurring isotopes of an element.

For example: Silicon is known to exist naturally as a mixture of three isotopes (Si-28, Si-29 and Si-30). The relative amount of each of the three different silicon isotopes is found to be 92.2297% with a mass of 27.97693, 4.6832% with a mass of 28.97649 and the remaining 3.0872% with a mass of 29.97377. The atomic weight of silicon is then determined as the weighted average (cf. GM 1.4.3 C) of each of the isotopes as follows:

Si mass = (27.97693 × 0.922297)
+ (28.97649 × 0.046832)
+ (29.97377 × 0.030872)
= 28.0854 g/mol.

It is also important to note that as the number of protons distinguishes *elements* from each other, it is their electronic configuration (CHM 2.1, 2.2, 2.3) that determines their *reactivity*.

The mass of a nucleus is always smaller than the combined mass of its constituent protons and neutrons. The difference in mass is converted to energy (E) which holds protons and neutrons together within the nuclear core.

Let's consider the number of protons and neutrons in two commonly discussed isotopes: carbon and hydrogen. Carbon C-12, C-13 and C-14 are isotopes with 12, 13 and 14 MN, respectively. The atomic number of carbon is 6, which means that every carbon atom has 6 protons, so that the number of neutrons of these isotopes must be 6, 7 and 8, respectively. Likewise, hydrogen (AN = 1 = 1 proton) has 3 isotopes: H-1 (0 neutrons), H-2 (= deuterium, D; 1 neuron); and H-3 (= tritium, T; 2 neutrons).

Mass number —— **A**
(# protons + # neutrons)

$_Z^A X$

The element's symbol; represents an atom like:
• hydrogen (H) • oxygen (O)
• carbon (C) • uranium (U)

Atomic number —— **Z**
(# protons; defines the element; AN)

neutrons = **A** - **Z**

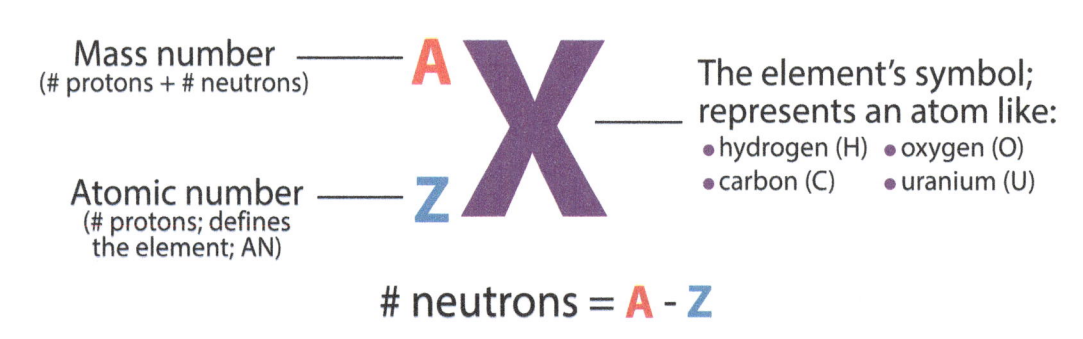

Figure III.B.12.1b: Atomic symbol anatomy.

PHY-174   CHAPTER 12: ATOMIC AND NUCLEAR STRUCTURE

12.3 Nuclear Forces, Nuclear Binding Energy, Stability, Radioactivity

Coulomb repulsive force (between protons) in the nuclei are overcome by nuclear forces. The nuclear force is a non-electrical type of force that binds nuclei together and is equal for protons and neutrons. The nuclear binding energy (E_b) is a result of the relation between energy and mass changes associated with nuclear reactions,

$$\Delta E = \Delta mc^2$$

in ergs in the CGS system, i.e. m = grams and c = cm/sec; ΔE = energy released or absorbed; Δm = mass lost or gained, respectively; c = velocity of light = 3.0×10^{10} cm/sec.

Conversions:
1 gram = 9×10^{20} ergs
1 a.m.u. = 931.4 MeV (Mev = 10^6 electron volts)
1 a.m.u. = 1/12 the mass of $_6C^{12}$.

The preceding equation is a statement of the law of conservation of mass and energy. The value of E_b depends upon the mass number (MN) as follows, (see Figure III.A.12.2):

The peak E_b/MN is at MN = 60. Also, E_b/MN is relatively constant after MN = 20. <u>Fission</u> is when a nucleus splits into smaller nuclei. <u>Fusion</u> is when smaller nuclei combine to form a larger nucleus. Energy is released from a nuclear reaction when nuclei with MN >> 60 undergo fission or nuclei with MN << 60 undergo fusion. Both fusion and fission release energy because the mass difference between the initial and the final nuclear states is converted into energy.

Not all combinations of protons are stable. The most stable nuclei are those with an even number of protons and an even number of neutrons. The least stable nuclei are those with an odd number of protons and an odd number of neutrons. Also, as the atomic number (AN) increases, there are more neutrons (N) needed for the nuclei to be stable.

According to the *Baryon number conservation*, the total number of protons and neutrons remains the same in a nuclear reaction even with the inter-conversions occurring between protons and neutrons.

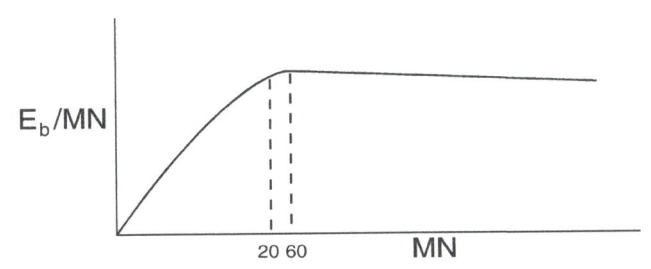

Figure III.A.12.2: Binding Energy per Nucleus. E_b/MN = binding energy per nucleus; this is the energy released by the formation of a nucleus.

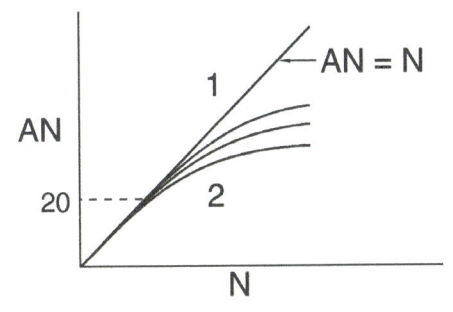

Figure III.A.12.3: Stability of Atoms. AN = atomic number and N = number of neutrons.

Up to AN = 20 (Calcium) the number of protons is equal to the number of neutrons, after this there are more neutrons. If an atom is in region #1 in Figure III.A.12.3, it has too many protons or too few neutrons and must decrease its protons or increase its neutrons to become stable. The reverse is true for region #2. All nuclei after AN = 84 (Polonium) are unstable.

Unstable nuclei become stable by fission to smaller nuclei or by absorption or emission of small particles. Spontaneous fission is rare. Spontaneous radioactivity (*emission of particles*) is common. The common particles are (*note that the superscripts are written on the right side, which is an alternative notation*):

(1) alpha (α) particle = $_2He^4$ (helium nucleus);

(2) beta (β) particle = $_{-1}e^0$ (an electron);

(3) a positron $_{+1}e^0$ (same mass as an electron but opposite charge);

(4) gamma (γ) ray = no mass and no charge, just electromagnetic energy (PHY 9.2.4, 11.1);

(5) orbital electron capture - nucleus takes electrons from K shell and converts a proton to a neutron. If there is a flux of particles such as neutrons ($_0n^1$), the nucleus can absorb these also.

> A neutron walks into a bar and asks the bartender: "How much for a beer?" The bartender answers: "For you, no charge."   :)

12.4 Nuclear Reaction, Radioactive Decay, Half-Life

Nuclear reactions are reactions in which changes in nuclear composition occur. An example of a nuclear reaction which involves uranium and hydrogen:

$$^{238}_{92}U + ^{2}_{1}H \rightarrow ^{238}_{93}Np + 2^{1}_{0}n$$

for $^{238}_{92}U$: 238 = mass number, 92 = atomic number. The sum of the lower (or higher) numbers on one side of the equation equals the sum of the lower (or higher) numbers on the other side of the equation. Another way of writing the preceding reaction is: $^{238}_{92}U(^{2}_{1}H, 2^{1}_{0}n)^{238}_{93}Np$. {# neutrons (i.e. $^{238}_{92}U$) = superscript (238) − subscript (92) = 146}

Radioactive decay is a naturally occurring spontaneous process in which the atomic nucleus of an unstable atom loses energy by the emission of ionising particles. Such unstable nuclei are known to spontaneously decompose and emit minute atomic sections to essentially gain some stability. The radioactive decay fragments are categorised into alpha, beta and gamma-ray decays. The radioactive decay can result in a nuclear change (*trans-*

mutation) in which the parent and daughter nuclei are of different elements. For example, a C-14 atom may undergo a beta decay and emit radiation and as a result, transform into a N-14 daughter nucleus. It is also possible that radioactive decay does not result in transmutation but only decreases the energy of the parent nucleus. As an example, a Ni-28 atom undergoing a gamma decay will emit radiation and then transform to a lower energy Ni-28 nucleus. The following is a brief description of the three principle types of radioactive decay.

(1) **Alpha (α) decay:** Alpha decay is a type of radioactive decay in which an atomic nucleus emits an alpha particle. An alpha particle is composed of two protons and two neutrons which is identical to a helium-4 nucleus. An alpha particle is the most massive of all radioactive particles. Because of its relatively large mass, alpha particles tend to have the most potential to interact with other atoms and/or molecules and ionise them as well as lose energy. As such, these particles have the lowest penetrating power (= *least ability to go straight through matter*, an object). If an atomic nucleus of an element undergoes alpha decay, this leads to a transmutation of that element into another element as shown below for the transmutation of Uranium-238 to Thorium-234:

$$^{238}_{92}U \rightarrow {}^{234}_{90}Th + {}^{4}_{2}He^{2+}$$
$$^{238}U \rightarrow {}^{234}Th + \alpha$$

(2) **Beta (β) decay:** Beta decay is a type of decay in which an unstable nucleus emits an electron or a positron. A positron is the antiparticle of an electron and has the same mass as an electron but opposite in charge. The electron from a beta decay forms when a neutron of an unstable nucleus changes into a proton and in the process, an electron is then emitted. The electron in this case is referred to as a beta minus particle or β−. In beta decays producing positron emissions, it is referred to as beta plus or β+. For an

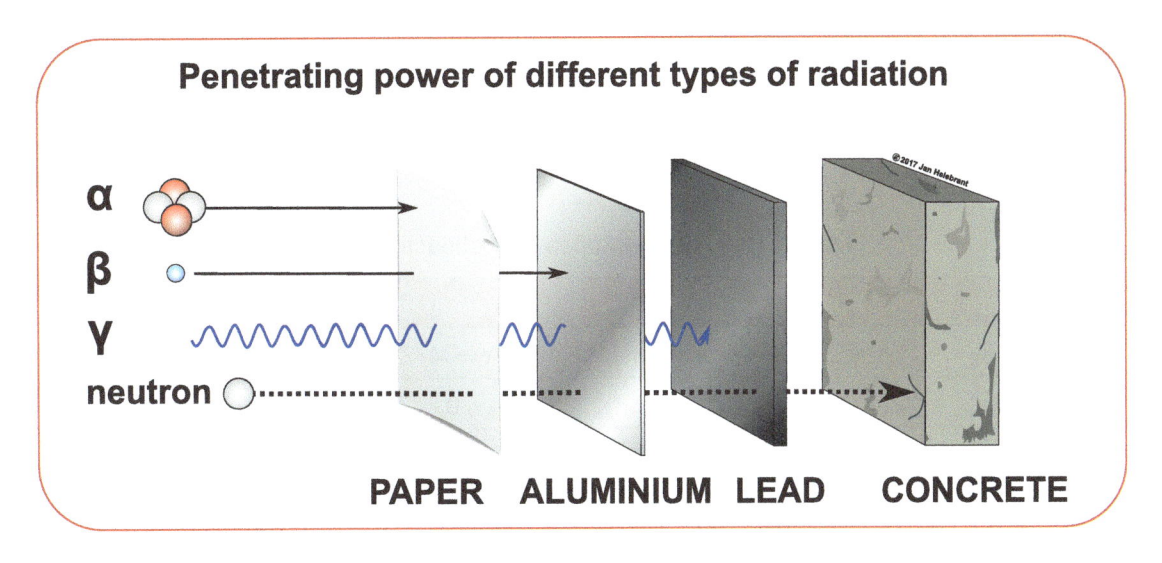

Penetrating power of different types of radiation

α
β
γ
neutron

PAPER   ALUMINIUM   LEAD   CONCRETE

atomic nucleus undergoing beta decay, the process leads to the transmutation of that element into another as shown for the transmutation of Cesium-137 for beta minus and Na-22 for beta plus emissions:

$$^{137}_{55}Cs \rightarrow {}^{137}_{56}Ba + \beta^-$$
$$^{22}_{11}Na \rightarrow {}^{22}_{10}Ne + \beta^+$$

(3) Gamma (γ) decay: Gamma decay is different from the other two types of decays. Gamma decay emits a form of electromagnetic radiation (PHY 9.2.4). Gamma rays are high energy photons known to penetrate matter very well and are symbolised by the Greek letter gamma (γ). A source of gamma decay could be a case in which an excited daughter nucleus - following an alpha or beta decay - lowers its energy state further by gamma-ray emission without a change in mass number or atomic number. The following is an example:

$$^{60}Co \rightarrow {}^{60}Ni^* + \beta^-$$

Co-60 decays to an excited Ni*-60 via beta decay and subsequently, the excited Ni*-60 drops to ground state and emits gamma (γ) rays as follows:

$$^{60}Ni^* \rightarrow {}^{60}Ni + \gamma$$

To summarise, a gamma ray has no charge and no mass since it is a form of electromagnetic radiation (PHY 9.2.4). As shown, gamma rays are usually emitted in conjunction with other radiation emissions.

Spontaneous radioactive decay is a first order process. This means that the rate of decay is *directly* proportional to the amount of material present:

$$\Delta m/\Delta t = \text{rate of decay}$$

where Δm = change in mass, Δt = change in time.

The preceding relation is equalised by adding a proportionality constant called the decay constant (k) as follows,

$$\Delta m/\Delta t = -km.$$

The minus sign indicates that the mass is decreasing. Also, $k = -(\Delta m/m)/\Delta t$ = fraction of the mass that decays with time.

The *half-life* ($T_{1/2}$) of a radioactive atom is the time required for one half of it to disintegrate. The half-life is related to k as follows,

$$T_{1/2} = 0.693/k.$$

Table III.A.11.1: Modes of Radioactive Decay

Decay Mode	Participating particles	Change in (A, Z)	Daughter Nucleus
Alpha decay	α	A = –4, Z = –2	(A – 4, Z – 2)
Beta decay	β⁻	A = 0, Z = +1	(A, Z + 1)
Gamma decay	γ	A = 0, Z = 0	(A, Z)
Positron emission	β⁺	A = 0, Z = –1	(A, Z – 1)

If the number of half-lives n are known we can calculate the percentage of a pure radioactive sample left after undergoing decay since the fraction remaining = $(1/2)^n$.

For example, given a pure radioactive substance X with $T_{1/2}$ = 9 years, calculating the percentage of substance X after 27 years is quite simple,

$27 = 3 \times 9 = 3\ T_{1/2}$

Thus

$n = 3$, $(1/2)^n = (1/2)^3 = 1/8$ or 13%.

After 27 years of disintegration, 13% of pure substance X remains. {Similarly, note that *doubling time* is given by $(2)^n$; see BIO 2.2}

12.5 Quantised Energy Levels For Electrons, Emission Spectrum

Work by Bohr and others in the early part of the last century demonstrated that the electron orbits are arranged in shells, and that each shell has a defined maximum number of electrons it can contain.

For example, the first shell can contain two electrons, the second eight electrons (*see* CHM 2.1, 2.2). The maximum number of electrons in each shell is given by:

$$N_{electrons} = 2n^2$$

$N_{electrons}$ designates the number of electrons in shell n.

The state of each electron is determined by the four quantum numbers:

- principal quantum number n determines the number of shells, possible values are: 1 (K), 2 (L), 3 (M), etc...
- angular momentum quantum number l, determines the subshell, possible values are: 0 (s), 1 (p), 2 (d), 3 (f), n-1, etc...

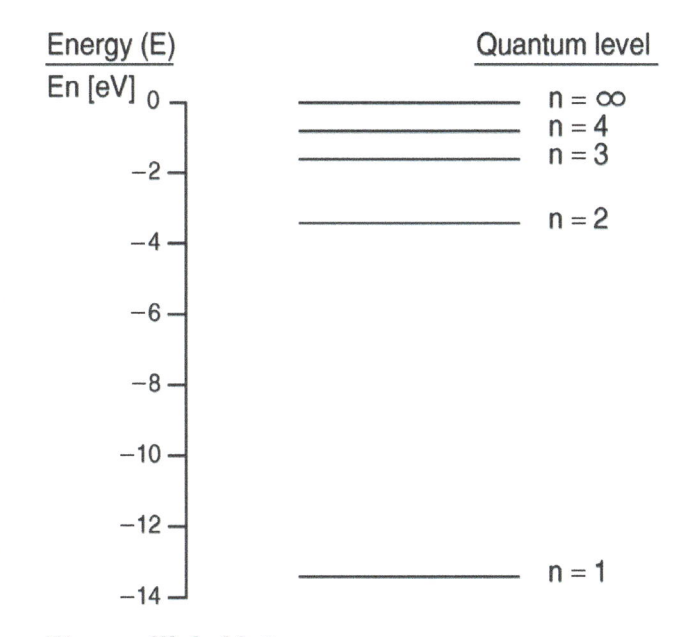

Figure III.A.11.4a: Energy levels. The energy E_n in each shell n is measured in electron volts.

- magnetic momentum quantum number m_l, possible values are: ±l, ... , 0
- spin quantum number m_s, determines the direction of rotation of the electron, possible values are: ±1/2.

{We will explore the quantum numbers in GAMSAT-level practice questions in CHM 2.}

GAMSAT-Prep.com
GOLD STANDARD PHYSICS

High-level Importance

Chemical reactions and electrical effects are all concerned with the behavior of electrons in the outer shell of any particular atom. If a shell is full, for example, the atom is unlikely to react with any other atom and is, in fact, one of the noble (inert) gases such as helium.

The energy that an electron contains is not continuous over the entire range of possible energy. Rather, electrons in a atom may contain only discrete energies as they occupy certain orbits or shells. Electrons of each atom are restricted to these discrete energy levels. These levels have an energy below zero.

This means energy is released when an electron moves from infinity into these energy levels.

If there is one electron in an atom, its ground state is n = 1, the lowest energy level available. Any other energy level, n = 2, n = 3, etc., is considered an excited state for that electron. The difference in energy (E) between the levels gives the absorbed (or emitted) energy when an electron moves to a higher orbit (or lower orbit, respectively) and therefore, the frequency (f) of light necessary to cause excitation.

$$E_2 - E_1 = hf$$

where E_1 = energy level one, E_2 = energy level two, h = planck's constant, and f = the frequency of light absorbed or emitted.

Therefore, if light is passed through a substance (e.g., gas), certain wavelengths will be absorbed, which correspond to the energy needed for the electron transition. An *absorption* spectrum will result that has dark lines against a light background. Multiple lines result because there are possible transitions from all quantum levels occupied by electrons to any unoccupied levels.

An *emission* spectrum results when an electron is excited to a higher level by another particle or by an electric discharge, for example. Then, as the electron falls from the

ABSORPTION SPECTRUM OF HYDROGEN

EMISSION SPECTRUM OF HYDROGEN

ABSORPTION SPECTRUM OF HELIUM

EMISSION SPECTRUM OF HELIUM

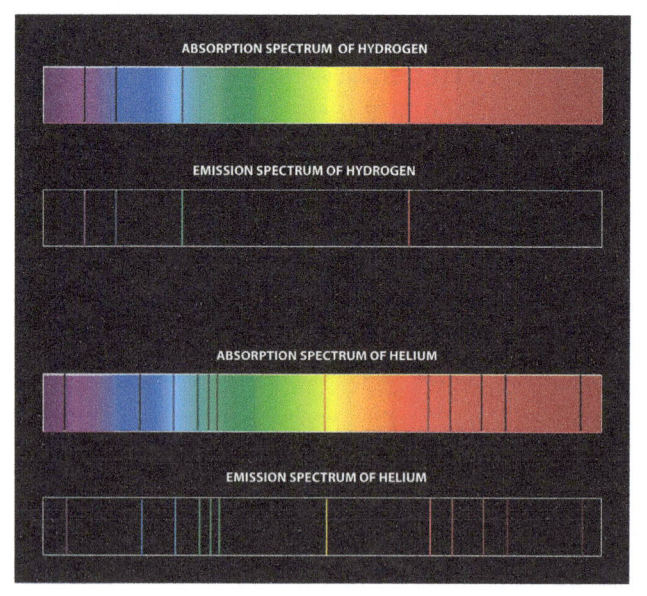

Figure III.A.11.4b: Absorption and emission spectra of the first two elements of the periodic table: hydrogen and helium. When electrons in an element become excited, for example by being heated, they enter higher energy orbits. When they return to their ground state, they release the extra energy as light radiation at a specific wavelength. The wavelengths emitted by an element are characteristic of that element. The dark lines within the absorption spectra show at what wavelengths light that passes through an element (when in its ground state) will be absorbed. As can be seen, the emission and absorption lines match. (Credit: Carlos Clarivan/Science Photo Library.)

excited state to lower states, light is emitted that has a wavelength (which is related to frequency) corresponding to the energy difference between the levels since: $E_1 - E_2 = hf$. The resulting spectrum will have <u>light lines</u> against a <u>dark background</u>.

The total energy of the electrons in an atom, where KE is the kinetic energy, can be given by:

$$E_{total} = E_{emission} \text{ (or } E_{ionisation}) + KE$$

12.6 Fluorescence

Fluorescence is an <u>emission process</u> that occurs after light absorption excites electrons to higher electronic and vibrational levels. The electrons spontaneously lose excited vibrational energy to the electronic states. There are certain molecular types that possess this property, e.g., some amino acids (tryptophan).

The fluorescence process is as follows:
- **step 1** - absorption of light;
- **step 2** - spontaneous deactivation of vibrational levels to zero vibrational level for electronic state;
- **step 3** - fluorescence with light emission (longer wavelength than absorption).

Figure III.B.12.5 shows diagrammatically the steps described above. Step 2 which is not shown in the figure is the intermediate step between light absorption and light emission. *See* BIO 1.5.1 for fluorescence as applied to microscopy.

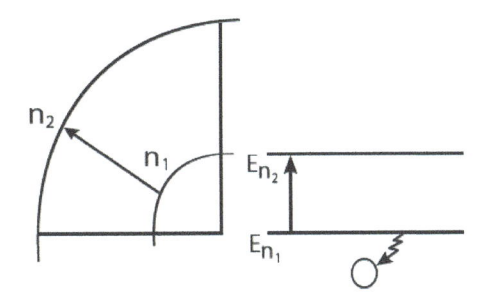

Step 1: light absorption

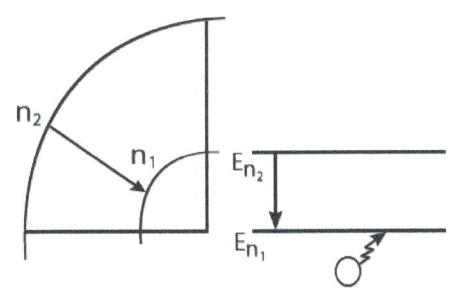

Step 3: light emission

Figure III.B.12.5: The fluorescence process. Represented is an atom with shells n_1, n_2 and their respective energy levels E_n.

CHAPTER 12: Atomic and Nuclear Structure

GOLD STANDARD FOUNDATIONAL GAMSAT PRACTICE QUESTIONS

1) Compared to the charge and mass of a proton, an electron has:

   A. the same charge and a smaller mass.
   B. an opposite charge and a smaller mass.
   C. the same charge and the same mass.
   D. an opposite charge and the same mass.

2) What is the mass number of an atom which contains 17 protons, 18 electrons, and 20 neutrons?

   A. 17
   B. 18
   C. 20
   D. 37

3) Which of the following statements about isotopes are correct?

   I. They have the same number of protons.
   II. They have the same number of electrons.
   III. They have the same number of neutrons.

   A. I and III only
   B. I and II only
   C. II and III only
   D. I, II and III

4) The isotope deuterium ($_1^2H$ or D) of hydrogen ($_1^1H$) has which of the following?

   A. No neutrons and one proton
   B. One electron and two neutrons
   C. One neutron and two protons
   D. One proton and one neutron

5) The isotope ^3H (tritium) has:

   A. three electrons.
   B. three neutrons.
   C. three protons.
   D. one proton and two neutrons.

6) Over time, the naturally occurring isotope of carbon ^{14}C breaks down to a different element, nitrogen ^{14}N. What net change must occur for this to happen?

   A. The ^{14}C gained a proton.
   B. The ^{14}C gained an electron.
   C. The ^{14}C lost an electron.
   D. The ^{14}C gained a neutron.

7) Among the particles released as a consequence of radioactive decay are:

   • beta (β) particle = $_{-1}e^0$ (an electron);
   • a positron $_{+1}e^0$ (same mass as an electron but opposite charge).

   When a $_5B^8$ atom decays by the emission of a positron, the resultant atom is:

   A. $_4Be^8$.
   B. $_6C^8$.
   C. $_5B^8$.
   D. $_3Li^4$.

8) A radioactive isotope has a half-life of 6 months. What fraction of the sample will be in original form after 2 years?

   A. 1/4
   B. 1/8
   C. 1/16
   D. 1/32

9) A Geiger counter is an instrument used for detecting and measuring radiation. A Geiger counter is placed in proximity to a radioactive isotope with significant background radiation from the environment (50 counts/second). The graph presenting the results over time is illustrated in Figure 1.

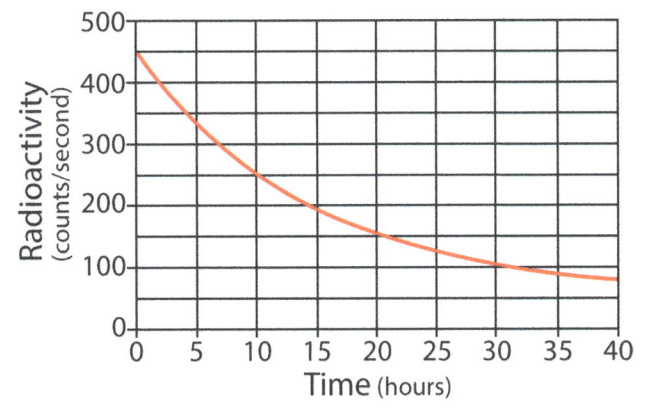

Figure 1

According to Figure 1, which of the following is the best determination of the half-life of the isotope?

A. 10 hours
B. 12.5 hours
C. 20 hours
D. More than 20 hours

10) The biological half-life (also known as the elimination half-life), of a medication or radionuclide is the time that it takes from its maximum concentration to half-maximum concentration in the human body. Consider a radionuclide administered to a patient. After 1 hour, it is found that the amount of the radionuclide in the body has fallen to approximately 6.25% of its original concentration. Find the approximate biological half-life.

A. Less than 4 minutes
B. 6.25 minutes
C. 10 minutes
D. More than 10 minutes

GOLD STANDARD GAMSAT-LEVEL PRACTICE QUESTIONS

Questions 11–12

Radiotherapy is the treatment of disease, especially cancer, with the use of radioactivity. Radioactivity is the term used to describe the natural process by which some atoms spontaneously disintegrate, emitting both particles and energy as they transform into different, more stable atoms, also called radioactive decay. Radioactivity is measured in terms of disintegrations, or decays. The following table contains the common units used in radioactivity and in radiation sciences.

Irradiance	W•m^{-2}	[Power]/[Area] for all kinds of energy deposition
Activity | Radioactivity	Bq	Bequerel: [Events]/[Time]
Absorbed dose	J•kg^{-1}, Gy	Gray: [Energy]/[Mass]
Absorbed dose rate	Gy•s^{-1}	[Absorbed dose]/[Time]
Absorbed dose equivalent	J•kg^{-1}, Sv	Sievert: [const][Energy]/[Mass]
Exposure	C•kg^{-1}	[Charge]/[Mass] for ionising radiation

11) Units can often be converted to basic SI units such as the metre (m) and seconds (s). Which of the following units is equivalent to m^{2}s^{-2}?

   A. Bequerel
   B. Gray
   C. (Sievert)(bequerel)
   D. (Sievert)/(bequerel)

12) A 50-kg female underwent radiotherapy for a 100-gram breast tumour. Which of the following most accurately reflects the absorbed dose after 0.05 kJ was delivered to the tumour?

   A. 0.5 kGy
   B. 50 Gy
   C. 1.0 Gy
   D. 5000 Gy

Questions 13–14

Exponential decay describes the process of reducing an amount by a consistent percentage rate over a period of time and can be expressed by the formula:

$$y = a(1-b)^x$$

where y is the final amount, a is the original amount, b is the decay factor, and x is the amount of time that has passed.

It is possible to determine the decay factor graphically. For example, consider Figure 1. The two diagonal lines permit a reasonably accurate assessment of the decay factor based on the number of half-lives elapsed. Note that a point along the left diagonal line is read along the left y-axis while along the right diagonal line is read along the right y-axis. For either line, 10 half-lives can be read as a decay factor of 10^{-3}.

Figure 1

[Graph showing Decay factor vs Number of half-lives elapsed, with two curves on log scale from 10^0 to 10^{-3} (left axis) and 10^{-3} to 10^{-6} (right axis).]

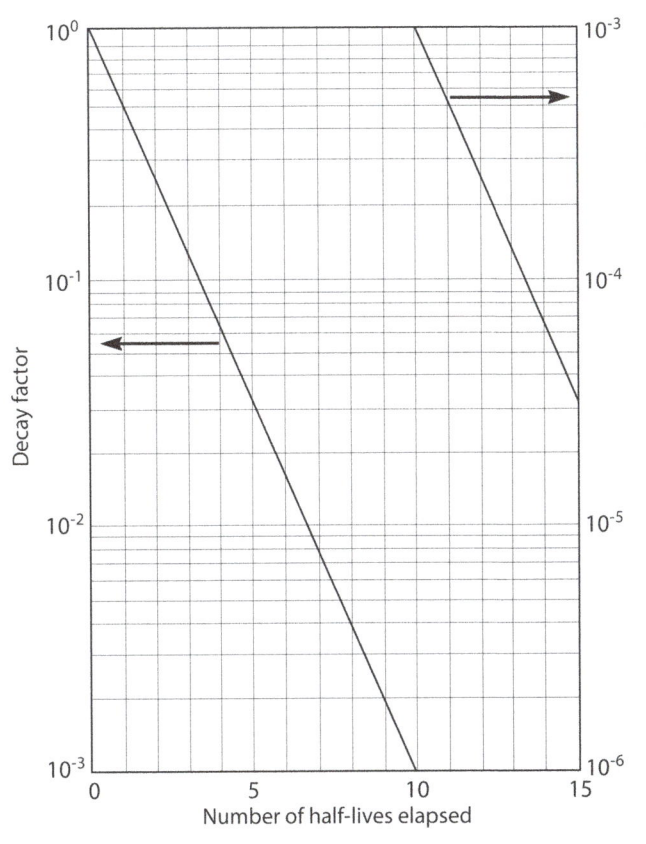

Figure 1

13) Based on Figure 1, identify the decay factor most consistent with 4 half-lives having been elapsed.

A. 0.5
B. 0.6
C. 0.056
D. 0.065

14) Based on Figure 1, a change in the number of half-lives elapsed from 1 to 11 would change the original decay factor (DF_o) by approximately what multiple?

A. $DF_o \times 1$
B. $DF_o \times 10^{-3}$
C. $DF_o \times 10^{-4}$
D. $DF_o \times 10^{-5}$

15) The dose equivalent is defined as the absorbed dose (in grays, Gy) $\times W_R$ (the radiation weighting factor, formerly known as the quality factor, Q). The result is measured in sieverts (Sv).

Radiation	W_R (formerly Q)
x-rays, gamma rays, beta particles, muons	1
protons, charged pions	2
alpha particles, nuclear fission products, heavy nuclei	20

Table 1: Radiation weighting factors W_R used to represent relative biological effectiveness.

A radiology nurse accidently receives an absorbed dose of 5 cGy in nuclear fission products and 20 cGy in gamma rays. Given the information provided, what is the dose equivalent for the nurse?

A. 1.0 Sv
B. 1.2 Sv
C. 2.2 Sv
D. 4.4 Sv

16) Naturally occurring boron (10.8 amu) consists of just two isotopes. One of the isotopes consists of atoms having a mass of 10 amu, the other of 11 amu. What is the percent natural abundance of the heavier isotope?

A. 10%
B. 20%
C. 50%
D. 80%

GAMSAT-Prep.com
GOLD STANDARD PHYSICS

Questions 17–20

In a nuclear decay experiment, two physicists recorded the radioactive emissions of Uranium 238. During the course of the experiment, the physicists recorded the following process:

$$^{238}_{92}U \xrightarrow{A} W \xrightarrow{B} X \xrightarrow{C} Y \xrightarrow{D} Z$$

At each step, A, B, C, D, radioactive emissions were observed as follows:

Step A: Alpha emission ($^4_2$He)

Step B: Beta minus ($^0_{-1}$e) and gamma emission (electromagnetic radiation)

Step C: Beta minus ($^0_{-1}$e) and gamma emission (electromagnetic radiation)

Step D: Alpha emission ($^4_2$He)

From this data, the physicists wish to determine what element the Uranium has transformed into at points W, X, Y, Z.

17) Into which of the following elements has the Uranium transformed by point X?

A. $^{235}_{92}$U
B. $^{234}_{92}$Th
C. $^{234}_{91}$Pa
D. $^{214}_{84}$Po

18) How much mass has each Uranium atom lost by point Z?

A. 4 mass units
B. 6 mass units
C. 7 mass units
D. 8 mass units

19) Which of the following is most consistent with the balanced decay for step C?

A. $^{234}_{90}$Th ⟶ $^0_{-1}$e + $^{234}_{91}$Th
B. $^{230}_{90}$Th ⟶ $^4_2$He + $^{226}_{86}$Ra
C. $^{230}_{90}$Th ⟶ $^4_2$He + $^0_0\gamma$ + $^{226}_{38}$Ra
D. $^{234}_{91}$Pa ⟶ $^0_{-1}$e + $^{234}_{92}$U

20) Into which element has the Uranium likely transformed by point Z?

A. $^{236}_{86}$Ac
B. $^{236}_{92}$U
C. $^{230}_{90}$Th
D. $^{230}_{88}$Ra

21) Carbon-14 is a radioactive isotope of carbon used for radiocarbon dating of ancient life forms. A living organism has a C-14 to C-12 ratio of 1/20 during its lifetime. Its remains now has a C-14 to C-12 ratio of 1/80. Approximately how old is this organism?

Note: Take the half-life of C-14 to be 6000 years.

A. It is 6000 years old.
B. It is 12 000 years old.
C. It is 18 000 years old.
D. It is 24 000 years old.

22) Consider Figure 1.

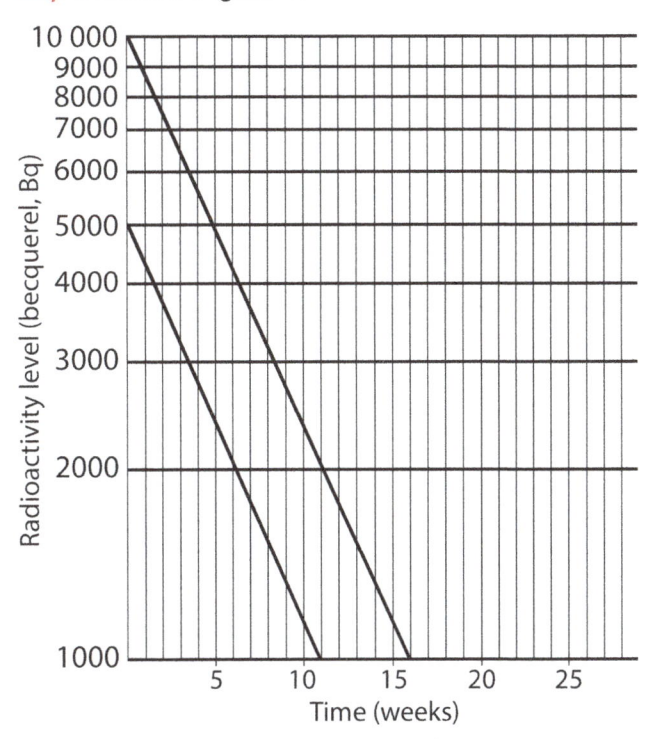

Figure 1: Radioactivity decay of Katai-68 under investigation for the treatment of metastatic cancer.

The half-life of Katai-68 is best approximated by which of the following?

A. 2.5 weeks
B. 5 weeks
C. 7.5 weeks
D. Cannot be determined as the two graphs illustrate significantly different half-lives.

---

23) A fossil was discovered in the forests of Africa and when examined, it was found that it had a carbon-14 activity of 10.8 disintegrations per minute per gram (dpm g^{-1}). If the average activity of carbon–14 in a living organism is 43.0 dpm g^{-1}, approximately how many half-lives have passed since the death of the organism?

A. 8
B. 4
C. 3
D. 2

24) The radioactive decay of Uranium-238 eventually leads to Lead-206. There are many steps along the way, but they all have very short half-lives compared to that of U-238, so they can be ignored on such a long (*geologic*) time scale.

Consider Figure 1.

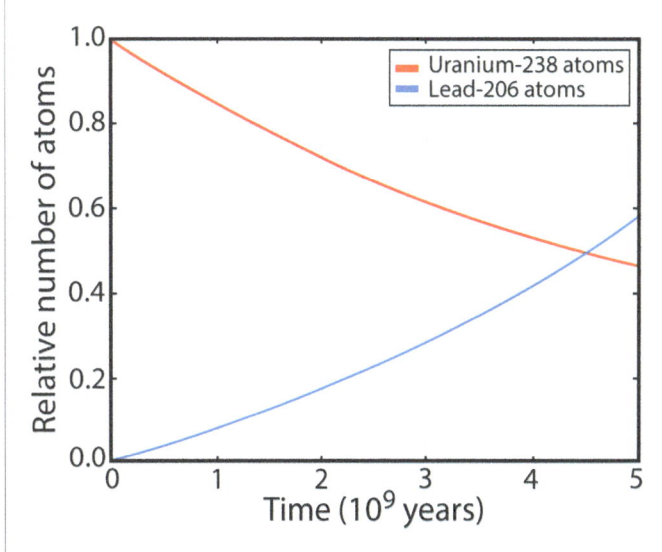

Figure 1: Radioactive decay of Uranium-238

Which of the following is **not** consistent with Figure 1?

A. The graph for Uranium-238 exhibits exponential decay.
B. The half-life for the decay of Lead-206 mirrors that of Uranium-238.
C. Using a log scale for the relative number of atoms would result in a straight line with a positive slope for Lead-206.
D. The half-life of Uranium-238 is 4.5 billion years.

25) For a number of radioisotopes of particular medical interest, the rate of excretion has been cast in the form of an effective biological half-life. The physical half-life and the biological half-life can be combined to provide the effective half-life of an isotope, according to the following:

$$\frac{1}{T_{Effective}} = \frac{1}{T_{Physical}} + \frac{1}{T_{Biological}}$$

Examples of half-lives show that biological clearing is sometimes dominant and sometimes physical decay is the dominant influence.

Isotope	Half-lives in days		
	$T_{Physical}$	$T_{Biological}$	$T_{Effective}$
^{3}H	4.5×10^3	12	12
^{32}P	14.3	1155	14.1
^{90}Sr	1.1×10^4	1.8×10^4	6.8×10^3
^{99m}Tc	0.25	–	0.20

Table 1

Based on the information provided, determine the biological half-life of ^{99m}Tc.

A. 12 hours
B. 1 day
C. 2 days
D. Cannot be determined from the information provided.

And in closing, a quote from a pioneering atomic physicist:

"All of physics is either impossible or trivial. It is impossible until you understand it, and then it becomes trivial."

– E. Rutherford

Good luck with your studies!

GAMSAT MASTERS SERIES

> **SPOILER ALERT** ⚠️
>
> Gold Standard has cross-referenced the content in this chapter to examples from ACER's official GAMSAT practice materials. It is for you to decide when you want to explore these questions since you may want to preserve some of ACER's materials for timed mock-exam practice.
>
> **Examples** – Although the topic is NMR (nuclear magnetic resonance, GAMSAT Organic Chemistry), the questions are strictly about the basic features of atoms presented in Chapter 12: Q26-28 of 1; very easy nuclear decay with balancing of reactions: Q28 and Q30 of 5 (Q29 is pure dimensional analysis; GM 2.2); classic radioactivity decay questions: Q103 and Q104 of 5. Note that "Q" is followed by the question number, and, for example, "of 1" refers to booklet number 1 which is referenced in the Spoiler Alert table at the end of Chapter 1. The 10 full-length HEAPS GAMSAT practice tests (by Gold Standard and MediRed), exams 1 through 10, contain specific cross-references to this chapter within the worked solutions. Note that 3 units are from our Gold Standard GAMSAT Virtual Reality on-campus mock exams: Radiotherapy and grays (dimensional analysis) is VR-1, the exponential-decay unit with graph and the dose-equivalent question are from VR-2.

High-level Importance

Chapter Checklist

- ☐ Access your online account to view answers, worked solutions and discussion boards.
- ☐ Reassess your 'learning objectives' for this chapter: Go back to the first page of this chapter and re-evaluate the top 3 boxes and the Introduction.
    - ☐ Please be sure that you have completed the *Need for Speed* exercises at the beginning of this chapter.
- ☐ Complete a maximum of 1 page of notes using symbols/abbreviations to represent the entire chapter based on your learning objectives. These are your Gold Notes.
- ☐ Consider your multimedia options based on your optimal way of learning:
    - ☐ Download the free Gold Standard GAMSAT app for your Android device or iPhone.
    - ☐ Create your own, tangible study cards or try the free app: Anki.
    - ☐ Record your voice reading your Gold Notes onto your smartphone (MP3s) and listen during exercise, transportation, etc.
    - ☐ Try out the Gold Standard GAMSAT online videos at gamsat-prep.com, or you can try other options on YouTube like Khan Academy or Crash Course Physics.
- ☐ Reassess your schedule for your full-length GAMSAT practice tests: ACER and/or HEAPS exams. Ensure that you have scheduled one full day to complete a practice test and 1-2 days for a thorough assessment of worked solutions while adding to your abbreviated Gold Notes.
- ☐ Reassess your progress in scheduling and/or evaluating stress reduction techniques such as regular exercise (sports), yoga, meditation and/or mindfulness exercises (*see* YouTube for suggestions).

High-level Importance

GOLD NOTES